Personalized Management of Gastric Cancer

Jia Wei • Baorui Liu
Editors

Personalized Management of Gastric Cancer

Translational and Precision Medicine

Springer

Editors
Jia Wei
The Comprehensive Cancer Center
Drum Tower Hospital
Medical School of Nanjing University
Nanjing
Jiangsu
China

Baorui Liu
The Comprehensive Cancer Center
Drum Tower Hospital
Medical School of Nanjing University
Nanjing
Jiangsu
China

ISBN 978-981-10-3977-5 ISBN 978-981-10-3978-2 (eBook)
DOI 10.1007/978-981-10-3978-2

Library of Congress Control Number: 2017940425

Printed on acid-free paper

This Springer imprint is published by Springer Nature
The registered company is Springer Nature Singapore Pte Ltd.
The registered company address is: 152 Beach Road, #21-01/04 Gateway East, Singapore 189721, Singapore

Preface

We are on the precipice of entering a stage of rapid development in the treatment of gastric cancer. For quite a long time, treatment progress was slow and stood in sharp contrast to the advances seen in lung cancer, colon cancer, and melanoma. However, a large reason for this slow progression was the reluctance of researchers to boldly apply the most advanced scientific concepts and technology to its treatment. With the vision of an emerging era of precise medicine, this book is based on the author's perception of both clinical experience and the most up-to-date scientific research. In so doing, the book describes and comments on the four fields most likely to significantly improve the therapeutic efficacy of gastric cancer treatment: personalized therapy, precision regional therapy, immunotherapy, and nanomedicine.

The first part of the book elaborates on personalized therapy in the treatment of gastric cancer. A comprehensive review is made from relevant aspects of molecular pathology, genetics and molecular signatures, circulating tumor cells, customized chemotherapy, and targeted gastric cancer therapy, thereby providing the latest research results for precise medication in the treatment of gastric cancer. The second part details precision regional therapy in gastric cancer. It is discussed through the following lenses: laparoscopic and robotic surgical approaches, radiotherapy, and personalized intraperitoneal strategies. The third part is focused on current "hotspots" in immunotherapy and is presented from the perspectives of checkpoint therapy, therapeutic vaccines, adoptive cell therapy, as well as combinational strategies. All of these approaches are explored with regard to their prospective applications in gastric cancer treatment. The final part is based on current research and focuses on nanomedicine and their delivery systems in the diagnosis and treatment of cancer. It has a specific focus on the translational significance of biomaterials and clinical medicine.

Collectively, these four parts seek to tackle the current hotspots in gastric cancer treatment as well as the remaining difficulties faced in the field. This is accomplished by combining translational research and clinical explorations, which together hold great promise in helping doctors and research fellows engaged in the necessary goal of gastric cancer treatment.

Nanjing, China

Jia Wei
Baorui Liu

Contents

Part I

Personalized Therapy in Gastric Cancer

Molecular Pathology of Heredity Gastric Cancer

1

Lin Li and Xiangshan Fan

1.1 Introduction

Gastric cancer (GC) affects nearly one million individuals every year, and most of them are from China, Japan, and Korea. It is the fifth most common malignant tumor worldwide and the third leading cause of malignant tumor mortality with more than 723,000 deaths [1]. About 70–85% of individuals with GC die within 5 years of diagnosis, and the high mortality associated with GC is mainly a result of limited therapeutic methods and lacking of early diagnosis. Aggregation within families occurs in almost 10% of patients (5–30%), although most GCs are sporadic. Now we know that hereditary germline mutations lead to half of these familial cases [2, 3]. In regions where the incidence of GC is low, heritable pathogenic mutations, which leads to most familial cases, increase risk from birth. Truly hereditary cases, as some studies pointed out, account for 1–3% of the global burden of GC [4], and most of those are hereditary diffuse gastric cancer (HDGC). It is reported that, in about 40% of families affected by HDGC, the E-cadherin/CDH1 germline mutations can been found. It is very important to identify the inherited factors among patients with family histories of GC, in order to diagnose early and manage effectively. We usually use symptoms, such as different family individuals are diagnosed with cancer, the histological types are diffused adenocarcinoma, and the patients are young and with multiple cancer syndromes, to identify HDGC. Some cases of other hereditary tumor syndromes may also present GC, and thus the risk of GC should be taken into account in these patients. The hereditary cancer syndromes include the gastric adenocarcinoma and proximal polyposis of the stomach (GAPPS), familial intestinal gastric cancer (FIGC), Lynch syndrome (LS) caused by germline mutations in DNA mismatch repair genes and microsatellite instability, familial adenomatous polyposis (FAP) associated with germline APC mutations, MUTYH-associated polyposis (MAP) associated with MUTYH mutation, Peutz-Jeghers syndrome (PJS) caused by germline STK11 mutations , juvenile polyposis syndrome (JPS) associated with germline mutations in the BMPR1A and SMAD4 genes, hereditary breast-ovarian cancer syndromes (HBCS) related to germline mutations of BRCA1 and BRCA2, Li-Fraumeni syndrome (LFS) due to germline p53 mutations, and so on [5].

Screening for familial gastric cancer (FGC) is an especially important procedure. Because it has a higher risk of GC incidence, to the individuals who have inherited the mutant gene, prophylactic

L. Li • X. Fan (✉)
Department of Pathology of Drum Tower Hospital, Medical School of Nanjing University, Nanjing 210008, China
e-mail: fxs23@hotmail.com

J. Wei, B. Liu (eds.), *Personalized Management of Gastric Cancer*,
DOI 10.1007/978-981-10-3978-2_1

gastrectomy is worthy of consideration [6]. It is an enormous fiscal expenditure of society to manage and control FGC each year. Thus, screening for prevention for it is a crucial step to decrease cancer incidence and mortality [7]. It is necessary to interview with pedigree precisely to find the familial syndromes, individuals at risk, and genotypes [8]. At present, it is in urgent need of guidelines for genetic detecting, counseling, and management of patients with HDGC. If we pay more attention on these syndromes, we may increase opportunities to detect and prevent GCs in these high-risk cases.

Hereditary gastric cancer syndromes are an infrequent but characteristic etiology of GCs. So far, we haven't clarified the genetic mutations attacking most affected families. Up to date, there are at least three main hereditary GC syndromes that have been reported: HDGC, GAPPS, and FIGC [5, 9]. In this chapter, we mainly discuss the available knowledge on HDGC, GAPPS, FIGC, and several other hereditary cancer syndromes associated with GC, with the aim of clarifying the molecular pathology and genesis of these heredity GCs.

1.2 Hereditary Diffuse Gastric Cancer

HDGC is an autosomal dominant disorder predisposition syndrome with obvious penetrance (about 80%) and characterized by an enhancive risk of early-onset, multigenerational, and signet ring cell GC (Lauren diffuse type) and lobular breast carcinoma.

A diagnosis of families with the HDGC syndrome can be established if one of the following clinical features are present. Firstly, at least two patients of documented diffuse GC in first- or second-degree family members, with one or more being diagnosed younger than 50 years old. Secondly, at least three documented patients of diffuse GC in first- or second-degree family members, ignoring of age of diagnosis. The checklist above was defined by the International Gastric Cancer Linkage Consortium (IGCLC) in 1999.

There was a renewed version for genetic testing in 2010 [10]. The families, which fulfill the following criteria for HDGC, would be recommended to consider genetic counseling and genetic testing for CDH1 gene mutations. Firstly, at least two patients of documented diffuse GC in first-degree family members, with one or more documented case of diffuse GC being diagnosed younger than 50 years old. Secondly, at least three documented patients of diffuse GC in first- or second-degree family members, ignoring of age of diagnosis. Thirdly, the diffuse GC case, with no family history, was diagnosed before the age of 40 years. Fourthly, families with patients of both lobular breast cancer and diffuse GC, with at least one diagnosed younger than the age of 50 years.

The age at onset of clinically significant diffuse GC may be extremely variable with the average onset in the fourth decade of life (14–85 years old), and the distribution of lesions also varies, involving all the topographic regions within the stomach. HDGC's genetic susceptibility and the molecular basis were first identified and then reinforced in Maori families and other populations, respectively, in 1998 [11, 12].

Heterozygous germline alterations in the E-cadherin gene (CDH1) result in HDGC [11]. There are five types of germline CDH1 mutations, including large rearrangements (4–8.7%), nonsense (17.3%) and missense (17.3%) mutations, splice site (23.1%), as well as small frameshifts (37.5%). They affect the protein's functional domains and the entire coding sequence [13–15]. 141 probands harboring more than one hundred different pathogenic germline CDH1 alterations have been described across multiple ethnicities so far [16, 17]. The production of this gene, which locates at 16q22.1, is E-cadherin. E-cadherin is a calcium-dependent transmembrane cellular adhesion protein. There are three parts of E-cadherin, including an intracellular domain which binds β-catenin and p120-catenin, the transmembrane domain, and the extracellular domain with five cadherin repeats (EC1–EC5). There is a highly phosphorylated region in the intracellular domain. Binding β-catenin with the intracellular domain is necessary for E-cadherin to regulate intracellular signaling. E-cadherin promotes tumor growth by interacting with cytoskeleton actin filaments through the Wnt signaling pathway. Downregulation of E-cadherin is observed in a lot of epithelial carcinomas of human and promotes invasion through loss of epithelial cell-cell adhesion. Being deprived of E-cadherin expression or function has been involved in cancer progression and metastasis. Around 40% of the families with HDGC have CDH1 germline mutations with high susceptibility to early development of diffuse-type GC [11]. The frequency of CDH1 germline mutations was found to be much lower in families from the high incidence of GC regions (i.e., the Eastern) (13.0%) than in countries with low incidence of GC (i.e., New Zealand, Northern Europe, and North America) (26.8%) [18]. About 45.6% cases of HDGC probands carried CDH1 germline alterations [14]. However, only 5.7% [14] to 13.8% [18] of FDGC probands displayed mutations of CDH1 but not large deletions. Very rarely, germline promoter methylation of CDH1 or inherited a-E-catenin mutations has been reported recently [19].

The cases, who just have a single wild-type CDH1 allele, are called heterozygous carriers. Usually these patients are commonly asymptomatic because the functional CDH1 gene produces sufficient amount of E-cadherin protein to maintain all normal functions in the stomach [20]. When the remaining wild-type allele of the E-cadherin gene is inactivated by a second-hit molecular mechanism until the second decade of life, HDGC develops. There are mainly three types of second-hit mechanism of inactivation in both inherited and sporadic diffuse cancers, including the epigenetic modification (promoter hypermethylation of CDH1), deletion (LOH or intragenic deletions), or a second mutation [21, 22]. The former is the most common one. Primary tumor and lymph node metastases may show different second-hit mechanisms or different tumorous lesions and even the same neoplastic lesion from the same patient. For example, LOH is often found in lymph node metastases (58.3%), whereas promoter hypermethylation of CDH1 mainly occurs in primary lesions [15]. Genetic testing of CDH1 is recommended in a patient fulfilling the HDGC diagnose checklist above. The other families that met the IGCLC criteria remained genetically unexplained. Recently, candidate mutations were identified in 11% (16/144) probands in those CDH1 mutation-negative index cases, including mutations within genes of moderate and high penetrance: STK11, SDHB, PRSS1, ATM, CTNNA1, MSR1, BRCA2, and PALB2 [23].

There are two major histological variants of GC: diffuse-type GC (35%) and intestinal-type GC (50%). CDH1 mutations have been found only in diffuse-type GCs. Microscopically, single or multiple foci of invasive signet ring cells just develop below the surface mucosal epithelium, retaining the construction. On the other hand, cancer cells may show a pattern of signet ring cell carcinoma in situ and pagetoid distribution below the conserved epithelium of foveolae and pits but still be restricted to the basement membrane. Usually advanced HDGC shows as a poorly cohesive malignant tumor, while the entire stomach wall being penetrated by signet ring cells, and also less frequently mixed with mucinous or tubular adenocarcinoma. The expression of E-cadherin protein is reduced or absent in the tumor cells, while it's normal in adjacent non-neoplastic mucosa, by immunohistochemical test.

Individuals with a heterozygous germline CDH1 mutation have a lifetime risk of 70% in male and 56% in female of developing diffuse GC, and women with the CDH1 mutation were found to have a 42% lifetime risk for lobular-type breast cancer [3, 23]. According to Cisco et al. [24], four fifths of females and two thirds of males who are carriers of CDH1 gene mutations will develop HDGC by the age of 80 years. Individuals who met the HDGC diagnose checklist but did not have CDH1 mutations had longer survival times than GC cases harboring germline CDH1 mutations (48% vs. 36% survived for one year and 13% vs. 4% survived for five years) [3]. In mutation-positive patients, prophylactic total gastrectomy is recommended. With early detection (i.e., confined to mucosa and submucosa), >90% of patients with GC will be alive at 5 years compared with 10–20% of patients with advanced GC, even after potentially curative surgery has been carried out. Patients with a clinical diagnosis of HDGC could be tested for the CDH1 gene mutation. While the patients with the CDH1 gene mutation should be managed with more frequent endoscopic surveillance and biopsies, their children and/or relatives could be tested for the carrier status of CDH1 and therefore receive appropriate clinical management.

1.3 Gastric Adenocarcinoma and Proximal Polyposis Syndrome

GAPPS is a recently described autosomal dominant inherited GC syndrome with increased risk of gastric carcinoma, specialized with unique proximal gastric fundic gland polyposis (often less than1cm in size), with areas of multi-atypical hyperplasia lesions and subsequent intestinal-type GC formation (about 12.7% in call cases) [25, 26]. The typical gastric phenotype and the earliest GC has been observed at 10 and 33 years of age, respectively [25].

The diagnosis can be set up only after excluding the use of proton pump inhibitors (PPIs) and other heritable gastric polyposis syndromes, such as attenuated FAP, FAP, MAP, PJS, and CS. Though cases with Peutz-Jeghers syndrome may also carry fundic gastric polyps and excluding GC, the distribution of polyp is different from that in GAPPS [27, 28].

There is a diagnostic checklist which should be considered. Firstly, we count the number of polyps. For example, an index case with more than 100 gastric polyps carpeting the proximal stomach should be considered as GAPPS. The other situation is that a first-degree family of a known case carries over 30 polyps. Secondly, the location of polyps should be taken into account. In a case with no evidence of colorectal or duodenal polyposis, we may put it into GAPPS if his/her gastric polyps are restricted to the fundus and body of the stomach. Thirdly, histological feature should be thought over. If there are local areas presenting dysplasia or gastric adenocarcinoma in fundic gland polyposis (FGPs), the case would be diagnosed with GAPPS. The last but not the least, the autosomal dominant pattern of inheritance should be taken into consideration. Macroscopically, the lesions of GAPPS present florid and usually less than 1cm. The number of polyps distributing in the gastric fundus and body is more than 100, with relative less along the lesser curve of the stomach and without effecting gastric antrum and pylorus [25, 26]. Histologically, most of the lesions present fundic gastric polyposis without or with regions of atypical hyperplasia. Occasionally, adenomatous and hyperplastic polyps can be found with pure features or mixed characteristics focally within the fundic gastric polyps [27, 29]. The cases who met GAPPS would develop GC of intestinal type. The etiology and genetic cause of GAPPS with incomplete penetrance is unclear. In 2016, one study revealed that point mutations in APC promoter 1B were at risk of gastric adenocarcinoma in patients with GAPPS. The families with familial adenomatous polyposis may also harbor point mutations in APC promoter 1B [30]. However, mutations in APC, BMPR1A, CDH1, MUTYH, PTEN, SMAD4, and STK11 were preclusive in some families [26, 28].

1.4 Familial Intestinal Gastric Cancer

FIGC is an autosomal dominant inherited disorder; however, the genetic cause involved is currently unknown. It's lacking the mutation of CDH1 and poorly characterized genetic predisposition for intestinal-type GC [5, 10].

The recommended diagnosis checklist varies in regions with different incidence of GC [31]. Diagnosis criteria similar to the Amsterdam criteria for colorectal carcinoma (CRC) have been applied in regions with high incidence. According to the Amsterdam criteria, only 0.9% cases (31/3632 families) in Japan met the diagnosis checklist for FIGC. 28.6% of patients develop GC younger than 50 years [4]. In regions with low incidence, guidelines include the following clinical criteria [4, 27]: (a) more than one case of

GC in first-degree or second-degree relatives, with one or more confirmed patient of intestinal type in someone before the age of 50, and (b) at least three confirmed individuals of intestinal GC in first-degree or second-degree relatives, independent of age.

The GC display the common general features observed in the sporadic setting. Histologically, the tumors show the characteristics of Lauren intestinal-type adenocarcinoma [27]. Genetically, we do not find TP53, DNA mismatch repair genes, or CDH1 mutation in these tumors so far. However, some research reported that almost 17% of cases present epigenetic methylation of CDH1. There are also 9.4% of cases attracting attention because of loss of heterozygosity [31].

1.5 Lynch Syndrome

LS, also known as hereditary nonpolyposis colorectal cancer syndrome (HNPCC), is an autosomal dominant syndrome. About 2–4% of all CRC are LS, which is the most common form of inherited CRC syndrome [4]. Now we know there are two types of Lynch syndrome according to the clinical feature. The type, which is predisposing primarily to colonic carcinoma, we definite it as Lynch syndrome I. Part of tumors arising in the genitourinary tract, prostate, pancreaticobiliary tract, stomach, and endometrium have been identified as part of the neoplasm spectrum in Lynch syndrome II. In Lynch syndrome II, the lifetime risk of LS patients is up to 80% for CRC, 20–60% for endometrial cancer, and 11–19% for GC [32]. The lifetime risk for developing GC varies in different regions. In the Eastern, the lifetime risk of GC in LS patients (30% in Korea and 44.4% in China) is higher than it is in some Western countries (11–19%, even 2.1% in the Netherlands) [4, 32]. In Finland, the cumulative incidence of GC in LS is 13% by 70 years of age, and 52% of GC in LS are diagnosed in individuals younger than 50 years [33, 34]. GC associated with LS is predominantly intestinal phenotype, and the prevalence of *Helicobacter pylori* infection in LS patients with GC does not differ from it in the general population [35].

The predisposition of LS to cancers is related to the mutations of mismatch repair (MMR) genes, which would accelerate DNA microsatellite instability (MSI). Abnormal MMR gene can be found in 90% of tumors from LS patients with germline mutations and in 10–15% of sporadic cancers [36]. MMR proteins include the MutS proteins (such as hMSH2, hMSH3, and hMSH6) and the MutL proteins (such as hMLH1, hPMS1, hPMS2, and hMLH3) [37]. At least five MMR genes have been identified in LS, with approximately 90% of gene mutations in MLH1 and MSH2, 7–10% in MSH6, less 5% in PMS2, and very rarely in PMS1 [38]. The identification of MMR genetic alterations has a considerable clinical significance on the screening, diagnosis, and prevention of LS [32, 39]. MSI is a marker of the presence of replication errors in simple repetitive microsatellite sequences due to DNA MMR deficiency. Tumors are classified as microsatellite stable (MSS), MSI-low (MSI-L), and MSI-high (MSI-H). Several studies have reported that MSI is present in both familial and sporadic GC and that about 20–30% of GC have MSI [40]. MSI occurs at the stage of chronic gastritis, a long time before the development of GC [41]. Therefore, MSI analysis is promising as a valuable marker of the risk of progression to GC.

In the past, both Amsterdam criteria and Bethesda criteria have ever been used to establish a diagnosis of LS. GC, however, is not a defining criterion for LS in either classification. In 2004, the revised Bethesda guidelines, instead of the Amsterdam I and II, was proposed as the clinical screening criteria that can be used to select individuals for MSI analysis. Firstly, the patients, who was diagnosed with CRC at less than 50 years of age, are suspected to have LS. Secondly, we take the cases, which meet the criteria that present synchronous, metachronous colorectal, or other LS-related tumors at any age, into account. Thirdly, we think over the individuals who suffer from CRC diagnosed before the age of 60 years, and its MSI phenotype was high. Fourthly, CRC patients, whose first-degree family member was diagnosed with a LS-related tumor at less than 50 years of age, should be taken into consideration or CRC patients, who has family history and the relative diagnosed with a LS-related tumor at any age. If a patient fulfills the above diagnosis checklist, the molecular (such as PCR and direct DNA sequencing) and/or immunohistochemical (MMR protein) testing for MSI should be performed, because certain cases may fulfill the clinical feature but are MMS on testing, an exclusionary feature [42]. The presence of MSI in a tumor specimen is not indicative of a particular gene defect, and neither MSI nor IHC can distinguish between sporadic and LS-related cancer. However, IHC results indicating the absence of a specific MMR protein can be used to determine which targeted mutation analysis should be performed [43]. A full-scale analysis of the entire MSH6, PMS2, MSH2, and MLH1 genes is commendatory for making a definite diagnosis of LS [4]. The most common abnormity is seen in MSH2 (about 60% of LS cases) and MLH1 (about 30% of the cases). The remaining rare types are PMS2, MSH6, TGFBR2, and MLH3 mutations (about 10% of the cases) [4]. Some method for MSI detection in GC has been proposed, but whether it will become the treatment standard remains unknown [44]. In addition, the relative rarity of GC in LS families makes the cost-effectiveness of endoscopic screening questionable [4].

1.6 Familial Adenomatous Polyposis/MUTYH-Associated Polyposis/Attenuated Familial Adenomatous Polyposis

FAP is an autosomal dominant disease classically characterized by hundreds to thousands of adenomas through the gastrointestinal tract. Its etiology is adenomatous polyposis coli (APC) germline mutation which is located on chromosome 5q21. There are three clinical features that help us diagnose FAP. We take the cases, which can be detected in more than 100 adenomatous colorectal polyps, into account. APC germline mutation may also be a clue. If young people, whose first-degree or second-degree family member was diagnosed with FAP, carry any number of adenomas, he/she would be considered as FAP. Nearly 8% of FAP cases are attenuated FAP (AFAP), which characteristic is less than100 adenomatous colorectal polyps. Usually these patients carry 10–99 adenomas at age older than 30 years and have one first-degree family member with CRC and few adenomas. The other situation is two or more relative with 10–99 adenomas at age older than 30 years old [45]. MAP is an autosomal recessive polyposis syndrome [37]. A diagnosis is established only after exclusion of FAP syndrome by demonstrating an absence of APC mutation and confirmation of the biallelic mutations of MUTYH gene, a mut Y homolog (*Escherichia coli*) gene located at chromosome loci 1p34.3-p32.1, in a suspected individual on the basis of the given circumstances. Firstly, we take the cases, whose family member was diagnosed with CRC accordingly with an autosomal recessive pattern of inheritance, into account. Secondly, those who can't be detected in the germline mutation of APC gene and carry more than 100 colon polyps would be thought over. The third situation is those who harbor 10–100 colon polyps, whatever adenomas or hyperplastic type. Fourthly, we would take an individual who carries 1–10 colon adenomas in the first decade into consideration. The fifth part includes the cases with specific somatic mutation of KRAS (c.34G→T) in codon 12 and suffering from CRC at the same time. Extra-colonic neoplasms are observed often in patients with FAP, but clinical features of GC associated with FAP are not clear at present. The presence of gastric polyps (from 51% to 88% in FAP [46, 47] and 93% in AFAP [48]) and even polyps associated with dysplasia or canceration is the known manifestation of FAP/AFAP in the Eastern [4]. The risk of GC in FAP varies in different regions. A high risk has been reported in the Eastern (3.8% in Japan [49] and 4.2% in Korea [50]) but low in the Western (0.6%) [51], and GC related to FAP often originated from fundic gland polyps or adenomatous polyps. Patients with FAP are 7–10 times more likely to affect gastric carcinoma than nonsyndromic patients in the Eastern [52]. For example, in Japan, FGP were significantly more common in FAP than in

AFAP; however, GC was significantly less common in FAP than in AFAP. Upper gastrointestinal tumors/polyps were frequently found in patients with FAP, but the frequency of GC in patients with FAP was similar to that in the general population [49]. The age of onset of stomach manifestations is variable, but GC typically develops long after colectomy. The types of benign gastric lesions detected include FGPS, GAs, and, infrequently, hyperplastic polyps and pyloric adenomas. Syndromic FGPs have a higher incidence of carrying beginning dysplasia (25–44%) than sporadic cases (~1%) [53, 54]. The dysplasia often present low grade, and the risk of malignant transformation is low. Gastric involvement in patients with MAP is uncommon. Although gastric lesions, such as adenomas and fundic gland polyps, have been found in up to 11% of patients with MAP, the risk of GC does not increase currently [55].

The FAP syndromes are autosomal dominant inherited disorders with a close to 100% penetrance. The involved gene is the tumor suppressor gene of adenomatous polyposis coli (APC) located on chromosomal 5q21, which harbor heterozygous mutation. About 90% of germline inactivation of APC lead to truncation of APC protein. APC mutations have been proved to be associated with some gastric lesions, such as gastric fundic gland polyposis, gastric adenomas, and dysplastic and malignant gastric polyps. MAP is an autosomal recessive polyposis syndrome caused by the MUTYH gene located on 1p34.1, which plays a significant role in DNA base-excision repair.

1.7 Peutz-Jeghers Syndrome

Peutz-Jeghers syndrome (PJS) is an autosomal dominant disorder and inherited cancer syndrome characterized by gastrointestinal hamartomatous polyposis (preferentially involving the small intestine) and mucocutaneous melanin pigmentation. Polyps in the stomach are detected in 25% of the patients with the median age of onset of 16 years. Although reported as early as 12 years of age [56], GC usually develops after a long time (often more than 25 years) with the estimated lifetime risk of nearly 30% in PJS patients with SMAD4 gene mutations, and the common histological type is intestinal-type adenocarcinoma [4, 57]. Classic PJS presents four important features. Firstly, the patient harbors at least three polyps which measure up the standard of Peutz-Jeghers polyps in histology. Secondly, the case, whose family member develops PJS, can be detected in Peutz-Jeghers polyps regardless of the number. Thirdly, the individuals with a family histology of PJS present distinctive, remarkable, mucocutaneous pigmentation. Fourthly, the patients present remarkable, mucocutaneous pigmentation and carry Peutz-Jeghers polyps, no matter the number. The diagnosis should meet two or more of the checklist above. PJS is an autosomal dominant trait with almost complete penetrance. About 70% of patients with PJS harbor the germline mutations of LKB1/STK11 which encode a serine threonine kinase [58]. LKB1/STK11 is located on chromosome 19p13.3 and is a tumor suppressor gene. There are usually two patterns of LKB1/STK11 gene mutations, including truncating mutations and missense mutations. The latter type develop a later onset of gastric polyps in comparison with the former or no mutations. Not only the type but also the site would influence the development of GC and gastric polyps [59].

1.8 Juvenile Polyposis Syndrome

JPS, now we know, is an autosomal dominant disease. The patients present multiple polyps throughout the digestive tract with an increased risk for GC. Stomachic polyps are usually diagnosed in adults (median age of 41 years). GC has been found in up to 21% of gastric polyps and is either intestinal- or diffuse-type adenocarcinomas.

The cases should meet the following checklist when diagnosed with JPS. Firstly, the individuals with one or more relatives who developed JPS can be detected in JP polyps regardless of the number. Secondly, the patients harbor at least five polyps which measure up the standard of JP polyps in the rectum or colon in histology. Thirdly, the cases carry JP polyps throughout the entire gastrointestinal tract [60].

Genetic abnormality involved in JPS is inherited germline mutation of multiple genes. Germline mutations in SMAD4 (DPC4) gene on chromosome18q21 present in about 20% of JPS cases. Germline mutations in BMPR1A gene on 10q23 present in similar proportion of JPS patients [61, 62]. Severe upper gastrointestinal polyposis has been associated with the former, but not the latter mutations [63, 64]. The role of germline mutations in ENG and PTEN (phosphatase and tensin homolog) has been debatable [65].

1.9 Li-Fraumeni Syndrome

LFS is an autosomal dominant inherited disorder with an increased risk of typically developing leukemias, sarcomas, brain tumors, and breast and adrenal cortical carcinomas in children and young adults and associated with germline TP53 gene mutation located on Chr 17p13.1. GC is detected in up to 4.9% of LFS carriers [66]. The mean and median age at diagnosis of GC is 43 and 36 years, respectively (range, 24–74 years), which is significantly younger compared with that of sporadic GC (71 years) [66]. Pediatric GC reveals an atypical presentation of Li-Fraumeni syndrome [67]. The youngest we know is only 12 years old [68]. About 50% of the tumors have been located in the proximal stomach, and nearly 70% show a phenotype of intestinal type [66].

1.10 BRCA1 and BRCA2 Hereditary Breast and Ovarian Cancer

BRCA1 and BRCA2 hereditary breast and ovarian cancer is an autosomal recessive syndrome caused by mutations in BRCA1 located on Chr 17q21.31 or BRCA2 on 13q13.1. GC has been accompanied by BRCA1 and BRCA2 syndromes [4]. BRCA1 mutation at c.3936 C→T [69] and BRCA2 mutation at 6174delT [70] have been reported in a higher frequency of gastric carcinoma. In comparison with BRCA1, BRCA2 is more tightly associated with gastric cancer. However, there is a study from Polish that suggested that BRCA1 founder mutations in patients with breast-ovarian cancer do not contribute to increased GC risk [71].

1.11 Cowden Syndrome

The Cowden syndrome (CS) is an autosomal dominant disease characterized by multiple hamartomas of the gastrointestinal tract, skin, and other organs. Because the susceptibility gene, PTEN, resides on 10q23.3, CS is also known as PTEN hamartoma syndrome. The patients with CS often have multiple hyperplastic gastric polyps, and some have multiple hamartomatous polyps in the stomach [72]. One study has ever reported that two synchronous gastric carcinomas, multiple hyperplastic polyps, and small, sessile polyps were found in the stomach of the 73-year-old white man with CS [73].

Conclusions

With the rapid development of the technology of molecular biology, GC has been investigated intensively and extensively at molecular levels. However, the genetic and pathogenic determinants of hereditary or familiar GC syndromes are not yet fully recognized. Familial GC comprises at least three major syndromes: HDGC, GAPPS, and FIGC. The lifetime risk of development of GC is high in families with these syndromes above, but only HDGC is genetically explained, which was caused by germline disorder of CDH1 (encoding E-cadherin protein), and much efforts need to be made to identify genetic alterations that may guide the clinical management and genetic testing of patients with GAPPS or FIGC. In addition, GC is also involved in a range of several other cancer-associated syndromes with clear genetic reasons, such as LS, FAP, MAP, PJS, JPS, HBCS, LFS, and so on. In recent years, the research into and understanding of the genetic changes and molecular pathogenesis underlying familial or hereditary GC has increased significantly. These genetic alterations are not only associated with oncogenesis but also very practical biomarkers for tumor diagnosis and prediction of therapeutic response and prognosis. Personalized tumor treatment in the coming future would also depend on the individualized genetic signature. Thus, deep understanding to the genetic alterations must open a new fascinating window related to the new genetic testing approaches and novel potential therapeutic strategies to the hereditary or familiar GC. A raised awareness to the syndromes above may allow for increased detection and prevention of GC in these high-risk individuals and their familiar members.

References

1. Torre LA, Bray F, Siegel RL, Ferlay J, Lortet-Tieulent J, Jemal A. Global cancer statistics, 2012. CA Cancer J Clin. 2015;65(2):87–108. doi:10.3322/caac.21262.
2. Richards FM, McKee SA, Rajpar MH, Cole TR, Evans DG, Jankowski JA, et al. Germline E-cadherin gene (CDH1) mutations predispose to familial gastric cancer and colorectal cancer. Hum Mol Genet. 1999;8(4):607–10.
3. van der Post RS, Vogelaar IP, Manders P, van der Kolk LE, Cats A, van Hest LP, et al. Accuracy of hereditary diffuse gastric cancer testing criteria and outcomes in patients with a germline mutation in CDH1. Gastroenterology. 2015;149(4):897–906. doi:10.1053/j.gastro.2015.06.003.
4. Setia N, Clark JW, Duda DG, Hong TS, Kwak EL, Mullen JT, et al. Familial gastric cancers. Oncologist. 2015;20(12):1365–77. doi:10.1634/theoncologist.2015-0205.
5. Oliveira C, Pinheiro H, Figueiredo J, Seruca R, Carneiro F. Familial gastric cancer: genetic susceptibility, pathology, and implications for management. Lancet Oncol. 2015;16(2):e60–70. doi:10.1016/S1470-2045(14)71016-2.
6. Chen Y, Kingham K, Ford JM, Rosing J, Van Dam J, Jeffrey RB, et al. A prospective study of total gastrectomy for CDH1-positive hereditary diffuse gastric cancer. Ann Surg Oncol. 2011;18(9):2594–8. doi:10.1245/s10434-011-1648-9.
7. Winawer SJ. Gastric cancer: worldwide burden and prevention opportunities. Chin J Dig Dis. 2005;6(3):107–9. doi:10.1111/j.1443-9573.2005.00211.x.
8. Etemadi M, Pourian M, Shakib A, Sabokbar T, Peyghanbari V, Shirkoohi R. A registry program for familial gastric cancer patients referred to Cancer Institute of Iran. Asian Pac J Cancer Prev. 2014;15(5):2141–4.
9. Donner I, Kiviluoto T, Ristimaki A, Aaltonen LA, Vahteristo P. Exome sequencing reveals three novel candidate predisposition genes for diffuse gastric cancer. Fam Cancer. 2015;14(2):241–6. doi:10.1007/s10689-015-9778-z.
10. Fitzgerald RC, Hardwick R, Huntsman D, Carneiro F, Guilford P, Blair V, et al. Hereditary diffuse gastric cancer: updated consensus guidelines for clinical management and directions for future research. J Med Genet. 2010;47(7):436–44. doi:10.1136/jmg.2009.074237.
11. Guilford P, Hopkins J, Harraway J, McLeod M, McLeod N, Harawira P, et al. E-cadherin germline mutations in familial gastric cancer. Nature. 1998;392(6674):402–5. doi:10.1038/32918.
12. Gayther SA, Gorringe KL, Ramus SJ, Huntsman D, Roviello F, Grehan N, et al. Identification of germ-line E-cadherin mutations in gastric cancer families of European origin. Cancer Res. 1998;58(18):4086–9.
13. Fitzgerald RC, Hardwick R, Huntsman D, Carneiro F, Guilford P, Blair V, et al. Hereditary diffuse gastric cancer: updated consensus guidelines for clinical management and directions for future research. J Med Genet. 2010;47(7):436–44.
14. Oliveira C, Senz J, Kaurah P, Pinheiro H, Sanges R, Haegert A, et al. Germline CDH1 deletions in hereditary diffuse gastric cancer families. Hum Mol Genet. 2009;18(9):1545–55.
15. Oliveira C, Senz J, Kaurah P, Pinheiro H, Sanges R, Haegert A, et al. Germline CDH1 deletions in hereditary diffuse gastric cancer families. Hum Mol Genet. 2009;18(9):1545–55. doi:10.1093/hmg/ddp046.
16. Oliveira C, Pinheiro H, Figueiredo J, Seruca R, Carneiro F. E-cadherin alterations in hereditary disorders with emphasis on hereditary diffuse gastric cancer. Prog Mol Biol Transl Sci. 2013;116:337–59. doi:10.1016/B978-0-12-394311-8.00015-7.
17. Carneiro F. Hereditary gastric cancer. Pathologe. 2012;33(Suppl 2):231–4. doi:10.1007/s00292-012-1677-6.
18. Carneiro F, Oliveira C, Suriano G, Seruca R. Molecular pathology of familial gastric cancer, with an emphasis on hereditary diffuse gastric cancer. J Clin Pathol. 2008;61(1):25–30.
19. Majewski IJ, Kluijt I, Cats A, Scerri TS, de Jong D, Kluin RJ, et al. An alpha-E-catenin (CTNNA1) mutation in hereditary diffuse gastric cancer. J Pathol. 2013;229(4):621–9. doi:10.1002/path.4152.
20. Oliveira C, de Bruin J, Nabais S, Ligtenberg M, Moutinho C, Nagengast FM, et al. Intragenic deletion of CDH1 as the inactivating mechanism of the wild-type allele in an HDGC tumour. Oncogene. 2004;23(12):2236–40. doi:10.1038/sj.onc.1207335.
21. Grady WM, Willis J, Guilford PJ, Dunbier AK, Toro TT, Lynch H, et al. Methylation of the CDH1 promoter as the second genetic hit in hereditary diffuse gastric cancer. Nat Genet. 2000;26(1):16–7. doi:10.1038/79120.

22. Wm G, Ak GPD, Tt T, Lynch HWG, Ferguson K, Eng C, et al. Methylation of the CDH1 promoter as the second genetic hit in hereditary diffuse gastric cancer. Nat Genet. 2000;26(1):16–7.
23. Hansford S, Kaurah P, Li-Chang H, Woo M, Senz J, Pinheiro H, et al. Hereditary diffuse gastric cancer syndrome: CDH1 mutations and beyond. JAMA Oncol. 2015;1(1):23–32. doi:10.1001/jamaoncol.2014.168.
24. Cisco RM, Ford JM, Norton JA. Hereditary diffuse gastric cancer: implications of genetic testing for screening and prophylactic surgery. Cancer. 2008;113(7 Suppl):1850–6. doi:10.1002/cncr.23650.
25. Worthley DL, Phillips KD, Wayte N, Schrader KA, Healey S, Kaurah P, et al. Gastric adenocarcinoma and proximal polyposis of the stomach (GAPPS): a new autosomal dominant syndrome. Gut. 2012;61(5):774–9. doi:10.1136/gutjnl-2011-300348.
26. Yanarufujisawa R, Nakamura S, Moriyama T, Esaki M, Tsuchigame T, Gushima M, et al. Familial fundic gland polyposis with gastric cancer. Gut. 2012;61(7):1103–4.
27. Oliveira C, Pinheiro H, Figueiredo J, Seruca R, Carneiro F. Familial gastric cancer: genetic susceptibility, pathology, and implications for management. Lancet Oncol. 2015;16(2):e60–70.
28. Worthley DL, Phillips KD, Wayte N, Schrader KA, Healey S, Kaurah P, et al. Gastric adenocarcinoma and proximal polyposis of the stomach (GAPPS): a new autosomal dominant syndrome. Gut. 2012;61(5):774–9.
29. Carneiro F, Oliveira C, Wen X, Seruca R. Familial gastric carcinoma. Diagn Histopathol. 2014;20(6):239–46.
30. Li J, Woods SL, Healey S, Beesley J, Chen X, Lee JS, et al. Point mutations in Exon 1B of APC reveal gastric adenocarcinoma and proximal polyposis of the stomach as a familial adenomatous polyposis variant. Am J Hum Genet. 2016;98(5):830–42. doi:10.1016/j.ajhg.2016.03.001.
31. Corso G, Carvalho J, Marrelli D, Vindigni C, Carvalho B, Seruca R, et al. Somatic mutations and deletions of the E-cadherin gene predict poor survival of patients with gastric cancer. J Clin Oncol Off J Am Soc Clin Oncol. 2013;31(7):868–75. doi:10.1200/JCO.2012.44.4612.
32. Lynch HT, Smyrk TC, Watson P, Lanspa SJ, Lynch JF, Lynch PM, et al. Genetics, natural history, tumor spectrum, and pathology of hereditary nonpolyposis colorectal cancer: an updated review. Gastroenterology. 1993;104(5):1535–49.
33. Aarnio M, Sankila R, Pukkala E, Salovaara R, Aaltonen LA, de la Chapelle A, et al. Cancer risk in mutation carriers of DNA-mismatch-repair genes. Int J Cancer. 1999;81(2):214–8.
34. Geary J, Sasieni P, Houlston R, Izatt L, Eeles R, Payne SJ, et al. Gene-related cancer spectrum in families with hereditary non-polyposis colorectal cancer (HNPCC). Fam Cancer. 2008;7(2):163–72. doi:10.1007/s10689-007-9164-6.
35. Soer EC, Leicher LW, Langers AM, van de Meeberg PC, van der Wouden EJ, Koornstra JJ, et al. Equivalent Helicobacter pylori infection rates in Lynch syndrome mutation carriers with and without a first-degree relative with gastric cancer. Int J Colorectal Dis. 2016;31(3):693–7. doi:10.1007/s00384-016-2524-7.
36. Boland CR, Koi M, Chang DK, Carethers JM. The biochemical basis of microsatellite instability and abnormal immunohistochemistry and clinical behavior in Lynch syndrome: from bench to bedside. Fam Cancer. 2008;7(1):41–52. doi:10.1007/s10689-007-9145-9.
37. Lipkin SM, Wang V, Jacoby R, Banerjee-Basu S, Baxevanis AD, Lynch HT, et al. MLH3: a DNA mismatch repair gene associated with mammalian microsatellite instability. Nat Genet. 2000;24(1):27–35. doi:10.1038/71643.
38. Peltomaki P. Role of DNA mismatch repair defects in the pathogenesis of human cancer. J Clin Oncol Off J Am Soc Clin Oncol. 2003;21(6):1174–9.
39. Syngal S, Fox EA, Eng C, Kolodner RD, Garber JE. Sensitivity and specificity of clinical criteria for hereditary non-polyposis colorectal cancer associated mutations in MSH2 and MLH1. J Med Genet. 2000;37(9):641–5.
40. Pinto M, Oliveira C, Machado JC, Cirnes L, Tavares J, Carneiro F, et al. MSI-L gastric carcinomas share the hMLH1 methylation status of MSI-H carcinomas but not their clinicopathological profile. Lab Invest. 2000;80(12):1915–23.
41. Kashiwagi K, Watanabe M, Ezaki T, Kanai T, Ishii H, Mukai M, et al. Clinical usefulness of microsatellite instability for the prediction of gastric adenoma or adenocarcinoma in patients with chronic gastritis. Br J Cancer. 2000;82(11):1814–8. doi:10.1054/bjoc.1999.1154.
42. Vasen HF. Clinical description of the Lynch syndrome [hereditary nonpolyposis colorectal cancer (HNPCC)]. Fam Cancer. 2005;4(3):219–25. doi:10.1007/s10689-004-3906-5.
43. Wahlberg SS, Schmeits J, Thomas G, Loda M, Garber J, Syngal S, et al. Evaluation of microsatellite instability and immunohistochemistry for the prediction of germ-line MSH2 and MLH1 mutations in hereditary nonpolyposis colon cancer families. Cancer Res. 2002;62(12):3485–92.
44. Musulen E, Moreno V, Reyes G, Sancho FJ, Peinado MA, Esteller M, et al. Standardized approach for microsatellite instability detection in gastric carcinomas. Hum Pathol. 2004;35(3):335–42.
45. Nielsen M, Hes FJ, Nagengast FM, Weiss MM, Mathus-Vliegen EM, Morreau H, et al. Germline mutations in APC and MUTYH are responsible for the majority of families with attenuated familial adenomatous polyposis. Clin Genet. 2007;71(5):427–33.
46. Attard TM, Cuffari C, Tajouri T, Stoner JA, Eisenberg MT, Yardley JH, et al. Multicenter experience with upper gastrointestinal polyps in pediatric patients with familial adenomatous polyposis. Am J Gastroenterol. 2004;99(4):681–6. doi:10.1111/j.1572-0241.2004.04115.x.
47. Bianchi LK, Burke CA, Bennett AE, Lopez R, Hasson H, Church JM. Fundic gland polyp dysplasia is com-

mon in familial adenomatous polyposis. Clin Gastroenterol Hepatol. 2008;6(2):180–5. doi:10.1016/j.cgh.2007.11.018.
48. Lynch HT, Smyrk T, McGinn T, Lanspa S, Cavalieri J, Lynch J, et al. Attenuated familial adenomatous polyposis (AFAP). A phenotypically and genotypically distinctive variant of FAP. Cancer. 1995;76(12):2427–33.
49. Yamaguchi T, Ishida H, Ueno H, Kobayashi H, Hinoi T, Inoue Y, et al. Upper gastrointestinal tumours in Japanese familial adenomatous polyposis patients. Jpn J Clin Oncol. 2016;46(4):310–5.
50. Park JG, Park KJ, Ahn YO, Song IS, Choi KW, Hong YM, et al. Risk of gastric cancer among Korean familial adenomatous polyposis patients. Dis Colon Rectum. 1992;35(10):996–8.
51. Da LMA, Church JM, Burke CA. The evolution of prophylactic colorectal surgery for familial adenomatous polyposis. Dis Colon Rectum. 2009;52(8):1481–6.
52. Vasen HF, Moslein G, Alonso A, Aretz S, Bernstein I, Bertario L, et al. Guidelines for the clinical management of familial adenomatous polyposis (FAP). Gut. 2008;57(5):704–13. doi:10.1136/gut.2007.136127.
53. Wu TT, Kornacki S, Rashid A, Yardley JH, Hamilton SR. Dysplasia and dysregulation of proliferation in foveolar and surface epithelia of fundic gland polyps from patients with familial adenomatous polyposis. Am J Surg Pathol. 1998;22(3):293–8.
54. Bertoni G, Sassatelli R, Nigrisoli E, Pennazio M, Tansini P, Arrigoni A, et al. Dysplastic changes in gastric fundic gland polyps of patients with familial adenomatous polyposis. Ital J Gastroenterol Hepatol. 1999;31(3):192–7.
55. Nielsen M, Morreau H, Vasen HF, Hes FJ. MUTYH-associated polyposis (MAP). Crit Rev Oncol Hematol. 2011;79(1):1–16.
56. Schneider C, Simon T, Hero B, Uphoff US, Drebber U, Alakus H, et al. [18F]Fluorodeoxyglucose positron emission tomography/computed tomography-positive gastric adenocarcinoma in a 12-year-old girl with Peutz-Jeghers syndrome. J Clin Oncol Off J Am Soc Clin Oncol. 2012;30(14):e140–3.
57. Lier MGFV, Wagner A, Mathus-Vliegen EMH, Kuipers EJ, Steyerberg EW, Leerdam MEV. High cancer risk in Peutz-Jeghers syndrome: a systematic review and surveillance recommendations. Am J Gastroenterol. 2010;105(6):1258–64.
58. Hemminki A, Avizienyte E, Roth S, Loukola A, Aaltonen LA, Järvinen H, et al. A serine/threonine kinase gene defective in Peutz-Jeghers syndrome. Nature. 1998;391(6663):184–7.
59. Amos CI, Keithericheteri MB, Sabripour M, Wei C, Mcgarrity TJ, Seldin MF, et al. Genotype-phenotype correlations in Peutz-Jeghers syndrome. J Med Genet. 2004;41(5):327–33.
60. Jass JR, Williams CB, Bussey HJ, Morson BC. Juvenile polyposis—a precancerous condition. Histopathology. 1988;13(6):619–30.
61. Howe JR, Sayed MG, Ahmed AF, Ringold J, Larsen-Haidle J, Merg A, et al. The prevalence of MADH4 and BMPR1A mutations in juvenile polyposis and absence of BMPR2, BMPR1B, and ACVR1 mutations. J Med Genet. 2004;41(7):484–91.
62. Sayed MG, Ahmed AF, Ringold JR, Anderson ME, Bair JL, Mitros FA, et al. Germline SMAD4 or BMPR1A mutations and phenotype of juvenile polyposis. Ann Surg Oncol. 2002;9(9):901–6.
63. Latchford AR, Neale K, Phillips RK, Clark SK. Juvenile polyposis syndrome: a study of genotype, phenotype, and long-term outcome. Dis Colon Rectum. 2012;55(55):1038–43.
64. Schreibman IR, Baker M, Amos C, Mcgarrity TJ. The hamartomatous polyposis syndromes: a clinical and molecular review. Am J Gastroenterol. 2005;100(2):476–90.
65. van Hattem WA, Brosens LA, de Leng WW, Morsink FH, Lens S, Carvalho R, et al. Large genomic deletions of SMAD4, BMPR1A and PTEN in juvenile polyposis. Gut. 2008;57(5):623–7. doi:10.1136/gut.2007.142927.
66. Masciari S, Dewanwala A, Stoffel EM, Lauwers GY, Zheng H, Achatz MI, et al. Gastric cancer in individuals with Li-Fraumeni syndrome. Genet Med. 2011;13(7):651–7. doi:10.1097/GIM.0b013e31821628b6.
67. Chang VY, Federman N, Martinez-Agosto J, Tatishchev SF, Nelson SF. Whole exome sequencing of pediatric gastric adenocarcinoma reveals an atypical presentation of Li-Fraumeni syndrome. Pediatr Blood Cancer. 2013;60(4):570–4. doi:10.1002/pbc.24316.
68. da Silva EM, Achatz MI, Martel-Planche G, Montagnini AL, Olivier M, Prolla PA, et al. TP53 mutation p. R337H in gastric cancer tissues of a 12-year-old male child: evidence for chimerism involving a common mutant founder haplotype: case report. BMC Cancer. 2011;11:449. doi:10.1186/1471-2407-11-449.
69. Chen XR, Zhang WZ, Lin XQ, Wang JW. Genetic instability of BRCA1 gene at locus D17S855 is related to clinicopathological behaviors of gastric cancer from Chinese population. World J Gastroe nterol. 2006;12(26):4246–9.
70. Figer A, Irmin L, Geva R, Flex D, Sulkes J, Sulkes A, et al. The rate of the 6174delT founder Jewish mutation in BRCA2 in patients with non-colonic gastrointestinal tract tumours in Israel. Br J Cancer. 2001;84(4):478–81. doi:10.1054/bjoc.2000.1605.
71. Lawniczak M, Jakubowska A, Bialek A, Lubinski J, Jaworska-Bieniek K, Kaczmarek K, et al. BRCA1 founder mutations do not contribute to increased risk of gastric cancer in the Polish population. Hered Cancer Clin Pract. 2016;14:3. doi:10.1186/s13053-015-0043-0.
72. Trufant JW, Greene L, Cook DL, Mckinnon W, Greenblatt M, Bosenberg MW. Colonic ganglioneuromatous polyposis and metastatic adenocarcinoma in the setting of Cowden syndrome: a case report and literature review. Hum Pathol. 2012;43(4):601–4.
73. Al-Thihli K, Palma L, Marcus V, Cesari M, Kushner YB, Barkun A, Foulkes WD. A case of Cowden's syndrome presenting with gastric carcinomas and gastrointestinal polyposis. Nat Clin Pract Gastroenterol Hepatol. 2009;6(3):184–9.

Genetics and Molecular Signature of Gastric Cancer

2

Meng Zhu and Guangfu Jin

2.1 Introduction

Gastric cancer (GC) is a major contributor to the global cancer burden. According to GLOBOCAN 2012, approximately 952,000 new cases of gastric cancer were diagnosed globally in 2012 (representing 6.8% of total cancer diagnoses), and 723,000 patients died as a result of gastric cancer (representing 8.8% of all cancer-related deaths) [1]. These statistics make gastric cancer the fifth most common malignant tumor in the world, behind cancers of the lung, breast, colon, rectum, and prostate. Of these cases, more than 70% occurred in developing countries, and half the total were diagnosed in Eastern Asia (with China reporting approximately 43%) [1]. Encouragingly, numerous studies have demonstrated a decrease in the incidence of gastric cancer over the past few decades [2–4]. Nevertheless, the total number of new gastric cancer cases has risen in recent years as a result of population growth and changing demographics.

M. Zhu • G. Jin (✉)
Department of Epidemiology and Biostatistics, School of Public Health, Nanjing Medical University, Nanjing 211166, China

Jiangsu Key Lab of Cancer Biomarkers, Prevention and Treatment, Collaborative Innovation Center for Cancer Medicine, Nanjing Medical University, Nanjing 211166, China
e-mail: guangfujin@njmu.edu.cn

Histologically, gastric cancer can be divided into two classes, diffuse (DGC) or intestinal type (IGC). IGC generally arises from chronic precancerous lesions. Such lesions usually develop from chronic inflammation caused by *H. pylori* infection, which then progresses to atrophic gastritis and eventually to intestinal metaplasia and dysplasia [5]. In contrast, DGC usually develops from normal gastric mucosa with no definitive premalignant stage and is often associated with a negative *H. pylori* status [6]. In IGC, but not in DGC, malignant cells resemble gland-like structures. IGC occurs more frequently in high-risk regions, while DGC is more common in low-risk areas. DGC is more frequently diagnosed in young patients and females and behaves more aggressively than IGC-type cancer. Although often reported as a single entity, gastric cancer can also be divided into two main categories according to their topography: cardia gastric cancer (CGC), which develops in the area of the stomach adjoining the esophageal-gastric junction, and non-cardia gastric cancer (NCGC), which is found in more distal regions of the stomach [7]. Both CGC and NCGC are thought to be influenced by a variety of factors such as infection with *H. pylori*, cigarette smoking, consumption of high-sodium foods, and low intake of fruits and vegetables [8–11]. However, other risk factors are subtype specific. For example, CGC shares specific risk

J. Wei, B. Liu (eds.), *Personalized Management of Gastric Cancer*,
DOI 10.1007/978-981-10-3978-2_2

factors with esophageal adenocarcinoma, such as obesity and gastroesophageal reflux disease (GORD) [12, 13]. Gastric cancer is a solid tumor developing as a consequence of a complex interplay between genetic and environmental factors (Fig. 2.1). In addition to these environmental risk factors, host genetic factors also determine an individual's predisposition to GC, and the heritability estimate is approximately 24.3% for GC [14].

Clinically, symptoms of gastric cancer often present late in the development of the disease, thus limiting the opportunity for early detection and diagnosis. A lack of effective treatment

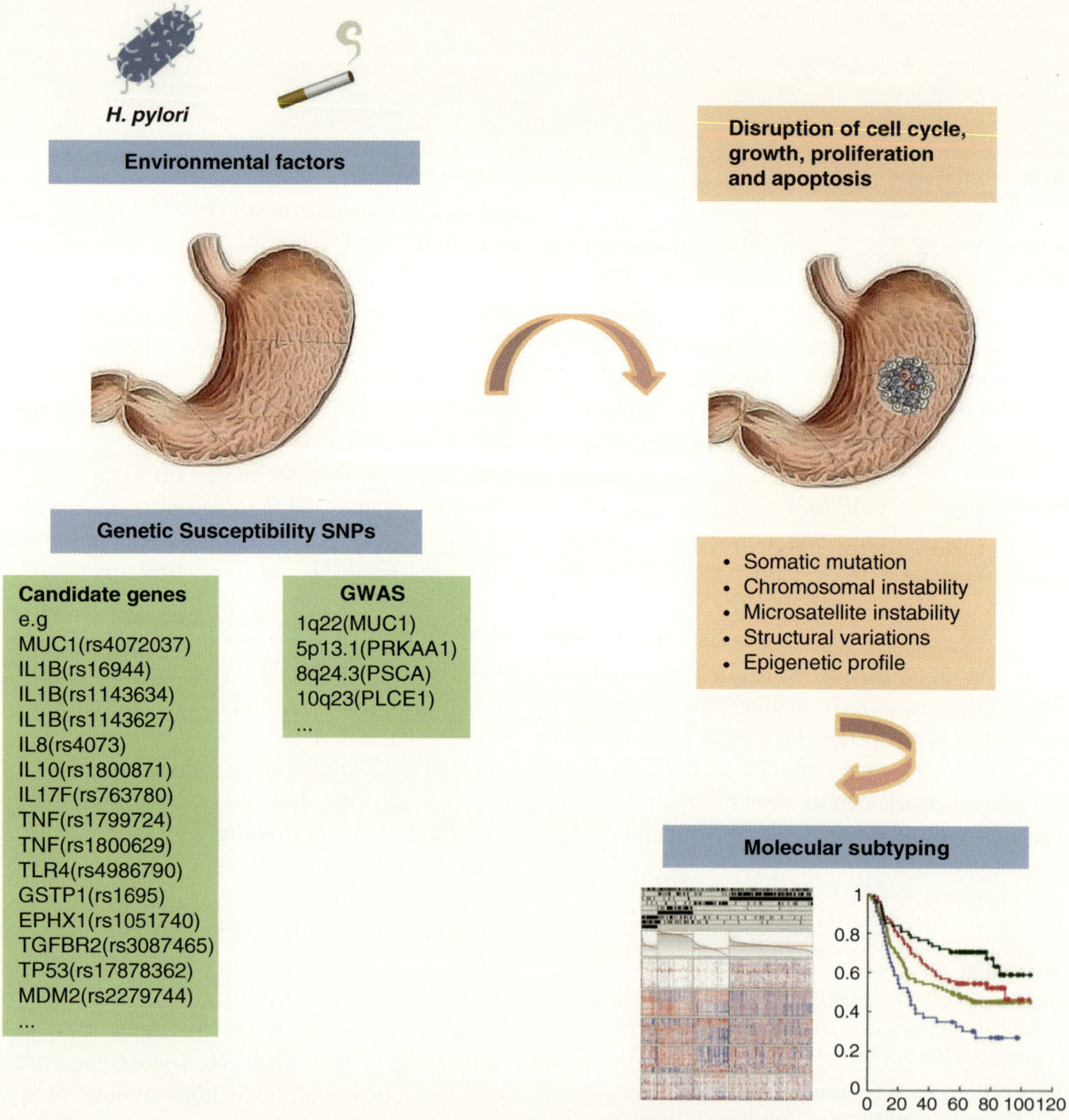

Fig. 2.1 Gastric cancer is a malignancy resulting from the complex interplay between genetic and environmental factors. The molecular alterations found in gastric cancer include somatic gene mutations, chromosomal instability, microsatellite instability, structure variants, and changes in epigenetic profile, which disrupt cell cycle, growth, proliferation, and apoptosis of gastric epithelial cells. These molecular alterations can be used for molecular subtyping, thus guiding clinical practice (Adapted from Nat Rev Gastroenterol Hepatol. 2014;11 [15])

options following diagnosis often leads to a poor prognosis. In order to address these issues, novel biomarkers and detailed description of molecular features of GC are paramount [15]. Over the past few decades, advances in technology and high-throughput sequencing analysis have enabled a greater understanding of the genetic and molecular aspects of gastric cancer pathogenesis. In this section, we will address the genetic basis that drives the disease and discuss genomic signatures that confer the specific molecular signature of gastric cancer.

2.2 The Genomic Susceptibility of Gastric Cancer

Only a subset of individuals exposed to environmental risk factors (such as *H. pylori* infection or smoke) ultimately develop GC, indicating that genetic variations might be a contributing factor. Single nucleotide polymorphisms (SNPs) are the most common genetic alterations naturally occurring, with variable frequencies within different ethnic populations. Particular SNPs can modify susceptibility to GC, either through altering the gene expression profile or by affecting gene function directly. With conferring increased susceptibility to GC, the risk alleles of SNPs often accumulate in GC cases, resulting in higher frequencies in GC cases compared to normal healthy individuals. Initially, the association between SNPs within key genes and GC susceptibility was explored using a hypothesis-driven candidate gene approach. Nowadays, with the advent of improved genotyping technologies, genome-wide association studies (GWAS) and high-throughput genetic analyses have become the main research strategy (Table 2.1). This new strategy is not hypothesis-driven and allows the simultaneous investigation of hundreds of thousands SNPs. The most significant advantage of this approach is the ability to identify new susceptibility genes, in turn offering crucial insights into the pathogenesis of gastric cancer.

Table 2.1 Summary of results from representative GWAS studies in gastric cancer

Region	Gene	Identified SNPs	Reference
Non-cardia gastric cancer			
1q22	ASH1L	rs80142782 T > C	Wang Z et al., 2015 [26]
3q13.31	ZBTB20	rs9841504 C > G	Shi Y et al., 2011 [52]
5q14.3	lnc-POLR3G-4	rs7712641 C > T	Wang Z et al., 2015 [26]
5p13.1	PTGER4-PRKAA1	rs13361707 T > C	Shi Y et al., 2011 [52]
6p21.1	UNC5CL	rs2294693 T > C	Hu N et al., 2016 [49]
8q24.3	PSCA	rs2294008 C > T	Wang Z et al., 2015 [26]
		rs2976392 A > G	Shi Y et al., 2011 [52]
Cardia gastric cancer			
10q23	PLCE1	rs2274223 A > G	Abnet CC et al., 2010 [48]
			Wang LD et al., 2010 [69]
20p13	C20orf54	rs1304295 C > T	Wang LD et al., 2010 [69]
Cardia and non-cardia gastric cancer			
1q22	MUC1	rs4072037 A > G	Hu N et al., 2016 [49]
5p13.1	PTGER4-PRKAA1	rs10074991 G > A	Hu N et al., 2016 [49]
Diffuse gastric cancer			
8q24.3	PSCA	rs2294008 C > T	Study Group of Millennium Genome Project for Cancer, 2008 [47]
1q22	MUC1	rs2070803G > A	Study Group of Millennium Genome Project for Cancer, 2008 [47]

2.3 SNPs in Candidate Genes

2.3.1 Mucins

Mucins are high molecular weight proteins modified with O-linked oligosaccharides and n-glycan chains, thus belonging to the class of glycoproteins. In the human genome, 21 mucin (MUC) genes have been described [16]. These genes encode two distinct groups of mucins involved in epithelial barrier protection between a host and its environment: secreted mucins and membrane-bound mucins. The major mucins expressed in the stomach are the membrane-bound *MUC1* as well as the secreted *MUC5AC* and *MUC6*. *MUC1* usually expressed in the gastric mucosa in the superficial and foveolar epithelium and mucous neck zone cells. In contrast, *MUC5AC* is often detected in the superficial epithelium, while *MUC6* is found in the deep glands. The specific expression pattern of *MUC1*, *MUC5AC*, and *MUC6* is altered in the carcinogenesis of gastric cancer, with de novo expression of secreted *MUC2*. Crucially, several studies have highlighted the important role of genetic variants in these mucin genes in the development of GC [16, 17].

Polymorphisms in *MUC1* associated with gastric carcinoma, as well as with chronic atrophic gastritis and incomplete intestinal metaplasia, were first identified in Europeans in the 1990s [18]. These polymorphisms mostly constituted variable number of tandem repeat (VNTR) [18–20]. In addition, using an LD-based tag SNP approach, a recent population-based case-control study in the Polish population linked SNP rs4072037 with a significantly increased risk of GC [21]. This association was subsequently replicated by several additional GWAS studies and candidate gene studies in different ethnicities [22–26], while other studies reported conflicting results [27, 28]. A further meta-analysis comprising 6580 cases and 10,324 controls confirmed that the A allele of rs4072037 was associated with an increased risk of GC progression, predominantly in Asians [29].

MUC5AC encodes a mucin secreted by the gastric mucosa which is thought to play a role in the colonization of *H. pylori* [30]. In patients with chronic *H. pylori* infection, the number of MUC5ACproducing cells as well as expression levels of MUC5AC may gradually decrease [31]. Currently, the number of studies investigating the association between *MUC5AC* polymorphisms and GC risk is limited. *Jia* et al. evaluated the association between eight tag SNPs of *MUC5AC* and the risk of GC in a Polish population and found one SNP—rs868903—to be significantly associated with GC risk while not related to the risk of *H. pylori* infection [21]. In another study, a total of 12 tag SNPs were assessed in a Chinese population, but none were associated with an increased risk of GC or *H. pylori* infection [32]. In summary, while these studies showed inconsistent results for GC risk, both suggested that the polymorphisms of *MUC5AC* are not associated with an increased risk of *H. pylori* infection [21, 33].

MUC6 encodes a secreted mucin which is highly expressed in normal gastric mucosa. Studies have shown that the unique glycan residues on *MUC6* inhibit the biosynthesis of a major cell wall component (cholesteryl-αD-glucopyranoside), thus playing an important role in the host defense against *H. pylori* infection [34, 35]. In GC tumors, the expression of *MUC6* has been shown to be significantly reduced [36]. The association between VNTR polymorphisms in *MUC6* and GC risk has been extensively studied. Small VNTR alleles of *MUC6* have been found to be associated with an increased risk of both *H. pylori* infection and GC [37, 38]. Kwon et al. identified short rare minisatellites-5 alleles of *MUC6* that influence susceptibility to gastric carcinoma by regulating the expression of *MUC6* [39]. However, no SNPs in *MUC6* were shown to be associated with GC risk thus far.

MUC2 is not expressed in normal gastric mucosa but is detected in intestinal metaplasia and GC. The expression of *MUC2* is thought to be activated by pro-inflammatory cytokines which are produced as a reaction to *H. pylori* infection. Similar to *MUC6*, while short rare minisatellites-6 alleles of *MUC2* have been shown to be associated with GC risk, no significantly associated SNPs have been identified [40].

2.4 Inflammatory Cytokines and Immune Response Genes

H. pylori infection is thought to be the most common environmental risk factor for GC and has been recognized as a class I carcinogen by the World Health Organization (WHO) [41]. Nearly 50% of the world population has contracted *H. pylori at one point*, and a three- to sixfold increased risk of GC has been observed in individuals infected with *H. pylori* [42]. Following infection with *H. pylori*, the host immune response modulates and mediates the inflammatory response, which determines the severity and scope of the tissue damage. Inflammatory cytokines (e.g., *IL1*, *IL8*, *IL10*, *IL17*, and *TNF*) and immune-related genes (e.g., *TLR4*) are the most common and pivotal genes involved in the host immune response to *H. pylori* infection. The association between genetic variants in these inflammatory cytokine and immune response genes and GC risk has been widely investigated in the past few years.

IL1B is the most powerful pro-inflammatory cytokine produced in response to *H. pylori* infection; in addition, it is also a potent inhibitor of gastric acid secretion [43]. In the absence of *H. pylori* infection, an overt malignant pathology was still observed in a transgenic mouse model with overexpression of *IL-1β* in the stomach through promoter targeted driven. When *H. pylori* colonization was introduced into this model, an accelerated pathological consequence was observed [44]. These results indicate that increased expression of *IL1B* is sufficient to induce gastric dysplasia or carcinogenesis. Furthermore, these results also reinforce the importance of host-environment interactions in the development of GC. Based on these biological findings, the impact of SNPs in the cluster of IL1 genes (encoding *IL-1RN*, *IL-1α*, *IL-1β*, and the naturally occurring receptor antagonist) on the risk of gastric cancer has been evaluated in various populations of different ethnicities. However, results from different studies have proven inconsistent. In a recent meta-analysis by Simone et al. [45], *IL1B*-511(rs16944) was identified and shown to be significantly associated with an increased risk of cardia GC, with an estimated OR of 1.20 (95%CI 1.06–1.35). In contrast, no association with diffuse-type GC was found. Furthermore, The SNP *IL1B* + 3954(rs1143634) significantly increased the risk of gastric cancer in *H. pylori*-positive cases and controls (OR = 1.72, 95%CI 1.32–2.24). Using a standard protocol, Persson and colleagues also conducted a series of meta-analyses on these inflammation-related genes in the human genome epidemiology (HuGE) review and found a consistent positive association between the VNTR IL1RN*2 and an increased risk of gastric cancer. This association was specific to non-Asian populations and was observed for both IGC and DGC, particularly in cancers with a distal location [46]. In contrast, the SNP IL1B-31(rs1143627) was associated with a significantly reduced risk of GC in Asian populations. While the quality of these associations was considered high or intermediate in the meta-analysis, these SNPs were not associated with the expression of *IL1B* in stomach tissues or peripheral blood according to GTEx. As yet, the exact mechanisms underlying these associations remain unclear.

In light of the associations in the IL1 gene cluster, there has been a growing interest in SNPs in other interleukin gene families (e.g., *IL-8*, which stimulates the proliferation of endothelial cells; *IL-10*, which downregulates cytotoxic responses; and *IL-17*, which alters the host inflammatory microenvironment) and whether these SNPs could alter the susceptibility of gastric cancer. Through a systematic meta-analysis, Simone et al. found that rs4073 and rs2227306 in *IL8* were significantly associated with an increased risk of GC (OR = 1.24 for rs4073; and OR = 1.23 for rs2227306). These two SNPs were in high linkage disequilibrium (LD), with R^2 of 0.81, and were shown to regulate the expression of IL8 in peripheral blood. In addition, rs1800871, which regulates the expression of *IL10*, was found to be significantly associated with a reduced risk of GC (OR = 0.57, 95%CI 0.37–0.88). While rs763780, a missense variant in *IL17F*, was significantly associated with an increased risk of

GC (OR = 1.29, 95%CI 1.34–1.46) specific to the Asian population [45].

Other genes involved in the host inflammatory response to *H. pylori* infections are *TNF* (primarily involved in the adaptive immune system) and *TLR4* (mainly involved in initiating the innate immune system). Several studies have assessed sequence variants in these two genes in the context of gastric cancer. According to a meta-analysis by Simone et al., rs1799724 and rs1800629 in *TNF* were significantly associated with increased risk of GC, and the association of rs1800629 was more prominent in Caucasian population as well in cardia and diffuse-type GC. Similarly, a missense variant in *TLR4*, rs4986790, showed a positive association with an increased risk of GC, especially in Caucasian population and non-cardia GC [45].

2.5 Other Genetic Variants

In addition to the two major gene sets described above, sequence variants in several other genes associated with pathophysiological mechanisms have been studied in the context of gastric cancer susceptibility. These genes include enzymes involved in the metabolism of chemical carcinogens (e.g., cytochrome P450 enzymes, *EPHX1*, *GSTM1*, *GSTP1*, and *GSTT1*), DNA repair (e.g., *ERCC* gene family and *XRCC* gene family), epithelial cell growth, proliferation, apoptosis, and protection (e.g., *FAS/FASL*, *TFF* gene family, and *TGFB* gene family), as well as ABO blood type and the most commonly mutated tumor suppressor gene *P53* and its negative regulator *MDM2*. Despite some inconsistent conclusions, Simone et al. found several reliable associations after a systematic review and subgroup meta-analysis: The SNP rs1695, a missense variant in *GSTP1*, was observed significantly associated with a 1.19-fold increased risk of GC specific to Asian populations; rs1051740, a missense variant in *EPHX1*, was correlated with the risk of GC with an estimated OR of 1.24 in a Caucasian population; the SNP rs3087465 in the promoter region of *TGFBR2* significantly reduced the risk of GC only in Asians, while rs8176719, which defines the O blood type, was associated with an 0.81-fold decreased risk of GC only in Caucasians. A 16 bp duplication in intron 3 of the *TP53* gene (PIN3 Ins16bp, rs17878362) was associated with an increased risk of GC, with estimated OR of 1.37, while SNP rs2279744 in *MDM2*, the negative regulator of *TP53*, was found to be significantly associated with an increased risk of cardia GC (OR = 1.38, 95%CI 1.13–1.69). These findings reinforce the relevance of certain candidate genes in the development of gastric cancer and provide an additional understanding of how a person's genetic background contributes to the susceptibility of GC. However, the exact mechanisms underlying these associations remain unexplored.

2.6 Susceptibility Regions Identified by GWAS

2.6.1 1q22

In 2008, Sakamoto and colleagues performed a GWAS study of diffuse gastric cancer and identified two significantly associated variants (rs2075570 in *MTX1* and rs2070803 in *TRIM46*) within chromosome 1q22 in a Japanese population [47]. In a subsequent study, these associations were confirmed in another Japanese population as well as in a Korean population [25, 47]. Furthermore, in another GWAS study on gastric adenocarcinoma and esophageal squamous cell carcinoma, Christian et al. also identified two variants (rs4072037 in *MUC1* and rs4460629 in the downstream of *KRTCAP2*) related to the susceptibility of gastric adenocarcinoma in a Chinese population [48]. Wang et al. confirmed the association of the *MUC1* variant rs4072037 in a GWAS meta-analysis [26]. In addition, stratification analysis revealed that this association was also significant in both cardia and non-cardia gastric cancer [49]. In a systematic meta-analysis by Simone et al., a total of eight variants in different genes on locus 1q22 were found significantly associated with the susceptibility of diffuse gastric cancer [45]. However, all these variants were in medium-high LD with each other ($R^2 > 0.5$).

A total of five genes (*KRTCAP2*, *TRIM46*, *MUC1*, *THBS3*, and *MTX1*) reside in the strong LD block harboring rs2070803, rs2075570, rs4072037, and rs4460629. *MUC1*, which has been closely investigated in candidate gene studies, is located at the center of this block and is thought to be responsible for conferring the increased cancer susceptibility. As described above, *MUC1* is a membrane-bound protein in the gastric mucosa and is involved in the epithelial barrier protection between a host and its environment. Besides its involvement in epithelial barrier formation, studies have also shown that phosphorylation of *MUC1* can affect many important cell functions through its multifaceted functional repertoire. For example, *MUC1* can stimulate the β-catenin-Wnt pathway, thus affecting cyclin D1 transcription and cell growth, and influence cell kinase-driven signaling pathways. Furthermore, MUC1 interacts with several pivotal transcription factors (including the STATs and NF-κB), thus affecting expression of downstream targets and influencing cell-cell adhesion [15]. Due to its versatile functions, *MUC1* is considered an oncoprotein implicated in a number of tumors and a potential therapeutic target.

The mechanisms by which these candidate genes affect cancer susceptibility have not been fully understood. There is evidence that rs4072037 (G > A) in exon 2 of the *MUC1* gene confers the disease risk, with the G allele being protective. Xu et al. assessed *MUC1* protein expression in gastric cancer specimens and found that the A allele of rs4072037 was associated with reduced protein levels [50]. In support of this result, rs4072037 was found to reduce the activity of the *MUC1* promoter in functional reporter assays [25]. Moreover, rs4072037 is located in the region spanning exons 1 and 2, which could potentially affect the splicing of the second exon. Further analysis showed that the risk allele A of rs4072037 leads to a 9-amino acid deletion in the second exon, causing modifications of both the signal peptide and the N-terminal amino acid of the mature protein by changing the signal peptide cleavage site [51]. This change may affect intracellular trafficking, as well as glycosylation, and protein folding, effecting alteration in the functions of the mature protein.

2.6.2 5p13.1

Through a three-stage analysis of 4294 non-cardia gastric cancer cases and 5882 controls, Shi et al. demonstrated a significant association of the C allele of rs13361707 with an increased risk of non-cardia gastric cancer in a Chinese population [52]. This variant is located within the intronic sequence of *PRKAA1* on locus 5p13.1. This association was further validated by several additional studies in Eastern Chinese, Korean, and European populations [53–55]. In a genome-wide study designed to compare the associations between cardia and non-cardia tumors, Hu et al. found a significant association between rs10074991 in *PRKAA1* and a reduced risk of both cardia and non-cardia gastric cancer [49]. The rs10074991 and rs13361707 sequence variants, both located in the intronic sequence of *PRKAA1*, were in perfect LD (R^2 = 1.00). In a systematic meta-analysis by Simone et al., rs13361707 was also found significantly associated with both cardia and non-cardia gastric [45].

The strong LD block containing rs13361707 chiefly spans three genes—*PTGER4*, *TTC33*, and *PRKAA1*—on 5p13.1. Interestingly, results from GTEx showed a significant association of rs13361707 with the expression of these three genes in stomach tissues. *PTGER4* encodes a member of the G protein-coupled receptors and is also one of the four receptors for prostaglandin E2 (PGE2). This receptor has been shown to induce expression of early growth response 1 (EGR1) and to regulate the level and stability of cyclooxygenase-2 (COX-2) mRNA [56, 57]. Studies have demonstrated that PGE2 signaling promotes the tumorigenesis of gastric cancer through *PTGER4*-activated epidermal growth factor receptor (*EGFR*) and metalloproteases (*ADAMs*). Additionally, it is involved in the gastric mucosal defense against *H. pylori* infection [58, 59]. Few studies on *TTC33* have been conducted so far, and the role of *TTC33* in tumorigenesis is yet unclear. The protein encoded by

PRKAA1 belongs to the ser/thr protein kinase family and is a catalytic subunit of the 5′-prime-AMP-activated protein kinase (AMPK). AMPK is a cellular energy sensor conserved in all eukaryotic cells and plays a crucial role in the regulation of a number of key metabolic enzymes through phosphorylation. Activation of AMPK is triggered by an increase in the cellular AMP/ATP ratio [60]. AMPK protects cells from stresses that cause ATP depletion by blocking ATP-consuming biosynthetic pathways. Recent studies suggest an involvement of AMPK in the inhibition of YAP activity, thus suppressing oncogenic transformation of Lats-null cells [61]. Although studies have suggested an involvement of *PTGER4* and *PRKAA1*in promoting tumorigenesis, the exact mechanisms underlying the associations in 5p13.1 and gastric cancer risk are not fully understood.

2.6.3 8q24.3

In 2008, the first GWAS study of gastric cancer linked rs2294008 and rs2976392 on locus 8q24.3 to an increased risk of diffuse-type gastric cancer in a Japanese population [47]. The rs2294008 and rs2976392 variants were in strong LD in Asians ($R^2 = 0.98$). This association was subsequently confirmed by several following studies in Chinese, South Korean, and Caucasian populations [62–66]. Despite variable frequencies between different ethnicities, the unexpected association was conserved. Moreover, these studies also expanded the significance to intestinal gastric cancer as well as non-cardia gastric cancer [65].

SNPs with high LD with rs2294008 ($R^2 > 0.8$) mainly span three genes (*JRK*, *PSCA*, and *LY6K*) based on LD structure of Asians in the 1000 Genomes Project. The rs2294008 sequence is located in the 5’UTR of the *PSCA* gene. In previous studies, *PSCA* was thought to be responsible for the observed association in this region. *PSCA* encodes a glycosylphosphatidylinositol-anchored cell membrane glycoprotein and was first identified as a prostate-specific antigen found overexpressed in prostate cancer [67]. Later it was shown to be expressed in a variety of tumors (such as cancers of the bladder and pancreas) as well as in some normal tissues (including stomach and bladder epithelial cells) [68]. In gastric cancer tissue specimens, *PSCA* is frequently downregulated at both the gene and protein level. To unravel the biological significance of *PSCA* in tumorigenesis, in vitro transfection studies were carried out. These studies revealed that *PSCA* is involved in the inhibition of gastric epithelial cell proliferation [47]. Furthermore, substitution of the C allele with the risk allele T at rs2294008 was shown to lead to a frameshift variation in the start codon of PSCA and was associated with reduced gene transcription activity [47].

2.6.4 10q23.33

Cardia gastric adenocarcinoma (GCA) and esophageal squamous cell carcinoma (ESCC) are not only closely related in terms of their anatomic locations but usually share many similarities in terms of concurrent geographic distribution and environmental risk factors. In 2010, Wang et al. identified a SNP rs2274223 on 10q23.33 that significantly associated with the susceptibility to ESCC in a Chinese population. This variant was also shown to be associated with GCA in a follow-up validation study with 2766 gastric cardia adenocarcinoma cases and 11,013 control subjects [69]. At the same time, Christian et al. also performed a GWAS study including ESCC, CGC, and NCGC using samples from Shanxi and Linxian (two areas in China with extremely high incidence rates of upper gastrointestinal cancer). Results from this study further validated the association of rs2274223 with ESCC and CGC, while no link to NCGC was established [48]. In addition to these two GWAS studies, several additional studies also supported this association in Chinese populations [45, 70, 71] but not in Caucasian populations [23].

SNPs in high LD ($R^2 > 0.8$) with rs2274223 are mainly located within *PLCE1* and *NOC3L*. Among these SNPs, the sequence variants rs2274223 and rs3765524 are missense mutations in the coding regions of *PLCE1*, resulting in R1927H and I1777T amino acid substitutions. The *PLCE1* gene encodes an enzyme named phospholipase C epsilon 1, which regulates intracellular signaling by catalyzing the hydrolysis of phosphatidylinositol-4,5-bisphosphate to 1,2-diacylglycerol and inositol 1,4,5-trisphosphate [69, 72]. *PLCE1* contains several Ras-binding domains for small G proteins and usually acts as an effector of GTPases Ras, Rap1, and Rap2. These GTPases have been shown to be involved in regulating cell growth, differentiation, apoptosis, and angiogenesis [73]. *PLCE1* plays a role in skin and intestinal carcinogenesis through modulating inflammation signaling pathways and promotes the progression of head and neck squamous cell carcinoma by binding members of the Ras family [74, 75]. Notably, studies have also shown *PLCE1* to be overexpressed in precancerous chronic atrophic gastritis tissues and stomach carcinoma compared to normal gastric tissues. Intriguingly a potential therapeutic benefit of inhibiting this enzyme was demonstrated in a xenograft model [69, 76]. Taken together, these results substantiate the finding that *PLCE1* contributes to the susceptibility to gastric cardia carcinoma, though the exact mechanisms remain unknown.

2.7 Other Regions

In addition to the loci described above, some GWA studies have detected several susceptibility regions that could not be replicated by other association studies. These loci include rs9841504 in *ZBTB20* (3q13.31), rs7712641 in *lnc-POLR3G-4* (5q14.3), and rs2294693 in *UNC5CL* (6p21.1) for non-cardia gastric cancer as well as rs1304295 in C20orf54 (20p13) for cardia gastric cancer [26, 49, 52, 69]. The lack of validation of these associations could possibly be due to the heterogeneity of the gastric cancer biopsies taken or the populations studied or could be the result of differences in the study design (e.g., sample size). Notably, in a recent GWAS pooled study by Wang et al., a new variant, rs80142782, in the *ASH1L* gene was reported to be independent from the previously reported SNP rs4072037 on 1q22 and was found to be associated with a reduced risk of non-cardia gastric cancer in a Chinese population [26]. While these results will require further validation and confirmation, potential new insights into the pathogenesis of gastric cancer have been inferred from these findings.

2.8 Molecular Signature of Gastric Cancer

2.8.1 Microsatellite Instability and Chromosomal Instability in Gastric Cancer

Microsatellite instability (MSI) is characterized by length alterations within simple repeated sequences called microsatellites. Deficient DNA mismatch repair genes (MMR) are thought to be the main reason for MSI. In sporadic gastric cancers, MSI is found in about 15% of tumors and was frequently the result of epigenetic changes of the mismatch repair gene MSH1 [77]. Hypermethylation of the promoter region is the most common reason for impaired DNA mismatch repair and results in multiple mutations within simple nucleotide repeats. These changes affect the expression levels of numerous downstream genes and exert profound functional consequences on a number of pathways such as cell signaling, cell cycle, and tumor suppression [15]. Gastric cancers can be divided into subgroups based on the levels of microsatellite instability, and overall survival is usually prolonged in patients with high levels of microsatellite instability compared to those with stable or low microsatellite instability. Microsatellite instability tumors are also more likely to exhibit an antral location and are found more frequently in intestinal gastric cancer [78].

Chromosomal instability (CIN) is another hallmark of multiple malignancies. This instability can manifest as a change on the chromosome level, leading to losses and gains of whole chromosomes or large portions thereof [79]. These chromosomal changes can cause the activation or loss of important gene families such as oncogenes, tumor suppressor genes, or genes involved in cell cycle checkpoints or DNA repair [15, 80]. Chromosomal instability can also be a consequence of gene deletion, amplification, translocation, or loss of heterozygosity (LOH). Chromosomal instability is frequently detected in gastric cancer and is often linked to histological type, patient survival, or other clinicopathological parameters [80].

2.9 Molecular Subtyping of GC

Advances in next-generation sequencing technologies have enabled us to produce a near-comprehensive catalogue of GC-associated "driver" alterations. These alterations include gene mutations, transcriptional changes, somatic copy number alterations (sCNAs), structural variants, and epigenetic changes. Based on this information, several studies have used molecular subtyping analysis to further stratify GC cases in order to complement the currently used histological classifications (Table 2.2). The Cancer Genome Atlas (TCGA) evaluated 295 tumors (mainly from Western

Table 2.2 Comparisons of molecular subtypes of gastric cancer

Study	Molecular subtype			
TCGA	GS	EBV	MSI	CIN
• Mainly from western Europe and the United States • Somatic mutation, sCNAs, mRNA and miRNA expression, DNA methylation, and phosphoprotein	• CDH1 and RHOA mutations • CLDN18-ARHGAP26 fusion • Cell adhesion pathways • Younger patients • Enrichment of the diffuse histological subtype	• DNA hypermethylation • PIK3CA mutation • PD-L1 and PD-L2 overexpression • Recurrent JAK2 and ERBB2 amplification • CDKN2A silencing • Immune cell signaling • Common in the fundus or body • Common in males • Frequent ARID1A and BCOR mutation • Rare TP53 mutation	• Hypermutation • MLH1 silencing • KRAS or NRAS activation • RASA1 and PTEN inactivation • Mitotic pathways • Older patients • Female patients • Less A- > C transversion	• RTK-RAS activation (ERBB2, EGFR, MET, VEGFA, and KRAS or NRAS) • TP53 mutation • Amplifications of cell cycle mediators (CCNE1, CCND1, and CDK6), GATA4 and GATA6 • Common in GOJ and cardia cancer
ACRG	MSS/EMT	MSS/TP53+	MSI	**MSS/TP53-**
• Mainly from Korean • Gene expression profiles	• CDH1 silencing • Younger patients • Worst prognosis • Enrichment of the diffuse histological subtype • Lower number of mutation events	• Intact TP53 • MDM2 amplification • EBV infection • Enrichment with PIK3CA,ARID1A, APC, KRAS, or SMAD4 mutation and cytokine signature in EBV+ tumor	• Common in the antrum • Common in intestinal subtype • Best prognosis • Hypermutation • MLH1 silencing • Frequent mutations in KRAS, MTOR, PTEN, PI3KCA, ASL, and ARID1A	• TP53 mutation • Genomic instability • Recurrent amplification (ERBB2, EGFR, GATA6, MYC, CCNE1, and CCND1)
Li et al., combined cohorts	Regular-C2	–	Hypermutated	**Regular-C1**
• Combined from several cohorts • Somatic mutation	• Frequently mutations in ARID1A, CDH1, PIK3CA, and RHOA • Even distribution of CIN and GS • Poor survival outcome compared to C2		• Hypermutation • Enriched with MSI • Frequent mutations in BRCA2, FANCM, PRKDC, and MSH3	• TP53 mutation • Frequently mutations in XIRP2, APC, ERBB4, and AKAP6 • Enriched with CIN • Better prognostic outcome compared to C2

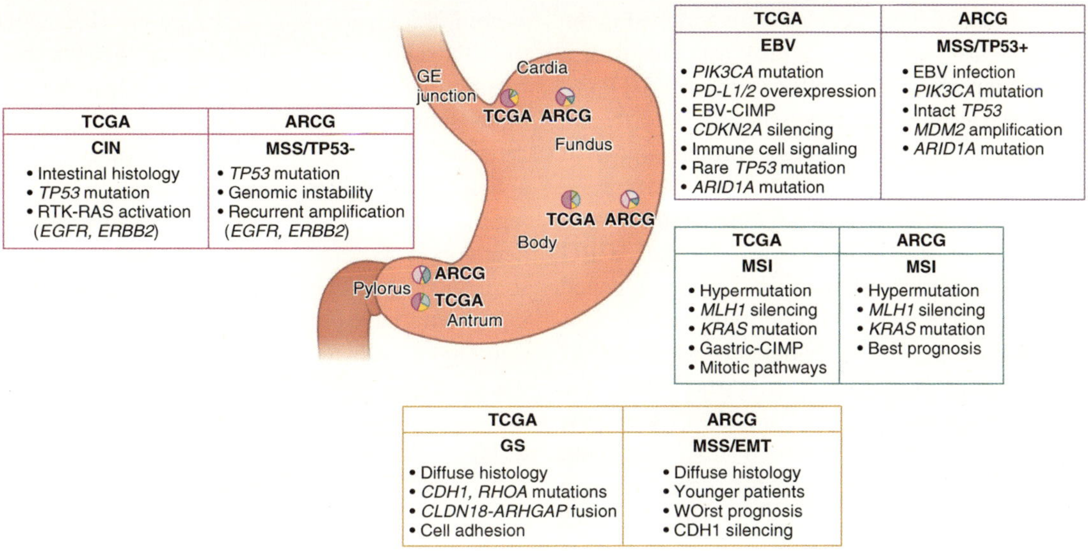

Fig. 2.2 Comparison of the key features between the TCGA and ARCG classification systems of gastric cancer (Adapted from Cancer Genome Atlas Research N. Comprehensive molecular characterization of gastric adenocarcinoma (2014), [81])

Europe and the United States) with data from whole exome sequencing, somatic copy number alterations (sCNAs), mRNA and miRNA sequencing, DNA methylation analysis, and phosphoprotein status and eventually identified four molecular subgroups [81]. Two of these subgroups were defined by the presence of Epstein-Barr virus (EBV) infection or microsatellite instability. The remaining tumors were classified into chromosome instability (CIN) and genome-stable (GS) tumors by evaluating the aneuploidy status of tumors. In another study, the Asian Cancer Research Group (ACRG), which mainly includes Korean GCs, also performed a classification analysis based on gene expression profiles [82]. Similarly to the findings published by the TCGA, ACRG also identified four subgroups, including MSS/EMT, MSS/TP53+, MSI, and MSS/TP53-. However, while the MSI group was identified in both studies, ACRG did not classify tumors according to EBV infection status. The ACRG study further divided tissue samples without any indication of MSI into three subtypes: the MSS/EMT subtype was significantly correlated with the expression of epithelial-mesenchymal transition (EMT) signature, while the remaining samples were further classified according to TP53 mutation status (MSS/TP53+ and MSS/TP53-).

The subgroups from both classification systems share significant similarities but also show considerable differences (Fig. 2.2). The TCGA GS, EBV+, MSI, and CIN subtypes were enriched in ACRG MSS/EMT, MSS/TP53+, MSI, and MSS/TP53- subtypes, respectively. For GS and MSS/EMT, the samples were both more common in younger patients and enriched in the diffuse histological subtype. Both EBV+ and MSS/TP53+ tissue samples showed frequent *PIK3CA* and *ARID1A* mutations with fewer aberrations in the *TP53* gene. The MSI groups in both datasets displayed higher mutation rates accompanied by *KRAS* or *NRAS* activation as well as *MLH1* silencing. In the CIN and MSS/TP53- subgroups, mutations in *TP53* were found more frequently compared to other groups, and several pivotal cell cycle genes such as *GATA6*, *CCNE1*, and *CCND1* were often amplified [81, 82]. However, despite these numerous similarities, several key differences were also observed between the two classification systems. *CDH1* and *RHOA* mutations were highly prevalent in the TCGA GS subtype but not in the ACRG MSS/EMT subtype.

Even though EBV+ samples were enriched in the MSS/TP53+ subtype, they only accounted for a small proportion of samples in the MSS/TP53+ subtype. Despite of their enrichment, the CIN and GS subtypes in the TCGA were present across all four ACRG subtypes [81, 82].

When overall survival was compared between the different subtypes classified by the ACRG system using survival analysis , results indicated that patients with the MSI subtype had the best prognosis followed by patients with the MSS/TP53+ and MSS/TP53- subtypes, while the MSS/EMT subtype was associated with the worst prognosis of the four (N = 251, log-rank, $P = 0.0004$). After adjusting for several clinical covariates with multivariable analysis, the association remained significant in the ACRG cohort (Cox $P = 0.019$). This trend was also validated in the Samsung Medical Center cohort 2 (N = 277, Cox $P = 0.0004$), the Singapore cohort (N = 200, Cox $P = 0.01$), and the TCGA gastric cohort (N = 205, Cox $P = 0.04$) [82]. In contrast, when applying the TCGA molecular subtyping system, initial outcome data from the TCGA cohort did not reveal survival differences between the four subgroups [81]. This indicates that the ACRG molecular subtyping system might have an application prospect for further clinical and preclinical translational research.

As a complement to the two classification systems, Li and colleagues also defined subtypes of gastric cancer based on somatic information (Table 2.2) [83]. Gastric cancer patients were first classified into regular- and hypermutated subgroups according to their "mutation burden," with the mutation rate of the regular-mutated group (median, 2.4mutations/Mb; range, 0–8.3) lower than in the hypermutated group (median, 20.5mutations/Mb; range, 9.6–200.2). Intriguingly, the hypermutated group was markedly enriched with microsatellite instability. In the regular-mutated group, two subgroups (referred to as C1 and C2) were further clustered using a NMF-based algorithm. The C1 subgroup was characterized by high mutation rates in *TP53*, *XIRP2*, *APC*, *ERBB4*, and *AKAP6*, while the C2 subgroup harbored mutations in *ARID1A*, *CDH1*, *PIK3CA*, and *RHOA* [83]. Compared to the TCGA classification system, the C1 subtype was more enriched with the CIN subtype, while C2 cases had an even distribution of CIN and GS [81, 83]. When linking these subgroups to clinical outcome, Li et al. determined that the C1 group was associated with a significantly better prognostic outcome, a finding that was further validated in another independent cohort. While these different studies yielded some inconsistent results, these molecular subtyping systems have provided us with a deeper understanding of the heterogeneity of gastric cancer.

2.10 "Driver" Alterations of Gastric Cancer

Mutations in somatic cells, i.e., non-germline cells, are called somatic mutations. In each case of GC (excluding hypermutated cases), 50–70 nonsynonymous mutations have accumulated according to current estimates based on NGS studies. These numbers are comparable to mutation rates in esophageal and colon cancer but less than in lung cancer and melanoma [84]. Similarly to other solid epithelial cancers, these somatically acquired mutations are usually distributed in various different genes. In addition to total mutation frequency, a number of studies have also examined the mutational signatures of gastric cancer. These signatures were described using base substitutions and additionally included information in the sequence context of each mutation [83–85]. Six classes of base substitutions—C > A, C > G, C > T, T > A, T > C, and T > G (all substitutions were flipped to pyrimidine)—as well as incorporated information on the immediately adjacent bases were used to generate a total of 96 possible mutation classifications ($4 \times 6 \times 4$). On the basis of this classification system, Lawrence and colleagues determined that gastrointestinal tumors (including esophageal, colorectal, and gastric tumors) often show unusually high frequencies of transition mutations at CpG dinucleotides [84]. In another study, Alexandrov et al. identified a total of 21 mutation signatures in 30 different malignant tumors, with seven of these signatures observed in gastric cancer. Of these seven signatures, two were significantly associated with both age (CpG) and APOBEC (TpCpW). The causes of others, however, remain unknown [85].

To date, more than 100 significantly mutated genes (SMGs) have been identified in GC. However, the concordance rate between different studies is remarkably low (Table 2.3). Among these SMGs, a total of 22 genes have been reported in at least two studies; these include *TP53*, *PTEN*, *ARID1A*, *RPL22*, *ACVR2A*, *CTNNB1*, *KRAS*, *PIK3CA*, *ERBB3*, *ERBB4*, *RHOA*, *CDH1*, *MUC6*, *BCOR*, *RNF43*, *FBXW7*, *SMAD4*, *APC*, *BNC2*, *ERBB2*, *ELF3*, and *TGFBR2* [81, 83, 86–89]. Found in nearly 50% of cases, *TP53* is the most frequently mutated gene in GC. Tumors with *TP53* mutations often exhibit high levels of sCNAs, supporting the gene's crucial role as a guardian of genomic integrity and cellular function [90]. While *KRAS*, *CTNNB1*, and *PIK3CA* are canonical oncogenes, *PTEN*, *SMAD4*, and *APC* are bona fide tumor suppressor genes. Activation of these oncogenes and inactivation of these tumor suppressor genes have been implicated in a number of different tumor type [5]. *ERBB2*, *ERBB3*, and *ERBB4* are members of the epidermal growth factor receptor (EGFR) family of receptor tyrosine kinases (RTKs) and play a crucial role in the RTK/RAS/MAPK signaling pathway [86]. *PIK3CA* mutations were frequently detected in EBV-positive gastric cancers, accounting for up to 80% of this subgroup [81]. Somatic mutations in the *CDH1* gene were found enriched in the diffuse-type gastric cancer. *ARID1A* encodes a component of the SWI/SNF chromatin remodeler complex and usually acts as a tumor suppressor by controlling the cell cycle regulators *CCNE1* and *E2F1* [88, 89]. Similarly to *ARID1A*, *RHOA* mutations occur in nearly 10–15% of gastric cancers. However, mutations in the *RHOA* gene, which affect downstream Rho signaling, are usually localized in an N-terminal hot spot region (Tyr42, Arg5, and Gly17) [87].

In addition to SMG, sCNAs and structural variations (SVs) are another mechanism involved in the activation of oncogenes and inactivation of tumor suppressor genes in GC. Studies by the TCGA and Wang et al. have systematically analyzed the sCNAs and SVs found in GC cases (Table 2.3) [81, 89]. Amplification of genes involved in the RTK/RAS/MAPK signaling pathway, including *HER2*, *EGFR*, *MET*, *FGFR2*, and *RAS*, were the most prevalent event in GC. Around 30–40% of gastric cancer patients harbor amplifications of one or several of these genes, and therapies targeting their protein products have entered clinical trials [81, 89, 90]. In EBV+ GCs, amplifications of *PD-L1* (*CD274*) and *PD-L2* (*PDCD1LG2*), which are widely targeted in immunotherapy, have also been frequently observed [81]. This finding suggests that PDL1/2 antagonists could be a potential therapeutic target for this subgroup. Additional gene clusters which are often found amplified in GC are related to cell cycle control, including *CCND1*, *CCNE1*, and *CDK6*. Moreover, amplifications of transcription factors (TFs) such as *GATA* factors (*GATA4/6*) and *MYC* are also observed in GC cases. These TFs might act as "lineage-survival" factors, functioning to reawaken early developmental programs that drive GC tumorigenesis [90]. In addition to amplifications of oncogenes, deletions of suppressor genes such as *PTEN*, *SMAD4*, *CDKN2A*, and *ARID1A* are another common feature of GCs [81, 89]. In addition to sCNAs, fusion genes stemming from genomic rearrangements are another candidate "driver" event in the development of GC. In two diffuse-type gastric cancer patients enrolled in the TCGA study, an interchromosomal translocation between *CLDN18* and *ARHGAP26* (*GRAF*) was observed, leading to the expression of a new fusion protein. CLDN18 is a component of tight junction adhesion structures, while ARHGAP26 is a GTPase-activating protein (GAP) of the Rho-effector pathway that has been implicated in enhancing cellular motility. The *CLN18-ARHGAP26* fusion gene was also observed in further nine GC cases, and its occurrence was mutually exclusive with mutations in *CDH1* and *RHOA* mutations [81]. A recent study suggested that the CLDN18-ARHGAP26 fusion protein is expressed in epithelial cells, where it reduces cell-cell and cell-extracellular matrix adhesion. This finding indicates that the fusion protein is involved in the epithelial-mesenchymal transition (EMT) [91]. Using a whole genome sequencing approach,

Table 2.3 "Driver alterations" identified by NGS studies of GC

Study[ref]	Year	Population	Sample size	SMG	Amplification	Deletion	Fusion genes	Hypermethylation
Wang et al. [88]	2011	Chinese	22 WES	TP53, PTEN, ARID1A, RPL22, TTK, FMN2, SPRR2B, PTN, ACVR2A, PMS2L3, DNAH7, TTN, FSCB, CTNNB1, SEMA3E, MCHR1, SPANXN2, METTL3, EIF3A, EPB41L3				
Miwako et al. [87]	2014	Japanese	30 WES and 57 validation	RHOA				
Wang et al. [89]	2014	Chinese	100 WGS	TP53, ARID1A, CDH1, MUC6, THBS1, SPTA1, CTNNA2, GLI3, ZIC4, SMAD4, RIMS2, RNF43, THSD7B, DCLK1, RHOA, ELF3, TGFBR2, ACVR2A, RPL22	CCND1, CCNE1, CDK6, EGFR, ERBB2, FGFR2, KRAS, MET, MYC	CDKN2A, PTEN	COL27A1-ZNF618, RHOA-COL7A1, RARA-ERBB2, EIF5-MAPK3, CDKL1-MAP4K5	MLH1, CHFR, BNIP3, MGMT, PARP6, TP73-AS1, CDX1, ASCL2, CDH17
TCGA [81]	2014	Combined	295 Multiple omics	TP53, KRAS, ARID1A, PIK3CA, ERBB3, PTEN, CHRD, HLA-B, CUL1, FBXW7, RNF43, CIC, LARP4B, FRMD4A, PTPN23, KIF13A, IWS1K, LMAN1, RBM28, IL2RG, VPS13A, IGF2BP3, ALPK2, IRF2, BCORL1, B2M, ZBTB20, HDAC4, MPG2, TBL1XR1, MYEOV, PAX6, GPR124, TMEM63A, NAA25, NF1, EP300, C13orf33, RNF111, MVK, CPD, SERPINB8, CTCF, CDH1, SMAD4, RHOA, MUC6, APC, BCOR, EYA4, BNC2, ABCA10, CTNNB1, MACF1, SMAD2, SOHLH2, RASA1, FAM46D, PLB1, CNGA4, EIF2C4, ERBB2, PTPRC	ERBB2, CCNE1, KRAS, MYC, EGFR, CDK6, GATA4, GATA6, ZNF217, CD44, 9p24.1/JAK2, 9p24.1/CD274, 9p24.1/PDCD1LG2	PTEN, SMAD4, CDKN2A, ARID1A	CLDN18-ARHGAP26	CDKN2A
Chen et al. [86]	2015	Chinese	78 WES and 2 WGS	TP53, ARID1A, CDH1, APC, RHOA, PIK3CA, SMAD4, MYC, KRAS				
Li et al. [83]	2016	Combined	544 Gastric patients	TP53, ARID1A, CDH1, PIK3CA, XIRP27, NBEA, APC, SMAD4, ERBB4, RHOA, KRAS, COL14A1, AKAP6, CDH11, CTNNB1, BNC2, ERBB2, ITGAV, TGFBR2, CNBD1, RNF43, FBXW7, MAP2K7, CDKN2A, SAMSN1, PIK3R1, ELF3, PIGR, THEMIS, AKAP2, ZHX3				

Wang et al. identified another fusion product in diffuse gastric cancer, resulting from the rearrangement of the RHOA and COL7A1 genes, suggesting that the occurrence of fusion proteins related to the RHO pathway constitutes another important genetic alteration in diffuse gastric cancer [89]. Wang et al. also identified an additional *COL27A1-ZNF618* fusion in two intestinal-type gastric cancer patients which resulted in elevated expression levels of *ZNF618*. Other putative genetic fusion products involve functionally important genes such as *EIF5-MAPK3*, *RARA-ERBB2*, and *CDKL1-MAP4K5*, which were identified in one patient [89].

Beside the "driver" alterations described above, several other aberrations are also thought to play crucial roles in the pathogenesis of GC. Aberrant methylation, especially of tumor suppressors silenced by promoter hypermethylation, is one of them. In the study conducted by Wang and colleagues, a list of putative tumor suppressors, including *MLH1*, *CHFR*, *BNIP3*, *MGMT*, *PARP6*, *TP73-AS1*, *CDX1*, *ASCL2*, and *CDH17*, was shown to be silenced as a result of promoter hypermethylation [89]. Interestingly, in the TCGA study, EBV-positive tumors exhibited the highest levels of DNA methylation, and all EBV+ GC cases displayed hypermethylation in the *CDKN2A* promoter region, possibly a consequence of the cellular reaction to viral infection [81].

Conclusion

Gastric cancer remains a lethal disease worldwide, with especially high rates in East Asians by now. While significant advances in biotechnology have improved our understanding of the molecular features of GC, few therapeutic avenues have emerged compared to other tumor types. Genetic analyses of GC patients, including both candidate gene studies and GWAS, have shed considerable light on disease pathogenesis. Combining results from these studies with an increased understanding of environmental risk factors (such as H. *pylori* infection, cigarette smoking, and drinking) can help us identify high-risk individuals prior to disease onset. Since gastric cancer is an infection-induced, inflammation-driven malignancy with a progression, early intervention—for example, by controlling or eradicating viral infection before they cause irreversible lesions—provides an opportunity to prevent this cancer. Applying this strategy in high-risk people will be a cost-effective approach. In addition, genetic screening of high-risk populations can facilitate the development of novel early detection methods for GC. High-throughput sequencing studies have helped formulate a comprehensive GC landscape on several levels. Based on these findings, new classification systems of GC have been proposed which provide us an improved understanding of the pathogenesis of gastric cancer. Even though these systems have not been tested in a clinical setting, they open the door for precision medicine. More importantly, several "driver alterations" of GC have been identified by these sequencing studies, offering a list of potential, unexplored therapeutic targets. At the same time, several "driver alterations," which are common in other tumors and have proven druggable with a targeted approach, are also observed in GC. This will help extend the application of these targeted drugs while improving the prognosis for GC patients harboring such genetic alterations. In the future, it will be easier, faster, and cheaper to sequence the whole genome of healthy individuals and GC patients. More and more genetic risk markers of GC will be found that will help define the risk degree of healthy individuals and determine early prevention and intervention approaches. Moreover, with the understanding of "driver alterations" in every GC patient, individualized treatment strategy will be formulated to achieve the best possible curative effect.

References

1. Ferlay J, Soerjomataram I, Ervik MDR, Eser S, Mathers C, Rebelo M, et al. GLOBOCAN 2012 v1.0, Cancer Incidence and Mortality Worldwide: IARC CancerBase No. 11 [Internet]. 2013.
2. Arnold M, Karim-Kos HE, Coebergh JW, Byrnes G, Antilla A, Ferlay J, et al. Recent trends in incidence of five common cancers in 26 European countries since

1988: analysis of the European cancer observatory. Eur J Cancer. 2015;51(9):1164–87. doi:10.1016/j.ejca.2013.09.002.
3. Chen W, Zheng R, Baade PD, Zhang S, Zeng H, Bray F, et al. Cancer statistics in China, 2015. CA Cancer J Clin. 2016;66(2):115–32. doi:10.3322/caac.21338.
4. Siegel RL, Miller KD, Jemal A. Cancer statistics, 2016. CA Cancer J Clin. 2016;66(1):7–30. doi:10.3322/caac.21332.
5. Grabsch HI, Tan P. Gastric cancer pathology and underlying molecular mechanisms. Dig Surg. 2013;30(2):150–8. doi:10.1159/000350876.
6. Yakirevich E, Resnick MB. Pathology of gastric cancer and its precursor lesions. Gastroenterol Clin N Am. 2013;42(2):261–84. doi:10.1016/j.gtc.2013.01.004.
7. Colquhoun A, Arnold M, Ferlay J, Goodman KJ, Forman D, Soerjomataram I. Global patterns of cardia and non-cardia gastric cancer incidence in 2012. Gut. 2015;64(12):1881–8. doi:10.1136/gutjnl-2014-308915.
8. Cook MB, Kamangar F, Whiteman DC, Freedman ND, Gammon MD, Bernstein L, et al. Cigarette smoking and adenocarcinomas of the esophagus and esophagogastric junction: a pooled analysis from the international BEACON consortium. J Natl Cancer Inst. 2010;102(17):1344–53. doi:10.1093/jnci/djq289.
9. Lunet N, Valbuena C, Vieira AL, Lopes C, Lopes C, David L, et al. Fruit and vegetable consumption and gastric cancer by location and histological type: case-control and meta-analysis. Eur J Cancer Prev. 2007;16(4):312–27. doi:10.1097/01.cej.0000236255.95769.22.
10. Limburg P, Qiao Y, Mark S, Wang G, Perez-Perez G, Blaser M, et al. Helicobacter pylori seropositivity and subsite-specific gastric cancer risks in Linxian, China. J Natl Cancer Inst. 2001;93(3):226–33.
11. Plummer M, Franceschi S, Vignat J, Forman D, de Martel C. Global burden of gastric cancer attributable to helicobacter pylori. Int J Cancer. 2015;136(2):487–90. doi:10.1002/ijc.28999.
12. Hoyo C, Cook MB, Kamangar F, Freedman ND, Whiteman DC, Bernstein L, et al. Body mass index in relation to oesophageal and oesophagogastric junction adenocarcinomas: a pooled analysis from the international BEACON consortium. Int J Epidemiol. 2012;41(6):1706–18. doi:10.1093/ije/dys176.
13. Ye W, Chow WH, Lagergren J, Yin L, Nyren O. Risk of adenocarcinomas of the esophagus and gastric cardia in patients with gastroesophageal reflux diseases and after antireflux surgery. Gastroenterology. 2001;121(6):1286–93.
14. Sampson JN, Wheeler WA, Yeager M, Panagiotou O, Wang Z, Berndt SI, et al. Analysis of heritability and shared heritability based on genome-wide association studies for thirteen cancer types. J Natl Cancer Inst. 2015;107(12):djv279. doi:10.1093/jnci/djv279.
15. McLean MH, El-Omar EM. Genetics of gastric cancer. Nat Rev Gastroenterol Hepatol. 2014;11(11):664–74. doi:10.1038/nrgastro.2014.143.
16. Boltin D, Niv Y. Mucins in gastric cancer—an update. J Gastrointest Dig Syst. 2013;3(123):15519. doi:10.4172/2161-069X.1000123.
17. Wen R, Gao F, Zhou CJ, Jia YB. Polymorphisms in mucin genes in the development of gastric cancer. World J Gastrointest Oncol. 2015;7(11):328–37. doi:10.4251/wjgo.v7.i11.328.
18. Carvalho F, Seruca R, David L, Amorim A, Seixas M, Bennett E, et al. MUC1 gene polymorphism and gastric cancer—an epidemiological study. Glycoconj J. 1997;14(1):107–11.
19. Silva F, Carvalho F, Peixoto A, Seixas M, Almeida R, Carneiro F, et al. MUC1 gene polymorphism in the gastric carcinogenesis pathway. Eur Journal of Hum Genet. 2001;9(7):548–52. doi:10.1038/sj.ejhg.5200677.
20. Carvalho F, Peixoto A, Steffensen R, Amorim A, David L, Sobrinho-Simoes M. MUC1 gene polymorphism does not explain the different incidence of gastric cancer in Portugal and Denmark. Ann Hum Genet. 1999;63(Pt 3):187–91.
21. Jia Y, Persson C, Hou L, Zheng Z, Yeager M, Lissowska J, et al. A comprehensive analysis of common genetic variation in MUC1, MUC5AC, MUC6 genes and risk of stomach cancer. Cancer Causes Control. 2010;21(2):313–21. doi:10.1007/s10552-009-9463-3.
22. Qiu LX, Hua RX, Cheng L, He J, Wang MY, Zhou F, et al. Genetic variant rs4072037 of MUC1 and gastric cancer risk in an eastern Chinese population. Oncotarget. 2016;7(13):15930–6. doi:10.18632/oncotarget.7527.
23. Palmer AJ, Lochhead P, Hold GL, Rabkin CS, Chow WH, Lissowska J, et al. Genetic variation in C20orf54, PLCE1 and MUC1 and the risk of upper gastrointestinal cancers in Caucasian populations. Eur J Cancer Prev. 2012;21(6):541–4. doi:10.1097/CEJ.0b013e3283529b79.
24. Li F, Zhong MZ, Li JH, Liu W, Li B. Case-control study of single nucleotide polymorphisms of PSCA and MUC1 genes with gastric cancer in a Chinese. Asian Pac J Cancer Prev. 2012;13(6):2593–6.
25. Saeki N, Saito A, Choi IJ, Matsuo K, Ohnami S, Totsuka H, et al. A functional single nucleotide polymorphism in mucin 1, at chromosome 1q22, determines susceptibility to diffuse-type gastric cancer. Gastroenterology. 2011;140(3):892–902. doi:10.1053/j.gastro.2010.10.058.
26. Wang Z, Dai J, Hu N, Miao X, Abnet CC, Yang M, et al. Identification of new susceptibility loci for gastric non-cardia adenocarcinoma: pooled results from two Chinese genome-wide association studies. Gut. 2015; doi:10.1136/gutjnl-2015-310612.
27. Zhang B, Hao GY, Gao F, Zhang JZ, Zhou CJ, Zhou LS, et al. Lack of association of common polymorphisms in MUC1 gene with H. Pylori infection and non-cardia gastric cancer risk in a Chinese population. Asian Pac J Cancer Prev. 2013;14(12):7355–8.
28. Frank B, Weck MN, Muller H, Klopp N, Illig T, Raum E, et al. Polymorphisms in MUC1, MUC2, MUC5B and MUC6 genes are not associated with the risk of chronic atrophic gastritis. Eur J Cancer. 2012;48(1):114–20. doi:10.1016/j.ejca.2011.04.016.
29. Zheng L, Zhu C, Gu J, Xi P, Du J, Jin G. Functional polymorphism rs4072037 in MUC1 gene contributes to the susceptibility to gastric cancer: evidence from

pooled 6,580 cases and 10,324 controls. Mol Biol Rep. 2013;40(10):5791–6. doi:10.1007/s11033-013-2682-4.
30. Van de Bovenkamp JH, Mahdavi J, Korteland-Van Male AM, Buller HA, Einerhand AW, Boren T, et al. The MUC5AC glycoprotein is the primary receptor for helicobacter pylori in the human stomach. Helicobacter. 2003;8(5):521–32.
31. Van De Bovenkamp JH, Korteland-Van Male AM, Buller HA, Einerhand AW, Dekker J. Infection with helicobacter pylori affects all major secretory cell populations in the human antrum. Dig Dis Sci. 2005;50(6):1078–86.
32. Zhou CJ, Zhang LW, Gao F, Zhang B, Wang Y, Chen DF, et al. Association analysis of common genetic variations in MUC5AC gene with the risk of non-cardia gastric cancer in a Chinese population. Asian Pac J Cancer Prev. 2014;15(10):4207–10.
33. Zhou CJ, Zhang LW, Gao F, Zhang B, Wang Y, Chen DF, et al. Common genetic variations in the MUC5AC gene are not related to helicobacter pylori serologic status. Asian Pac J Cancer Prev. 2014;15(24):10719–22.
34. Kawakubo M, Ito Y, Okimura Y, Kobayashi M, Sakura K, Kasama S, et al. Natural antibiotic function of a human gastric mucin against helicobacter pylori infection. Science. 2004;305(5686):1003–6. doi:10.1126/science.1099250.
35. Byrd JC, Yan P, Sternberg L, Yunker CK, Scheiman JM, Bresalier RS. Aberrant expression of gland-type gastric mucin in the surface epithelium of helicobacter pylori-infected patients. Gastroenterology. 1997;113(2):455–64.
36. Zheng H, Takahashi H, Nakajima T, Murai Y, Cui Z, Nomoto K, et al. MUC6 down-regulation correlates with gastric carcinoma progression and a poor prognosis: an immunohistochemical study with tissue microarrays. J Cancer Res Clin Oncol. 2006;132(12):817–23. doi:10.1007/s00432-006-0135-3.
37. Nguyen TV, Janssen Jr M, Gritters P, te Morsche RH, Drenth JP, van Asten H, et al. Short mucin 6 alleles are associated with H pylori infection. World J Gastroenterol. 2006;12(37):6021–5.
38. Garcia E, Carvalho F, Amorim A, David L. MUC6 gene polymorphism in healthy individuals and in gastric cancer patients from northern Portugal. Cancer Epidemiol Biomark Prev. 1997;6(12):1071–4.
39. Kwon JA, Lee SY, Ahn EK, Seol SY, Kim MC, Kim SJ, et al. Short rare MUC6 minisatellites-5 alleles influence susceptibility to gastric carcinoma by regulating gene. Hum Mutat. 2010;31(8):942–9. doi:10.1002/humu.21289.
40. Jeong YH, Kim MC, Ahn EK, Seol SY, Do EJ, Choi HJ, et al. Rare exonic minisatellite alleles in MUC2 influence susceptibility to gastric carcinoma. PLoS One. 2007;2(11):e1163. doi:10.1371/journal.pone.0001163.
41. Schistosomes, liver flukes and Helicobacter pylori. IARC Working Group on the Evaluation of Carcinogenic Risks to Humans. Lyon, 7–14 June 1994. IARC monographs on the evaluation of carcinogenic risks to humans/World Health Organization, International Agency for Research on Cancer. 1994;61:1–241.
42. Helicobacter, Cancer Collaborative Group. Gastric cancer and helicobacter pylori: a combined analysis of 12 case control studies nested within prospective cohorts. Gut. 2001;49(3):347–53.
43. El-Omar EM. The importance of interleukin 1beta in helicobacter pylori associated disease. Gut. 2001;48(6):743–7.
44. Tu S, Bhagat G, Cui G, Takaishi S, Kurt-Jones EA, Rickman B, et al. Overexpression of interleukin-1beta induces gastric inflammation and cancer and mobilizes myeloid-derived suppressor cells in mice. Cancer Cell. 2008;14(5):408–19. doi:10.1016/j.ccr.2008.10.011.
45. Mocellin S, Verdi D, Pooley KA, Nitti D. Genetic variation and gastric cancer risk: a field synopsis and meta-analysis. Gut. 2015;64(8):1209–19. doi:10.1136/gutjnl-2015-309168.
46. Persson C, Canedo P, Machado JC, El-Omar EM, Forman D. Polymorphisms in inflammatory response genes and their association with gastric cancer: a HuGE systematic review and meta-analyses. Am J Epidemiol. 2011;173(3):259–70. doi:10.1093/aje/kwq370.
47. Study Group of Millennium Genome Project for Cancer, Sakamoto H, Yoshimura K, Saeki N, Katai H, Shimoda T, et al. Genetic variation in PSCA is associated with susceptibility to diffuse-type gastric cancer. Nat Genet. 2008;40(6):730–40. doi:10.1038/ng.152.
48. Abnet CC, Freedman ND, Hu N, Wang Z, Yu K, Shu XO, et al. A shared susceptibility locus in PLCE1 at 10q23 for gastric adenocarcinoma and esophageal squamous cell carcinoma. Nat Genet. 2010;42(9):764–7. doi:10.1038/ng.649.
49. Hu N, Wang Z, Song X, Wei L, Kim BS, Freedman ND, et al. Genome-wide association study of gastric adenocarcinoma in Asia: a comparison of associations between cardia and non-cardia tumours. Gut. 2016;65(10):1611–8. doi:10.1136/gutjnl-2015-309340.
50. Xu Q, Yuan Y, Sun LP, Gong YH, Xu Y, Yu XW, et al. Risk of gastric cancer is associated with the MUC1 568 a/G polymorphism. Int J Oncol. 2009;35(6):1313–20.
51. Ng W, Loh AX, Teixeira AS, Pereira SP, Swallow DM. Genetic regulation of MUC1 alternative splicing in human tissues. Br J Cancer. 2008;99(6):978–85. doi:10.1038/sj.bjc.6604617.
52. Shi Y, Hu Z, Wu C, Dai J, Li H, Dong J, et al. A genome-wide association study identifies new susceptibility loci for non-cardia gastric cancer at 3q13.31 and 5p13.1. Nat Genet. 2011;43(12):1215–8. doi:10.1038/ng.978.
53. Qiu LX, He J, Cheng L, Zhou F, Wang MY, Sun MH, et al. Genetic variant of PRKAA1 and gastric cancer risk in an eastern Chinese population. Oncotarget. 2015;6(40):42661–6. doi:10.18632/oncotarget.6124.
54. Helgason H, Rafnar T, Olafsdottir HS, Jonasson JG, Sigurdsson A, Stacey SN, et al. Loss-of-function variants in ATM confer risk of gastric cancer. Nat Genet. 2015;47(8):906–10. doi:10.1038/ng.3342.
55. Kim YD, Yim DH, Eom SY, Moon SI, Yun HY, Song YJ, et al. Risk of gastric cancer is associated with

PRKAA1 gene polymorphisms in Koreans. World J Gastroenterol. 2014;20(26):8592–8. doi:10.3748/wjg.v20.i26.8592.
56. Sales KJ, Katz AA, Davis M, Hinz S, Soeters RP, Hofmeyr MD, et al. Cyclooxygenase-2 expression and prostaglandin E(2) synthesis are up-regulated in carcinomas of the cervix: a possible autocrine/paracrine regulation of neoplastic cell function via EP2/EP4 receptors. J Clin Endocrinol Metab. 2001;86(5):2243–9. doi:10.1210/jcem.86.5.7442.
57. Fujino H, Xu W, Regan JW. Prostaglandin E2 induced functional expression of early growth response factor-1 by EP4, but not EP2, prostanoid receptors via the phosphatidylinositol 3-kinase and extracellular signal-regulated kinases. J Biol Chem. 2003;278(14):12151–6. doi:10.1074/jbc.M212665200.
58. Oshima H, Popivanova BK, Oguma K, Kong D, Ishikawa TO, Oshima M. Activation of epidermal growth factor receptor signaling by the prostaglandin E(2) receptor EP4 pathway during gastric tumorigenesis. Cancer Sci. 2011;102(4):713–9. doi:10.1111/j.1349-7006.2011.01847.x.
59. Oshima H, Oshima M. Mouse models of gastric tumors: Wnt activation and PGE2 induction. Pathol Int. 2010;60(9):599–607. doi:10.1111/j.1440-1827.2010.02567.x.
60. Zaha VG, Young LH. AMP-activated protein kinase regulation and biological actions in the heart. Circ Res. 2012;111(6):800–14. doi:10.1161/CIRCRESAHA.111.255505.
61. Mo JS, Meng Z, Kim YC, Park HW, Hansen CG, Kim S, et al. Cellular energy stress induces AMPK-mediated regulation of YAP and the hippo pathway. Nat Cell Biol. 2015;17(4):500–10. doi:10.1038/ncb3111.
62. Wang S, Wu S, Zhu H, Ding B, Cai Y, Ni J, et al. PSCA rs2294008 polymorphism contributes to the decreased risk for cervical cancer in a Chinese population. Sci Rep. 2016;6:23465. doi:10.1038/srep23465.
63. Qiu LX, Cheng L, He J, Zhou ZR, Wang MY, Zhou F, et al. PSCA polymorphisms and gastric cancer susceptibility in an eastern Chinese population. Oncotarget. 2016;7(8):9420–8. doi:10.18632/oncotarget.7137.
64. Song HR, Kim HN, Piao JM, Kweon SS, Choi JS, Bae WK, et al. Association of a common genetic variant in prostate stem-cell antigen with gastric cancer susceptibility in a Korean population. Mol Carcinog. 2011;50(11):871–5. doi:10.1002/mc.20796.
65. Sala N, Munoz X, Travier N, Agudo A, Duell EJ, Moreno V, et al. Prostate stem-cell antigen gene is associated with diffuse and intestinal gastric cancer in Caucasians: results from the EPIC-EURGAST study. Int J Cancer. 2012;130(10):2417–27. doi:10.1002/ijc.26243.
66. Lochhead P, Frank B, Hold GL, Rabkin CS, Ng MT, Vaughan TL, et al. Genetic variation in the prostate stem cell antigen gene and upper gastrointestinal cancer in white individuals. Gastroenterology. 2011;140(2):435–41. doi:10.1053/j.gastro.2010.11.001.
67. Reiter RE, Gu Z, Watabe T, Thomas G, Szigeti K, Davis E, et al. Prostate stem cell antigen: a cell surface marker overexpressed in prostate cancer. Proc Natl Acad Sci U S A. 1998;95(4):1735–40.
68. Bahrenberg G, Brauers A, Joost HG, Jakse G. Reduced expression of PSCA, a member of the LY-6 family of cell surface antigens, in bladder, esophagus, and stomach tumors. Biochem Biophys Res Commun. 2000;275(3):783–8. doi:10.1006/bbrc.2000.3393.
69. Wang LD, Zhou FY, Li XM, Sun LD, Song X, Jin Y, et al. Genome-wide association study of esophageal squamous cell carcinoma in Chinese subjects identifies susceptibility loci at PLCE1 and C20orf54. Nat Genet. 2010;42(9):759–63. doi:10.1038/ng.648.
70. Zhang H, Jin G, Li H, Ren C, Ding Y, Zhang Q, et al. Genetic variants at 1q22 and 10q23 reproducibly associated with gastric cancer susceptibility in a Chinese population. Carcinogenesis. 2011;32(6):848–52. doi:10.1093/carcin/bgr051.
71. Wang M, Zhang R, He J, Qiu L, Li J, Wang Y, et al. Potentially functional variants of PLCE1 identified by GWASs contribute to gastric adenocarcinoma susceptibility in an eastern Chinese population. PLoS One. 2012;7(3):e31932. doi:10.1371/journal.pone.0031932.
72. Rhee SG. Regulation of phosphoinositide-specific phospholipase C. Annu Rev Biochem. 2001;70:281–312. doi:10.1146/annurev.biochem.70.1.281.
73. Bunney TD, Baxendale RW, Katan M. Regulatory links between PLC enzymes and Ras superfamily GTPases: signalling via PLCepsilon. Adv Enzym Regul. 2009;49(1):54–8. doi:10.1016/j.advenzreg.2009.01.004.
74. Bai Y, Edamatsu H, Maeda S, Saito H, Suzuki N, Satoh T, et al. Crucial role of phospholipase Cepsilon in chemical carcinogen-induced skin tumor development. Cancer Res. 2004;64(24):8808–10. doi:10.1158/0008-5472.CAN-04-3143.
75. Li M, Edamatsu H, Kitazawa R, Kitazawa S, Kataoka T. Phospholipase Cepsilon promotes intestinal tumorigenesis of Apc(Min/+) mice through augmentation of inflammation and angiogenesis. Carcinogenesis. 2009;30(8):1424–32. doi:10.1093/carcin/bgp125.
76. Wadhwa R, Song S, Lee JS, Yao Y, Wei Q, Ajani JA. Gastric cancer-molecular and clinical dimensions. Nat Rev Clin Oncol. 2013;10(11):643–55. doi:10.1038/nrclinonc.2013.170.
77. Yamamoto H, Imai K, Perucho M. Gastrointestinal cancer of the microsatellite mutator phenotype pathway. J Gastroenterol. 2002;37(3):153–63.
78. Falchetti M, Saieva C, Lupi R, Masala G, Rizzolo P, Zanna I, et al. Gastric cancer with high-level microsatellite instability: target gene mutations, clinicopathologic features, and long-term survival. Hum Pathol. 2008;39(6):925–32. doi:10.1016/j.humpath.2007.10.024.

79. Lengauer C, Kinzler KW, Vogelstein B. Genetic instabilities in human cancers. Nature. 1998;396(6712):643–9. doi:10.1038/25292.
80. Hudler P. Genetic aspects of gastric cancer instability. Scientific World J. 2012;2012:761909. doi:10.1100/2012/761909.
81. Cancer Genome Atlas Research N. Comprehensive molecular characterization of gastric adenocarcinoma. Nature. 2014;513(7517):202–9. doi:10.1038/nature13480.
82. Cristescu R, Lee J, Nebozhyn M, Kim KM, Ting JC, Wong SS, et al. Molecular analysis of gastric cancer identifies subtypes associated with distinct clinical outcomes. Nat Med. 2015;21(5):449–56. doi:10.1038/nm.3850.
83. Li X, Wu WK, Xing R, Wong SH, Liu Y, Fang X, et al. Distinct subtypes of gastric cancer defined by molecular characterization include novel mutational signatures with prognostic capability. Cancer Res. 2016;76(7):1724–32. doi:10.1158/0008-5472.CAN-15-2443.
84. Lawrence MS, Stojanov P, Polak P, Kryukov GV, Cibulskis K, Sivachenko A, et al. Mutational heterogeneity in cancer and the search for new cancer-associated genes. Nature. 2013;499(7457):214–8. doi:10.1038/nature12213.
85. Alexandrov LB, Nik-Zainal S, Wedge DC, Aparicio SA, Behjati S, Biankin AV, et al. Signatures of mutational processes in human cancer. Nature. 2013;500(7463):415–21. doi:10.1038/nature12477.
86. Chen K, Yang D, Li X, Sun B, Song F, Cao W, et al. Mutational landscape of gastric adenocarcinoma in Chinese: implications for prognosis and therapy. Proc Natl Acad Sci U S A. 2015;112(4):1107–12. doi:10.1073/pnas.1422640112.
87. Kakiuchi M, Nishizawa T, Ueda H, Gotoh K, Tanaka A, Hayashi A, et al. Recurrent gain-of-function mutations of RHOA in diffuse-type gastric carcinoma. Nat Genet. 2014;46(6):583–7. doi:10.1038/ng.2984.
88. Wang K, Kan J, Yuen ST, Shi ST, Chu KM, Law S, et al. Exome sequencing identifies frequent mutation of ARID1A in molecular subtypes of gastric cancer. Nat Genet. 2011;43(12):1219–23. doi:10.1038/ng.982.
89. Wang K, Yuen ST, Xu J, Lee SP, Yan HH, Shi ST, et al. Whole-genome sequencing and comprehensive molecular profiling identify new driver mutations in gastric cancer. Nat Genet. 2014;46(6):573–82. doi:10.1038/ng.2983.
90. Tan P, Yeoh KG. Genetics and molecular pathogenesis of gastric adenocarcinoma. Gastroenterology. 2015;149(5):1153–62. doi:10.1053/j.gastro.2015.05.059.
91. Yao F, Kausalya JP, Sia YY, Teo AS, Lee WH, Ong AG, et al. Recurrent fusion genes in gastric cancer: CLDN18-ARHGAP26 induces loss of epithelial integrity. Cell Rep. 2015;12(2):272–85. doi:10.1016/j.celrep.2015.06.020.

3 Circulating Tumor Cells in Gastric Cancer

Jie Shen and Lifeng Wang

3.1 Introduction

Historically, tumor tissue has been the major source of material used for cancer biomarker evaluation. However, several situations arise where there is a shortage of tissue needed for such tumor tissue-based detection strategies. First, it may be impossible to obtain tissue from advanced case patients. Tissues from biopsy may not always be enough for gene detection. Second, tumor tissue obtained at the time of the initial diagnosis might not reflect alterations of genetic profile observed at the time of clinical progression, because primary and metastatic tumors from the same person can be diffident at levels of genomic, transcriptomic, and epigenetic. Moreover, chemotherapy or targeted therapy may alter gene expression level itself. In such cases, circulating tumor cells could be a noninvasive and useful tool for tracking changes and providing useful and timely information for determining the best course of treatment. It could also be useful for those who do not have enough tissue for adequate gene detection when neoadjuvant or adjuvant chemotherapy needs to be chosen.

J. Shen (✉) • L. Wang
The Comprehensive Cancer Centre of Drum Tower Hospital, Medical School of Nanjing University and Clinical Cancer Institute of Nanjing University, 321 Zhongshan Rd, Nanjing 210008, China
e-mail: shenjie2008nju@163.com

3.2 Biology of Circulating Tumor Cells

Tumor cells that escape their primary microenvironment and enter the blood are termed "circulating tumor cells" (CTCs). CTCs can be thought of as the message of metastasis. When individual cancer cells or cancer cell clusters gain the ability to separate and run away from the primary mass of tumor, they acquire certain ability to migrate through surrounding tissue before penetrating local blood circulation (Fig. 3.1) [1, 2]. Arriving the bloodstream, CTCs may face some natural obstacles, including the enormous shearing forces present in the cardiovascular system [3], anoikis [4], and the actions of the immune system [5]. Thus, even though tens of thousands of tumor cells are dispersed throughout the body continuously, only very few of them may be able to evade the immune system and systemic therapy. If this occurs, it could then reach a distant organ and eventually grow into an overt metastasis.

According to their biology characteristics, CTCs can be subdivided into two groups: epithelial-like and EMT-associated. Epithelial-like CTCs usually form from the primary tumor and enter circulation directly by forces from external side, such as friction, mechanical forces, or tumor growth [2]. This type of CTCs derived is more possible to remain its original phenotype. In this way, epithelial-specific marker detection such as the EpCAM (the epithelial cell adhesion

J. Wei, B. Liu (eds.), *Personalized Management of Gastric Cancer*,
DOI 10.1007/978-981-10-3978-2_3

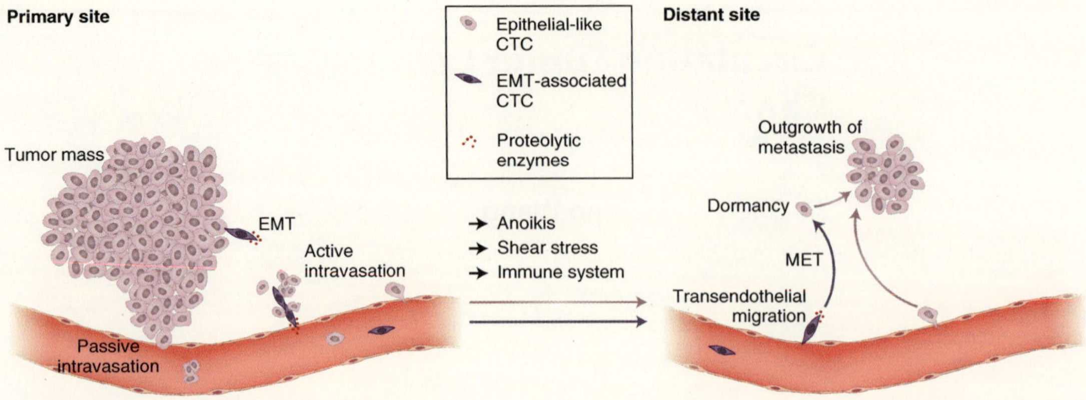

Fig. 3.1 The intravasation and migration of CTC (Adapted from detection and clinical implications of circulating tumor cells (2015), Joosse SA et al. [1])

molecule) will be feasible [6]. During the process of invasion, CTCs may undergo EMT (epithelial-to-mesenchymal transition), which increases their aggression and metastatic abilities. As such, this type of CTC has been classified as an EMT-associated CTC. Cells within this group have lost cell-to-cell adherence proteins such as cadherin and have subsequently gained the ability to migrate and invade [7].

3.3 Detection of Circulating Tumor Cells

3.3.1 Enrichment of Circulating Tumor Cells

CTCs are quite rare in circulating, making their exact quantification difficult. We may find only one CTC against the background of 10^6–10^7 normal peripheral mononuclear blood cells. In the patient without obvious metastatic mass, this occurrence rate may even be much lower. Such low numbers mean that systematic removal of PBMCs and selective enrichment of CTC are required when detecting CTCs in the blood. To date, more than 40 techniques have been developed for CTC detection, and novel strategies are still being published to date [8]. Generally speaking, there are five types of CTC isolation methods: (1) enrichment by density gradient centrifugation, (2) immune-magnetic separation (3) size-based isolation, (4) CTC-Chip, and (5) in vivo isolation (Fig. 3.2). We will now discuss each of these in more specific detail.

3.3.1.1 Enrichment by Density Gradient Centrifugation

Density gradient centrifugation was the earliest technique to be developed. It remains the simplest way to isolate CTCs through the use of special centrifugation liquid. However, this method yields low rates of CTC enrichment. CD45 depletion can be combined with density gradient depending centrifugation to increase the yield of CTCs. It should be noted that density gradient depending centrifugation and lysis of red blood cell may cause the loss of tumor cell.

3.3.1.2 Immune-Magnetic Separation

A great many CTC detection technologies are immune-magnetic based, which can be divided into those that rely on positive selection and those that rely on negative selection. EpCAM is the most commonly used label in positive selection methodologies. CellSearch system is one of the EpCAM-based CTC detection technologies and is the only approved CTC detection apparatus by FDA (US Food and Drug Administration). By using this approach, CTC has been proven as an independent prognostic biomarker on PFS (progression-free survival) and OS (overall survival) in a variety of cancers, including lung, liver, colon, breast, and prostate [8, 10–14]. The AdnaTest is also epithelial marker-based and can enrich CTCs positively. A study on metastatic breast cancer used this method

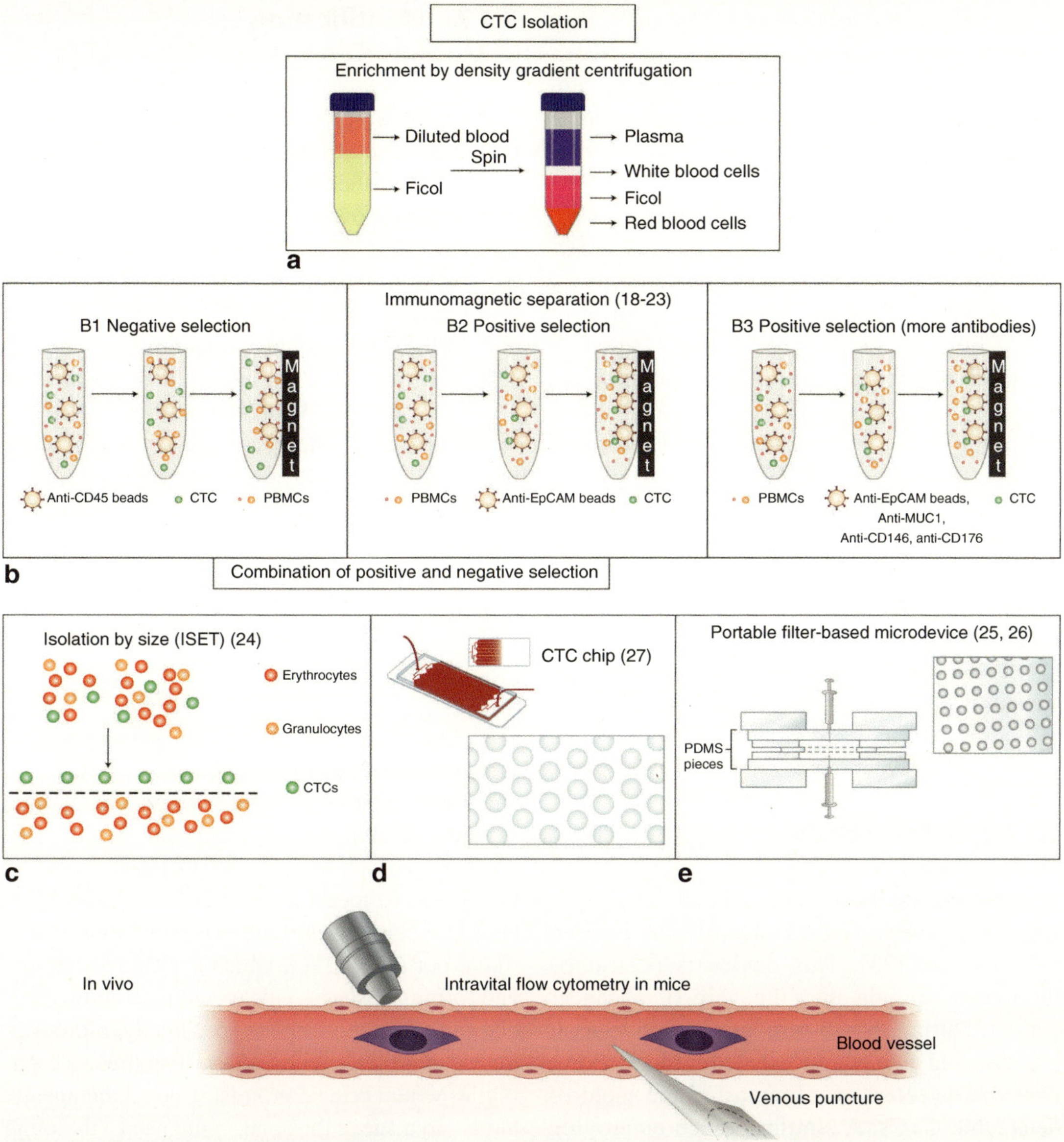

Fig. 3.2 In vitro and in vivo CTC isolation methods (Adapted from Circulating tumor cells in breast cancer: detection systems, molecular characterization, and future challenges (2011), Lianidou ES, Markou A [9])

and proved that CTC presence or absence was a valid prognostic and predictive marker [15]. A major drawback of this method is that it is not perfect in detecting MET-associated CTCs, since these have either downregulated EpCAM or a complete loss of it [16].

CD45 is the most commonly used label for negative selection approaches. Depletion of leukocytes with CD45-positive markers is the favorite approach for capturing CTCs that have downregulated or an absence of EpCAM expression [17]. CD45 depletion could also be used together with other label-independent method, such as density gradient depending centrifugation to increase the yield.

3.3.1.3 Size-Based Isolation

The ISET system is a typical size-based CTC isolation device. In general, this approach is designed to gain CTCs at a high enrichment rate. However, a major drawback of this method is that EMT-associated CTC might bc larger than leukocytes or not solid enough. As such, they may get loss by the size-based filter. What's more, even though CTC is captured on the membrane, it might be difficult to detect and examine for further genetic analysis.

3.3.1.4 CTC-Chip

Microfluidic device platforms like the CTC-Chip are promising alternatives to selectively capture CTCs [18]. Quite a large number of CTC-Chips are currently available, including the IsoFlux for EpCAM-positive tumor selection [19], CTC-iChip (a size-based filtration and affinity-based enrichment strategy) for systematic removal of PBMCs and RBCs [20], JETTATM microfluidic chip (a size- and deformability-based capture scheme) enabling single-cell analysis [21], and the spiral biochip (a size-based and EpCAM-independent separation method) with low leukocyte contamination [22]. Generally speaking, CTC-Chips are advantageous in that they have high recovery rates; however they are inconvenient to use and come at a high cost.

3.3.1.5 In Vivo Isolation

To circumvent sample volume limitations, an EpCAM-coated wire named CellCollector™ was designed by GILUPI GmbH for in vivo CTC capture [23]. This device is positioned through a cannula into the vein of a cancer patient. During the 30-min application time, it is estimated that up to 1.5 L of blood flows over the detector, thus increasing the yield of detectable CTCs. A similar device employing 3-aminopropyltriethoxysilane (γ-APS) as the coupling reagent and CBMA-grafted anti-EpCAM antibody-immobilized Nylon as cannula has also been developed. This method has also been shown to be a promising new material for in vivo CTC capture [24].

In general, CTC isolation can be achieved with different strategies. A great number of approaches for CTC enrichment are currently under development and may be on the market in the near future. However, both independent and large clinical studies will be needed to determine the robustness and clinical validity of these new methods.

3.3.2 Identification and Characterization of CTCs

CTCs could provide important information regarding disease progression as well as useful guidance for therapeutic strategies. Differential methods can now be applied to identify different types of CTC. To our knowledge, those methods include immunocytochemistry-based identification [25, 26], PCR-based identification [27–29], and EPISPOT-based identification [30, 31]. To this end, each strategy has its own advantages and disadvantages. As such, a combination of different analytical methodologies is likely to be beneficial and could allow for a better understanding of the role CTCs play in metastasis formation.

3.4 Ex Vivo and In Vivo Culture of CTCs

Past studies have shown that CTC is valuable predictive marker for disease recurrence prediction and useful prognostic marker for patient survival in quite a number of solid tumors [32–34]. However, it is also emphasized that not every CTC could lead to metastatic mass. Given this difference in metastatic capacity, it is quite important to figure out those CTCs which are able to migrate and form metastasis. This would then allow clinicians to target the formers specifically. Moreover, identifying CTCs with metastasis-initiating capabilities would bring a promising novel therapeutic target. To achieve this, one would need a thorough molecular and genetic characterization of CTCs from early cancers [35]. Moreover, if CTCs could be isolated, cultured, genotyped, and characterized through the whole course of therapeutic progress, they would allow clinicians to identify the most effective treatment strategy [36, 37].

3.4.1 Ex Vivo Culture of CTCs

Ten years ago, development of the EPISPOT assay allowed for the possibility of short-term cultures of CTCs. This assay is designed to detect specific proteins that are produced by CTCs

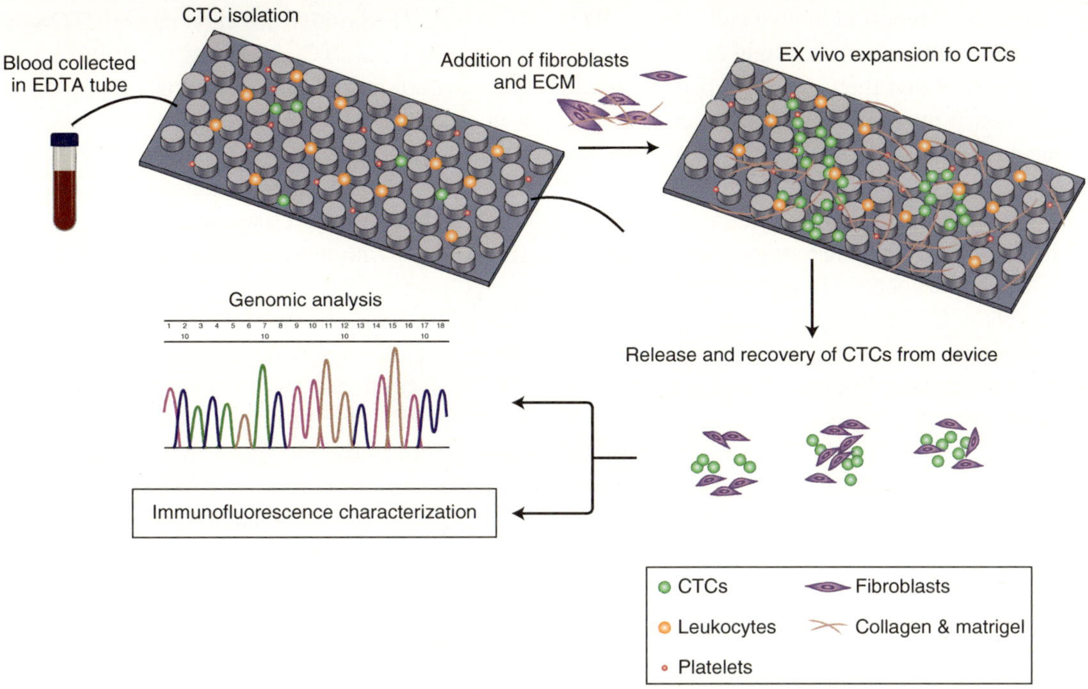

Fig. 3.3 Strategy for co-culture environment in vitro expansion of CTC (Adapted from Expansion of CTCs from early stage lung cancer patients using a microfluidic co-culture model (2014), Zhang Z et al. [41])

during the culture in vitro. Studies in colon and breast tumor have indicated that the number of CTC is correlated with worse outcome for patients [31]. The culture of CTCs in vitro was first described by Zhang et al. in breast cancer [38].

In the study conducted by Zhang et al. [38], researchers characterized and developed an invasive and metastatic type of CTC in vitro, named BMSM, from breast cancer patients. In their study, they successfully isolated and cultured CTCs for long term and demonstrated CTC's competency in the brain metastases [39]. In the Yu et al. study [40], a microfluidic technology termed CTC-iChip was reported. Using this chip and multiple rounds of testing with different culture conditions, they found that CTCs can proliferate better if cultured in serum-free media at tumor spheres, when supplemented with EGF (epidermal growth factor) and FGF (basic fibroblast growth factor) under hypoxic conditions.

In another study [41], a device based on immunoaffinity and microfluid was utilized and applied for lung cancer in early stage. In this study, researchers isolated and cultured CTC in the chip directly. And different culture environment was adopted to get the best conditions for the CTC's growing. As a result, it is observed that CTCs grown at the co-culture environment in 3D could exhibit the best levels of expansion (Fig. 3.3). Given this finding, fibroblasts together with ECM (extracellular matrix) protein were applied to establish a tumor-related microenvironment to facilitate CTCs' expansion. This study demonstrated that CTCs even in rare number got from cancer in early stage can also proliferate for further studies. Moreover, they could be used for the cancer-related gene sequencing without amplification previously, thus making gene study of CTCs more convenient.

3.4.2 In Vivo Culture of CTC

Another method to enlarge the number of CTC is the xenotransplantation of CTCs derived from patients into immunodeficient mice. This method was first reported by Baccelli's team and demonstrated that after xenotransplantation of CTCs from breast cancer patients into the bone of immunocompromised mice, they could grow and metastasize, with a phenotype of $CD47^{+}$, $CD44^{+}$, $EpCAM^{-}$, and $C\text{-}met^{+}$ [38].

The second report of in vivo cultured of CTCs was carried out on small-cell lung cancer patients. It was proved that the CTC from patients could be successfully xenotransplanted and tumorigenic in immunodeficient mice. Moreover, the CTC-derived explants could mirror the patients' responses to etoposide and platinum chemosensitivity, which may help to provide useful information for chemo agents' selection [42].

Recently, Cayrefourcq et al. reported the construction of CTC culture environment in vivo and their tumor-related characteristics in immunocompromised mice. CTCs from 71 colon cancer patients were tested by CellSearch device. Long-term CTC cultures were successfully enriched from two colon patients with a CTC number of more than 300. This was the first published report demonstrating that CTC detected in the peripheral blood of patients with metastatic colon cancer can be expanded and established as a stable colon cancer cell line. Further characteristic at the genomic and post-genomic level of this colon cell line revealed a special feature with attractive potent [43].

3.5 Clinical Implications of Circulating Tumor Cells

3.5.1 Prognostic Potentials of CTC in Gastric Cancer

Past studies have indicated that CTC is an important predictive and prognostic biomarker for the survival and recurrence of solid tumor patients. CTCs were proved to be a reliable biomarker for monitoring the recurrence earlier than radiographic image. By the time metastasis is significant radiographically, the size of tumor will be much larger to treat. Studies of advanced gastric cancer and other malignant tumor have shown that increased number of CTCs was correlated with worse survival [44]. To this end, a certain number of researchers are currently discovering and demonstrating the value of CTCs in clinical treatment and tumor burden monitoring.

One such study prospectively evaluated CTCs using CellSearch in advanced gastric cancer samples from 136 patients to decide the CTCs' positivity frequency. The positive detection rate of CTC was 18.4%. Positive CTC count was much more frequent in the tumor of diffuse histologic genotype, as well as distant metastasis. A multivariate analysis revealed that CTCs could be regarded as independent factors for PFS in gastric tumor [44].

In another study, CTCs were isolated from 100 patients with advanced gastric cancer using the CTC-Profiler (Veridex). This isolation method is magnetic particle-based and uses a coating of anti-EpCAM antibody. The positive CTC detection rate was 28%. The treatment response, PFS, and OS in the CTC-positive group were significantly less than that of the CTC-negative group. Further multivariate analysis proved that CTCs were independent factors for PFS or OS in advanced gastric cancer [45].

A study conducted by Kolostova et al. established a new size-based separation enrichment (MetaCell®) and CTC cultivation approach. The positive CTC detection rate using this method was found to be 59% (n = 13/22). In addition to further cytomorphological analysis of the enriched CTCs, a gene expression analysis of tumor-associated genes was also performed [46].

Finally, another study has focused on the capacity of CTCs' tumorigenicity in 42 patients with advanced gastric cancer. CTCs were separated and xenotransplanted into immunocompromised mice. After five months, nine tumor-like structures derived from six patients were established. These structures were also durable for passages [47].

3.5.2 Genetic Analysis of CTC

The analysis of CTCs' molecular characterization could be useful in identifying therapeutic targets, thereby contributing to a more tailored, anti-metastatic therapy for each patient. These CTC-specific analyses included tumor-associated amplification, genomic tumor mutation profiling, detection of tumor-associated mRNA, and single-cell RNA sequencing. Single-cell-RNA sequencing of CTC has been reported in both breast [48] and pancreatic cancers [49]. Until now, there has been no single-cell RNA sequencing of either CTC clusters or single CTCs in gastric cancer.

3.5.2.1 Detection of Tumor-Associated Amplification in CTC

Recently, a new cellular- and molecular-based method of subtraction enrichment and immunostaining-based FISH (iFISH) was successfully established. The method promised effective enrichment, phenotypic identification in situ, and CTCs' subtype characterization. This fine-grained information is critical, since different CTCs' subtypes might contribute different clinical significances to tumor growth, relapse, metastasis, and treatment resistance [50].

A similar study was also carried out by Shen et al. Briefly, iFISH was also used to determine CTCs' number and characteristics in advanced gastric cancer patients. The status of HER2 expression and the aneuploidy of the chromosome 8 in CTCs got from the patients were tested. Their results showed that examination of the CTC chromosome 8 copy number provided an important method for predicting chemosensitivity and monitoring treatment efficiency [51]. A similar study has also been conducted in breast cancer [52].

3.5.2.2 Genomic Tumor Mutation Profile Assessed in CTC

CTC analysis gnomically can also provide genetic mutation related to therapeutic resistance. For example, the mutations of KRAS were known to affect the efficiency of EGFR inhibitors in colorectal and lung cancer patients. An analysis of intrapatient KRAS [53] and BRAF mutation [54] heterogeneities in individual CTCs has been reported in colon cancer. The testing methods used included HRM, ASPCR, and ddPCR. The heterogeneity of PIK3CA mutation status was also investigated through single CTC detection in metastasis breast cancer patients [55]. Evaluation of PIK3CA mutational status in CTC could be a potential clinical method for tumor and treatment monitoring [56].Yet till now, no similar mutation reports are currently available in gastric cancer.

3.5.2.3 Detection of Tumor-Associated mRNA in CTC

Studies that have examined tumor-associated mRNA in CTC are rare. In a recent colon cancer study, CTC-specific mRNAs were investigated and shown to have higher expression in patients with $\geq$3 CTCs. mRNA expression levels of KRT19, KRT20, and AGR2 have also been reported in mCRC, but no similar results have been available in gastric cancer until recently [57].

3.6 Perspectives

In conclusion, CTCs obtained from circulation could be regarded as liquid biopsy and have important potential for the understanding of tumor metastasis biology. Moreover, using CTCs also lends itself to future improvements in the management of metastatic diseases.

References

1. Joosse SA, Gorges TM, Pantel K. Biology, detection, and clinical implications of circulating tumor cells. EMBO Mol Med. 2015;7(1):1–11. doi:10.15252/emmm.201303698.
2. Joosse SA, Pantel K. Biologic challenges in the detection of circulating tumor cells. Cancer Res. 2013;73(1):8–11. doi:10.1158/0008-5472.CAN-12-3422.
3. Mitchell MJ, King MR. Computational and experimental models of cancer cell response to fluid shear stress. Front Oncol. 2013;3:44. doi:10.3389/fonc.2013.00044.
4. Douma S, Van Laar T, Zevenhoven J, Meuwissen R, Van Garderen E, Peeper DS. Suppression of anoikis and induction of metastasis by the neurotrophic receptor TrkB. Nature. 2004;430(7003):1034–9. doi:10.1038/nature02765.
5. Steinert G, Scholch S, Niemietz T, Iwata N, Garcia SA, Behrens B, et al. Immune escape and survival mechanisms in circulating tumor cells of colorectal cancer. Cancer Res. 2014;74(6):1694–704. doi:10.1158/0008-5472.CAN-13-1885.
6. McDonald DM, Baluk P. Significance of blood vessel leakiness in cancer. Cancer Res. 2002;62(18):5381–5.
7. Pantel K, Passlick B, Vogt J, Stosiek P, Angstwurm M, Seen-Hibler R, et al. Reduced expression of plakoglobin indicates an unfavorable prognosis in subsets of patients with non-small-cell lung cancer. J Clin Oncol Off J Am Soc Clin Oncol. 1998;16(4):1407–13.
8. Parkinson DR, Dracopoli N, Petty BG, Compton C, Cristofanilli M, Deisseroth A, et al. Considerations in the development of circulating tumor cell technology for clinical use. J Transl Med. 2012;10:138. doi:10.1186/1479-5876-10-138.

9. Lianidou ES, Markou A. Circulating tumor cells in breast cancer: detection systems, molecular characterization, and future challenges. Clin Chem. 2011;57(9):1242–55. doi:10.1373/clinchem.2011.165068.
10. Cristofanilli M. Circulating tumor cells, disease progression, and survival in metastatic breast cancer. Semin Oncol. 2006;33(3 Suppl 9):S9–14. doi:10.1053/j.seminoncol.2006.03.016.
11. de Bono JS, Scher HI, Montgomery RB, Parker C, Miller MC, Tissing H, et al. Circulating tumor cells predict survival benefit from treatment in metastatic castration-resistant prostate cancer. Clin Cancer Res. 2008;14(19):6302–9. doi:10.1158/1078-0432.CCR-08-0872.
12. Dotan E, Alpaugh RK, Ruth K, Negin BP, Denlinger CS, Hall MJ, et al. Prognostic significance of MUC-1 in circulating tumor cells in patients with metastatic pancreatic adenocarcinoma. Pancreas. 2016; doi:10.1097/MPA.0000000000000619.
13. Bidard FC, Peeters DJ, Fehm T, Nole F, Gisbert-Criado R, Mavroudis D, et al. Clinical validity of circulating tumour cells in patients with metastatic breast cancer: a pooled analysis of individual patient data. Lancet Oncol. 2014;15(4):406–14. doi:10.1016/S1470-2045(14)70069-5.
14. Sun YF, Xu Y, Yang XR, Guo W, Zhang X, Qiu SJ, et al. Circulating stem cell-like epithelial cell adhesion molecule-positive tumor cells indicate poor prognosis of hepatocellular carcinoma after curative resection. Hepatology. 2013;57(4):1458–68. doi:10.1002/hep.26151.
15. Tewes M, Aktas B, Welt A, Mueller S, Hauch S, Kimmig R, et al. Molecular profiling and predictive value of circulating tumor cells in patients with metastatic breast cancer: an option for monitoring response to breast cancer related therapies. Breast Cancer Res Treat. 2009;115(3):581–90. doi:10.1007/s10549-008-0143-x.
16. Gasch C, Bauernhofer T, Pichler M, Langer-Freitag S, Reeh M, Seifert AM, et al. Heterogeneity of epidermal growth factor receptor status and mutations of KRAS/PIK3CA in circulating tumor cells of patients with colorectal cancer. Clin Chem. 2013;59(1):252–60. doi:10.1373/clinchem.2012.188557.
17. Deneve E, Riethdorf S, Ramos J, Nocca D, Coffy A, Daures JP, et al. Capture of viable circulating tumor cells in the liver of colorectal cancer patients. Clin Chem. 2013;59(9):1384–92. doi:10.1373/clinchem.2013.202846.
18. Nagrath S, Sequist LV, Maheswaran S, Bell DW, Irimia D, Ulkus L, et al. Isolation of rare circulating tumour cells in cancer patients by microchip technology. Nature. 2007;450(7173):1235–9. doi:10.1038/nature06385.
19. Harb W, Fan A, Tran T, Danila DC, Keys D, Schwartz M, et al. Mutational analysis of circulating tumor cells using a novel microfluidic collection device and qPCR assay. Transl Oncol. 2013;6(5):528–38.
20. Ozkumur E, Shah AM, Ciciliano JC, Emmink BL, Miyamoto DT, Brachtel E, et al. Inertial focusing for tumor antigen-dependent and -independent sorting of rare circulating tumor cells. Sci Transl Med. 2013;5(179):179ra47. doi:10.1126/scitranslmed.3005616.
21. Riahi R, Gogoi P, Sepehri S, Zhou Y, Handique K, Godsey J, et al. A novel microchannel-based device to capture and analyze circulating tumor cells (CTCs) of breast cancer. Int J Oncol. 2014;44(6):1870–8. doi:10.3892/ijo.2014.2353.
22. Hou HW, Warkiani ME, Khoo BL, Li ZR, Soo RA, Tan DS, et al. Isolation and retrieval of circulating tumor cells using centrifugal forces. Sci Rep. 2013;3:1259. doi:10.1038/srep01259.
23. Saucedo-Zeni N, Mewes S, Niestroj R, Gasiorowski L, Murawa D, Nowaczyk P, et al. A novel method for the in vivo isolation of circulating tumor cells from peripheral blood of cancer patients using a functionalized and structured medical wire. Int J Oncol. 2012;41(4):1241–50. doi:10.3892/ijo.2012.1557.
24. Wang H, Yue G, Dong C, Wu F, Wei J, Yang Y, et al. Carboxybetaine methacrylate-modified nylon surface for circulating tumor cell capture. ACS Appl Mater Interfaces. 2014;6(6):4550–9. doi:10.1021/am500394j.
25. Lu J, Fan T, Zhao Q, Zeng W, Zaslavsky E, Chen JJ, et al. Isolation of circulating epithelial and tumor progenitor cells with an invasive phenotype from breast cancer patients. Int J Cancer. 2010;126(3):669–83. doi:10.1002/ijc.24814.
26. Hausen BM. Hydrangenol, a strong contact sensitizer found in hydrangea (Hydrangea sp.; Hydrangeaceae). Contact Dermatitis. 1991;24(3):233–5.
27. Kasimir-Bauer S, Hoffmann O, Wallwiener D, Kimmig R, Fehm T. Expression of stem cell and epithelial-mesenchymal transition markers in primary breast cancer patients with circulating tumor cells. Breast Cancer Res. 2012;14(1):R15. doi:10.1186/bcr3099.
28. Strati A, Kasimir-Bauer S, Markou A, Parisi C, Lianidou ES. Comparison of three molecular assays for the detection and molecular characterization of circulating tumor cells in breast cancer. Breast Cancer Res. 2013;15(2):R20. doi:10.1186/bcr3395.
29. Stathopoulou A, Gizi A, Perraki M, Apostolaki S, Malamos N, Mavroudis D, et al. Real-time quantification of CK-19 mRNA-positive cells in peripheral blood of breast cancer patients using the lightcycler system. Clin Cancer Res. 2003;9(14):5145–51.
30. Alix-Panabieres C, Vendrell JP, Pelle O, Rebillard X, Riethdorf S, Muller V, et al. Detection and characterization of putative metastatic precursor cells in cancer patients. Clin Chem. 2007;53(3):537–9. doi:10.1373/clinchem.2006.079509.
31. Alix-Panabieres C. EPISPOT assay: detection of viable DTCs/CTCs in solid tumor patients. Recent Results Cancer Res. 2012;195:69–76. doi:10.1007/978-3-642-28160-0_6.
32. Pachmann K, Camara O, Kavallaris A, Krauspe S, Malarski N, Gajda M, et al. Monitoring the response of circulating epithelial tumor cells to adjuvant chemotherapy in breast cancer allows detection of patients at risk of early relapse. J Clin Oncol Off J Am Soc Clin Oncol. 2008;26(8):1208–15. doi:10.1200/JCO.2007.13.6523.

33. Cristofanilli M, Hayes DF, Budd GT, Ellis MJ, Stopeck A, Reuben JM, et al. Circulating tumor cells: a novel prognostic factor for newly diagnosed metastatic breast cancer. J Clin Oncol Off J Am Soc Clin Oncol. 2005;23(7):1420–30. doi:10.1200/JCO.2005.08.140.
34. Cohen SJ, Punt CJ, Iannotti N, Saidman BH, Sabbath KD, Gabrail NY, et al. Relationship of circulating tumor cells to tumor response, progression-free survival, and overall survival in patients with metastatic colorectal cancer. J Clin Oncol Off J Am Soc Clin Oncol. 2008;26(19):3213–21. doi:10.1200/JCO.2007.15.8923.
35. Fusi A, Metcalf R, Krebs M, Dive C, Blackhall F. Clinical utility of circulating tumour cell detection in non-small-cell lung cancer. Curr Treat Options Oncol. 2013;14(4):610–22. doi:10.1007/s11864-013-0253-5.
36. Hoshimoto S, Faries MB, Morton DL, Shingai T, Kuo C, Wang HJ, et al. Assessment of prognostic circulating tumor cells in a phase III trial of adjuvant immunotherapy after complete resection of stage IV melanoma. Ann Surg. 2012;255(2):357–62. doi:10.1097/SLA.0b013e3182380f56.
37. Hofman V, Ilie M, Long E, Guibert N, Selva E, Washetine K, et al. Detection of circulating tumor cells from lung cancer patients in the era of targeted therapy: promises, drawbacks and pitfalls. Curr Mol Med. 2014;14(4):440–56.
38. Baccelli I, Schneeweiss A, Riethdorf S, Stenzinger A, Schillert A, Vogel V, et al. Identification of a population of blood circulating tumor cells from breast cancer patients that initiates metastasis in a xenograft assay. Nat Biotechnol. 2013;31(6):539–44. doi:10.1038/nbt.2576.
39. Zhang L, Ridgway LD, Wetzel MD, Ngo J, Yin W, Kumar D, et al. The identification and characterization of breast cancer CTCs competent for brain metastasis. Sci Transl Med. 2013;5(180):180ra48. doi:10.1126/scitranslmed.3005109.
40. Yu M, Bardia A, Aceto N, Bersani F, Madden MW, Donaldson MC, et al. Cancer therapy. Ex vivo culture of circulating breast tumor cells for individualized testing of drug susceptibility. Science. 2014;345(6193):216–20. doi:10.1126/science.1253533.
41. Zhang Z, Shiratsuchi H, Lin J, Chen G, Reddy RM, Azizi E, et al. Expansion of CTCs from early stage lung cancer patients using a microfluidic co-culture model. Oncotarget. 2014;5(23):12383–97. doi:10.18632/oncotarget.2592.
42. Hodgkinson CL, Morrow CJ, Li Y, Metcalf RL, Rothwell DG, Trapani F, et al. Tumorigenicity and genetic profiling of circulating tumor cells in small-cell lung cancer. Nat Med. 2014;20(8):897–903. doi:10.1038/nm.3600.
43. Cayrefourcq L, Mazard T, Joosse S, Solassol J, Ramos J, Assenat E, et al. Establishment and characterization of a cell line from human circulating colon cancer cells. Cancer Res. 2015;75(5):892–901. doi:10.1158/0008-5472.CAN-14-2613.
44. Okabe H, Tsunoda S, Hosogi H, Hisamori S, Tanaka E, Tanaka S, et al. Circulating tumor cells as an independent predictor of survival in advanced gastric cancer. Ann Surg Oncol. 2015;22(12):3954–61. doi:10.1245/s10434-015-4483-6.
45. Lee SJ, Lee J, Kim ST, Park SH, Park JO, Park YS, et al. Circulating tumor cells are predictive of poor response to chemotherapy in metastatic gastric cancer. Int J Biol Markers. 2015;30(4):e382–6. doi:10.5301/jbm.5000151.
46. Kolostova K, Matkowski R, Gurlich R, Grabowski K, Soter K, Lischke R, et al. Detection and cultivation of circulating tumor cells in gastric cancer. Cytotechnology. 2015; doi:10.1007/s10616-015-9866-9.
47. Toyoshima K, Hayashi A, Kashiwagi M, Hayashi N, Iwatsuki M, Ishimoto T, et al. Analysis of circulating tumor cells derived from advanced gastric cancer. Int J Cancer. 2015;137(4):991–8. doi:10.1002/ijc.29455.
48. Aceto N, Bardia A, Miyamoto DT, Donaldson MC, Wittner BS, Spencer JA, et al. Circulating tumor cell clusters are oligoclonal precursors of breast cancer metastasis. Cell. 2014;158(5):1110–22.
49. Ting DT, Wittner BS, Ligorio M, Vincent Jordan N, Shah AM, Miyamoto DT, et al. Single-cell RNA sequencing identifies extracellular matrix gene expression by pancreatic circulating tumor cells. Cell Rep. 2014;8(6):1905–18.
50. Ge F, Zhang H, Wang DD, Li L, Lin PP. Enhanced detection and comprehensive in situ phenotypic characterization of circulating and disseminated heteroploid epithelial and glioma tumor cells. Oncotarget. 2015;6(29):27049–64.
51. Li Y, Zhang X, Ge S, Gao J, Gong J, Lu M, et al. Clinical significance of phenotyping and karyotyping of circulating tumor cells in patients with advanced gastric cancer. Oncotarget. 2014;5(16):6594–602.
52. Riethdorf S, Muller V, Zhang L, Rau T, Loibl S, Komor M, et al. Detection and HER2 expression of circulating tumor cells: prospective monitoring in breast cancer patients treated in the neoadjuvant GeparQuattro trial. Clin Cancer Res. 2010;16(9):2634–45.
53. Mohamed Suhaimi NA, Foong YM, Lee DY, Phyo WM, Cima I, Lee EX, et al. Non-invasive sensitive detection of KRAS and BRAF mutation in circulating tumor cells of colorectal cancer patients. Mol Oncol. 2015;9(4):850–60.
54. Reid AL, Freeman JB, Millward M, Ziman M, Gray ES. Detection of BRAF-V600E and V600K in melanoma circulating tumour cells by droplet digital PCR. Clin Biochem. 2015;48(15):999–1002.
55. Pestrin M, Salvianti F, Galardi F, De Luca F, Turner N, Malorni L, et al. Heterogeneity of PIK3CA mutational status at the single cell level in circulating tumor cells from metastatic breast cancer patients. Mol Oncol. 2015;9(4):749–57.
56. Markou A, Farkona S, Schiza C, Efstathiou T, Kounelis S, Malamos N, et al. PIK3CA mutational status in circulating tumor cells can change during disease recurrence or progression in patients with breast cancer. Clin Cancer Res. 2014;20(22):5823–34.
57. Mostert B, Sieuwerts AM, Bolt-de Vries J, Kraan J, Lalmahomed Z, van Galen A, et al. mRNA expression profiles in circulating tumor cells of metastatic colorectal cancer patients. Mol Oncol. 2015;9(4):920–32.

Customized Chemotherapy in Advanced Gastric Cancer

4

Jia Wei and Nandie Wu

4.1 Introduction

Currently, the therapeutic management of gastric cancer is based largely on clinical data and histological features. Numerous promising markers have been studied in an effort to identify those that will enable an accurate prediction of prognosis or response to chemotherapy. Such markers would allow for the identification of patient subgroups that might benefit from specific treatment regimens. In this chapter, we highlight novel biomarkers for that can be used for recommending chemotherapeutic agents to be used for the treatment of gastric cancer. While these types of new treatment options have been introduced recently, interindividual variability of response and drug resistance remains a challenge. Thus, promising biomarkers should be evaluated in clinical trials in order to establish customized therapeutic approaches.

J. Wei (✉) • N. Wu
The Comprehensive Cancer Centre of Drum Tower Hospital, Medical School of Nanjing University and Clinical Cancer Institute of Nanjing University, Nanjing 210008, China
e-mail: weijia01627@hotmail.com

4.2 Chemotherapy in Advanced Gastric Cancer

Chemotherapy can relieve symptoms, increase survival, and improve the quality of life in patients with advanced gastric cancer. A recent phase III trial (REGATTA) demonstrated that chemotherapy alone remains the standard method of treatment for patients with advanced gastric cancer, even in the case of those with a single non-curable factor [1]. Fluorouracil, platinum, and new-generation chemotherapeutic regimens including oral fluorouracil (S-1 and capecitabine), oxaliplatin, irinotecan, and taxanes have demonstrated positive effects in gastric cancer treatment.

Several different chemotherapy regimens have been used in the treatment of patients with advanced gastric cancer. However, the median survival of these patients remains low, around 1 year [2]. Biweekly combination of fluorouracil, leucovorin, and oxaliplatin (FLO or FOLFOX) has been demonstrated to be a well-tolerated alternative to cisplatin and fluorouracil in patients with local advanced or metastatic gastric cancer, with patients having a median survival time of 9.6–11.4 months [3–7]. A phase III trial showed that FLO exhibited a trend of improved progression-free survival (PFS) and significant less toxicity compared with fluorouracil, leucovorin, and cisplatin (FLP) [7]. In addition, FLO was associated a significant superior response rate, PFS, and overall survival (OS) in patients greater than 65 years of age.

J. Wei, B. Liu (eds.), *Personalized Management of Gastric Cancer*,
DOI 10.1007/978-981-10-3978-2_4

ECF (epirubicin, cisplatin, and fluorouracil) was widely used in the treatment of advanced gastric cancer beginning in the 1990s due to patients' superior survival and quality of life when compared with FAMTX (fluorouracil, Adriamycin, and methotrexate) and MCF (methotrexate, cisplatin, and fluorouracil) treatment. The phase III trial, Randomized ECF for Advanced and Locally Advanced Esophagogastric Cancer 2 (REAL-2) [8], was designed to determine whether fluorouracil can be replaced by capecitabine and cisplatin by oxaliplatin in the ECF regimen. The primary goal of the study was to understand whether capecitabine and oxaliplatin were as effective as fluorouracil and oxaliplatin treatment, respectively. The results from this study suggested that capecitabine and oxaliplatin were as effective as fluorouracil and cisplatin treatment, respectively. Compared to cisplatin, oxaliplatin was associated with lower incidences of grade 3 or 4 neutropenia, alopecia, renal toxicity, and thromboembolism. However, it was associated with a slightly higher incidence of grade 3 or 4 diarrhea and neuropathy [8].

Another phase III trial (ML 17032) was carried out to compare capecitabine and cisplatin (XP) and fluorouracil and cisplatin (FP) as the first line of treatment in advanced gastric cancer patients. This study suggested XP was associated with a better overall response rate (ORR) and OS [9]. A meta-analysis of the REAL-2 and ML17032 trials was carried out to evaluate the use of capecitabine-based combination chemotherapy and infused 5-fluorouracil-based combination chemotherapy for the treatment of advanced esophagogastric cancer. The results from this study demonstrated a superior OS in 654 patients that were treated with capecitabine combinations, compared 664 patients treated with 5-FU combinations [10].

Another triple chemotherapeutic regimen combining docetaxel, cisplatin, and fluorouracil (DCF) was evaluated in a randomized phase III study (V325) [11]. In this study, the time to progression (TTP) was found to be significantly longer with DCF treatment compared with cisplatin and fluorouracil (CF) treatment (5.6 months vs. 3.7 months, $p < 0.001$). The median OS was found to also be significantly longer with DCF treatment compared with CF treatment (9.2 months vs. 8.6 months, $p = 0.02$). In addition, the ORR was found to be significantly longer with DCF treatment compared with CF treatment (37% vs. 25%, $p = 0.01$). However, DCF was associated with increased hematologic and digestive toxicity of grade 3 or 4. Numerous modifications of the DCF regimen are currently undergoing clinical trials to improve the tolerability of this treatment regimen. A randomized phase II trial of docetaxel plus oxaliplatin with or without fluorouracil or capecitabine showed that docetaxel, oxaliplatin, and fluorouracil were associated with improved TTP, ORR, and OS, with an improved safety profile compared with that of docetaxel and oxaliplatin and docetaxel, oxaliplatin, and capecitabine treatment in advanced GC [12].

Another oral fluoropyrimidine S-1 has also demonstrated promising effects in the treatment of advanced gastric cancer when used alone or in combination with cisplatin. The phase III SPIRITS trial randomized advanced gastric cancer patients to S-1 and S-1 plus cisplatin (CS) groups. The median OS (13 months vs. 11 months) and PFS (6.0 months vs. 4 months) were significantly longer for the S-1 plus cisplatin group compared to the S-1 alone group [13]. The following phase III FLAGS trial demonstrated similar median OS in CS and cisplatin plus fluorouracil (CF) arms of the study (8.6 months vs. 7.9 months) [14]. However, CS was associated with a significantly improved safety profile and better survival in patients with a diffuse type of histology. However, there is doubt surrounding the conclusions from these studies due to the fact that the dose of cisplatin and S-1 was lower than that which is recommended by the Japanese study.

The phase III V-306 trial demonstrated that irinotecan, fluorouracil, and folinic acid (IF) treatments were non-inferior to CF treatment in terms of PFS, but not for OS and TTP. However, IF was associated with a more favorable toxicity profile [15]. Therefore, IF treatment may provide a viable, platinum-free, front-line treatment alternative for metastatic gastric cancer patients.

Another recent French phase III trial compared fluorouracil, leucovorin, and irinotecan (FOLFIRI) treatment with epirubicin, cisplatin, and capecitabine (ECX) treatment. FOLFIRI treatment was found to be better tolerated by patients and was associated with a longer time to treatment failure (5.1 months vs. 4.2 months, $p = 0.008$). However, there was no significant difference observed in PFS and OS [16]. Irinotecan used alone or in combination with other cytotoxic agents has not produced high-level evidence for the prolongation of survival in patients with advanced gastric cancer and was thus not recommended as a second-line treatment.

For advanced gastric cancer patients, only three targeted therapies, trastuzumab, ramucirumab, and apatinib, have demonstrated positive results in prospective phase III trials, leaving these as the main chemotherapy treatment options for gastric cancer patients. With recent developments in molecular biology, cancer treatment is beginning to move from the traditional "trial-and-error" approach to a position which involves a personalized approach. The aim of this chapter is to review how advances in prognostic, predictive, and toxicity markers are leading to a personalized approach for cancer management.

4.3 Customized Chemotherapy in Advanced Gastric Cancer

4.3.1 Platinum

DNA repair systems enable cells to identify and correct damage to DNA molecules, including those induced by chemotherapeutic agents. The activation of repair mechanisms is a common player in the acquired drug resistance. Thus, the identification of biomarkers involved in repair pathways could be useful for the stratification of patients according to prognosis and the likelihood of response to a chemotherapy treatment.

Cisplatin-induced DNA adducts in *S. cerevisiae* are processed by components of the nucleotide excision repair, recombination repair, and translesion synthesis pathways. The excision repair cross-complementing 1 (ERCC1) is a single-strand DNA endonuclease that functions to repair bulky lesions, such as those produced by platinum adducts, and thus contributes to platinum resistance. The expression of ERCC1, measured at either the mRNA or protein level, has been negatively correlated with patient survival and response to cisplatin- or oxaliplatin-based chemotherapy [17–20]. Breast cancer susceptibility gene 1 (BRCA1), which is involved in recombination repair mechanisms [21, 22], could act as a stronger predictive marker than ERCC1. BRCA1 functions as a differential modulator of survival with cisplatin and anti-microtubule drugs. This clinical effect is based on preclinical findings, which show that BRCA1 induces a 10- to 1000-fold increase in resistance to DNA-damaging agents and, in contrast, an 800- to greater than 1000-fold increase in sensitivity to anti-microtubule drugs [23, 24]. In our previous study [25], we demonstrated that BRCA1 mRNA levels were negatively associated ($R = -0.624$; $p = 0.002$) with cisplatin sensitivity but positively associated ($R = 0.468$; $p = 0.032$) with docetaxel sensitivity in gastric cancer patients [25].

Recent studies have demonstrated a more complex network involved in the response to DNA damage. In the process of DNA damage repair, mediator of DNA damage checkpoint protein 1 (MDC1) has been shown to serve as an upstream molecule which promotes H2AX phosphorylation. This results in the amplification of ataxia-telangiectasia mutated (ATM) signaling through sequential assembly of repair proteins, including BRCA1 and p53 binding protein 1 (53BP1). This process controls damage-induced cell cycle arrest checkpoints [26, 27]. The function of 53BP1 in DNA repair is abrogated upon BRCA1 depletion [28, 29]. Impaired accumulation of 53BP1 at DNA damage sites was also observed, along with depletion of PIAS4, and ubiquitin conjugating enzyme 9 (UBC9), the E3 and E2 ubiquitin ligases that function in the small ubiquitin-related modifier (SUMO)-conjugation system [30]. UBC9 functions to transport BRCA1 protein into the nucleus. Knockdown of UBC9 resulted in the cytoplasmic localization of BRCA1 proteins, which impaired their capacity to inhibit ovarian cancer cells growth [31]. The methyltransferase multiple myeloma SET domain (MMSET) plays a central role in the recruitment of 53BP1 to DNA damage sites [32]. Depletion of MMSET has been shown to confer hypersensitivity to ionizing radiation [32]. MMSET is highly expressed in several tumor types relative to normal tissue [33, 34]. Because high MMSET expression contributes to increased cell viability and growth, it is correlated with poor prognosis [35]. In addition, MMSET knockdown resulted in a decrease in transcript levels of several cell cycle genes, including BRCA1 [36]. MMSET has been shown to interact with MDC1 in a DNA-damage-inducible manner, with the downregulation of MMSET resulting in a significant decrease in histone methylation and the subsequent accumulation of 53BP1 [32]. A similar effect of MMSET was also observed in class switch recombination [37]. Downregulation of MMSET has been shown to confer hypersensitivity to DNA damage [32].

In addition, there are some components that are thought to interact with BRCA1 to modulate its function. For example, receptor-associated protein 80 (RAP80), also known as ubiquitin interaction motif containing 1 (UIMC1), is a ubiquitin-binding protein that has been shown to be essential for BRCA1's activity [38, 39]. In addition, BRCA1 is also modified by small ubiquitin-related modifier (SUMO) in response to genotoxic damage. Protein inhibitor of activated STAT (PIAS) SUMO ligase activity is required for proficient double-strand break repair mechanisms [30]. Following chemotherapy-induced DNA damage, PIAS1 and PIAS4 are needed for the accumulation of DNA repair proteins, including BRCA1, to the DNA damage site [30, 38]. PIAS1 has been shown to be required for the complete recruitment of BRCA1 to the DNA damage site, potentially through interaction with BRCA1 and RAP80, while PIAS4 is required earlier in the DNA damage repair cascade to recruit other DNA repair proteins [40], as depicted in Fig. 4.1.

In previous studies, we have analyzed mRNA expression levels of BRCA1, RAP80, PIAS1, PIAS4, MDC1, UBC9, 53BP1, and MMSET in advanced gastric cancer patients [41, 42]. All patients received first-line FOLFOX chemotherapy treatment and exhibited disease progression,

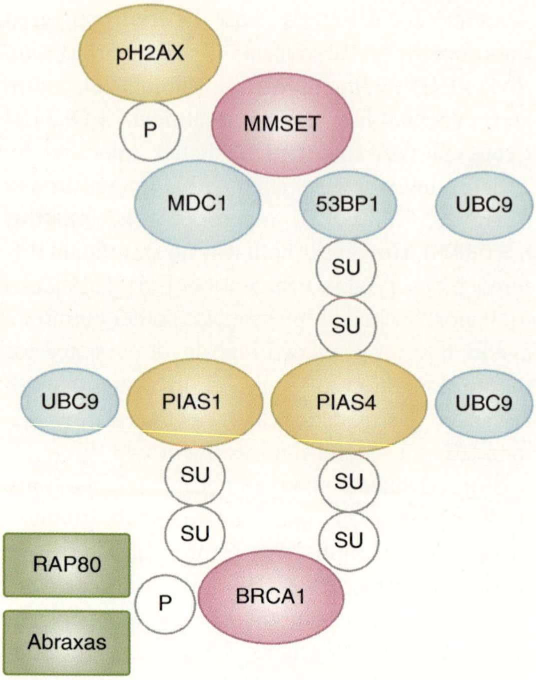

Fig. 4.1 The BRCA1 pathway in response to DNA double-stand breaks. SU: SUMOylation; P: Phosphorylation (Adapted from Differential effect of MMSET mRNA levels on survival to first-line FOLFOX and second-line docetaxel in gastric cancer (2014), Wei J et al. [42])

with 59 patients treated with second-line docetaxel-based chemotherapy. Among those patients that received only first-line oxaliplatin-based chemotherapy, the median survival was determined to be 12.3 months for those with low levels of MMSET, compared to 8.8 months for those with high levels of MMSET ($p = 0.04$). The median survival time was found to be 12.4 months for patients with low levels of UBC9 and 8.8 months for patients with high levels of UBC9 ($p = 0.01$). Longer survival was also observed in patients with low levels of BRCA1 ($p = 0.20$), MDC1 ($p = 0.49$), and 53BP1 ($p = 0.09$). However, the differences were not found to be significant. Among patients with low MMSET expression levels, the median survival time was 19.9 months for patients with low 53BP1 levels and 5.9 months for those with high 53BP1 levels ($p = 0.02$). Multivariable analyses were carried out in patients that received only first-line treatment. A decreased mortality risk was observed in patients with low MMSET levels (HR, 0.59; 95% CI, 0.35–0.98; $p = 0.04$) and in patients with low UBC9 levels (HR, 0.52; 95% CI, 0.31–0.88; $p = 0.01$). Differential modulators of survival were observed in several genes and gene combinations, an observation which will be discussed in the section regarding taxanes.

In addition to DNA repair genes, certain miRNAs impact the sensitivity of a patient toward chemotherapy treatment if their levels are artificially upregulated. This is similar to the data regarding miRNAs with diagnostic potential. An upregulation of miR-21 or miR-106a was demonstrated to result in an increase in cisplatin resistance of GC cells [43, 44]. However, the upregulation of miR-449 was demonstrated to have a positive impact on sensitivity toward cisplatin [45].

4.3.2 5-Fluorouracil (5-FU)/Capecitabine/S-1

5-FU and its oral forms are the primary chemotherapeutic drugs used in the treatment of gastric cancer patients. Capecitabine is hepatically metabolized and thus ultimately converted into 5-FU at the tissue level [46]. Another oral fluoropyrimidine, notably S-1, possesses tegafur as the active moiety. This is transformed to 5-FU by cytochrome p450 in the liver [47]. 5-FU is an S phase-specific agent which exhibits cytotoxicity through the incorporation of fluoronucleotides into RNA and DNA molecules. 5-FU is converted into its active metabolite, fluorodeoxyuridine monophosphate (FdUMP), by thymidine phosphorylase (TP) and orotate phosphoribosyltransferase (OPRT). FdUMP exhibits a high affinity for thymidylate synthase (TS), the primary target of fluoropyrimidines. Methylenetetrahydrofolate reductase (MTHFR) plays a critical role in both fluoropyrimidine synthesis and the regulation of folate intracellular flow. In addition, 5-FU is phosphorylated by orotate phosphoribosyl transferase, resulting in the inhibition of RNA synthesis. The rate-limiting enzyme in 5-FU catabolism is dihydropyrimidine dehydrogenase (DYPD). DYPD is also involved in the conversion of the oral prodrug capecitabine to 5-FU at the cellular level. TP activity in cancer cells has been correlated with the intra-tumoral 5-FU concentration following capecitabine administration [48]. Research studies related to 5-FU pharmacogenetics and pharmacogenomics primarily focused on several genes, including TS, TP, MTHFR, OPRT, and DYPD.

TS is the most extensively studied enzyme. A seminal study carried out in 1996 demonstrated that TS mRNA levels influence the response to 5-FU-based chemotherapy, and thus survival, in a cohort of patients with primary gastric cancer [49]. Numerous following studies validated this negative predictive role for TS expression in response to fluoropyrimidines [48]. However, in nonmetastatic cases, some studies have not identified any correlation between low TS expression and a response to 5-FU. This has been explained by a possible prognostic role of TS, which could be involved in tumor progression rather than the chemotherapy response in the case of these negative studies [50–52].

A meta-analysis demonstrated that polymorphisms in TS and MTHFR were closely associated with the clinical outcomes of GC patients treated with 5-FU-based chemotherapy [53]. However, the effect of TS polymorphisms could vary through ethnicity stratification due to different allelic distributions [54].

The biomarker study carried out in the SPIRITS trial demonstrated the effect of fluorouracil-metabolizing enzymes on the outcomes of patients treated with S-1 alone or S-1 plus cisplatin (CS) as the first-line treatment in advanced gastric cancer. The mRNA levels of TS, TP, OPRT, DYPD, vascular endothelial growth factor-A (VEGFRA), and epidermal growth factor receptor (EGFR) were studied in paraffin-embedded specimens isolated from primary tumors. Multivariate survival analysis in patients that received S-1 monotherapy demonstrated that low TP expression, low TS, and high OPRT were significant predictors of long overall survival. In patients with lower expression levels of both TP and TS, the S-1 alone group demonstrated longer overall survival compared to the CS group. However, the frequency of overall adverse events in the S-1 treatment alone group tended to be lower than that in CS treatment group [55].

Another study which examined biomarkers related to capecitabine, platinum, and taxane therapy has demonstrated the role of four key target or metabolic enzymes: class III β-tubulin (TUBB3),

TS, TP, and ERCC1. As described earlier, both TS and TP are key metabolic enzymes of capecitabine. TUBB3 and ERCC1 overexpression was shown to indicate a resistance to taxanes and platinum, respectively. The response rates of patients to capecitabine plus paclitaxel or capecitabine plus cisplatin treatment were observed to be markedly different between patients exhibiting low TUBB3/high TP expression levels (87.5%) compared with those exhibiting high TUBB3/low TP expression levels (14.3%) ($p = 0.01$). Similarly, the response rate was determined to be 57.9% for the low TS/high TP subgroup and 15.8% for the high TS/low TP subgroup ($p = 0.007$) [56].

In addition to 5-FU metabolic enzymes, the regenerating gene family (REG) was reported to play a role in chemosensitivity. In vitro studies have demonstrated that induction of REG Iα gene expression confers resistance to 5-FU or CDDP treatment in GC cells. In patients with stage IV GC, REG Iα could be a potential biomarker for predicting resistance to S-1/CDDP treatment [57]. In addition, high REG IV serum levels in gastric cancer patients was identified as predictive measure for the resistance to 5-fluorouracil-based chemotherapy [58].

4.3.3 Taxanes

Taxanes, as its name indicates, were first derived from the plants, *Taxus*. Taxane agents bind and stabilize microtubule, leading to tumor cell cycle arrest at the G2-M phase [59]. Taxanes have achieved definitive curative effects either alone or in combination with other chemotherapy drugs as both first- and second-line therapy in the treatment of gastric cancer. There are four primary types of taxane agents, including paclitaxel, docetaxel, nanoparticle albumin-bound paclitaxel (nab-paclitaxel), and cabazitaxel. Paclitaxel and docetaxel belong to the taxane family, as their chemical structures contain a common three-phenol ring. Nab-paclitaxel is a novel drug that is a biologically interactive form of paclitaxel. Cabazitaxel is second-generation taxane which is currently being used in ongoing phase II trials (NCT01757171, NCT01956149) to illustrate its role in the treatment of gastric cancer.

According to published reports, sensitivity to taxanes involves multiple mechanisms, including drug efflux, mutations in tubulin, altered microtubule dynamics, and impaired cell death signaling [60].

Overexpression of the multidrug resistance (MDR) gene like MDR1, which encodes P-glycoprotein, resulted in taxane efflux, decreasing drug retention and thus causing taxane resistance [61].

Because taxane targets microtubules, attention has been directed toward the study of tubulin and microtubule-associated proteins. Mutations [62] and polymorphisms [63, 64] in β-tubulin have been shown to be associated with taxane resistance. The overexpression of β-tubulin isotypes was identified as another mechanism of resistance [65]. Numerous studies have validated the fact that taxane treatment is inversely correlated with mRNA and protein expression levels of βIII-tubulin in gastric cancer [66–68]. Furthermore, a recent report suggested that the interaction of vascular endothelial growth factor (VEGF) with βIII-tubulin through hypoxia-inducible factor (HIF-alpha) was associated with taxane sensitivity. VEGF inhibition, which blocks both VEGFR-1 and VEGFR-2, has been demonstrated to reverse paclitaxel sensitivity in gastric cancer cells [69]. In addition, the sensitivity of gastric cancer patients to paclitaxel treatment was found to be inversely correlated with mRNA and protein expression levels of the microtubule-associated protein, tau (MAPT) [66, 70]. Chemokine receptor-4 (CXCR4) was identified to play a role in microtubule dynamics. CXCR4 mRNA levels in gastric cancer tissues were also found to correlate with docetaxel sensitivity [71].

The induction of apoptosis by taxanes has been shown to be mediated through the mitochondrial apoptotic pathway, typically by members of the Bcl2 family [72]. The pro-apoptotic protein, BIM, has been demonstrated to translocate from microtubules to mitochondria following taxane treatment [73]. Thus, cancer cell lines with higher BIM expression levels were found to be more sensitive to taxanes compared to cells that expressed lower levels of BIM [60]. In addition to antiapoptotic properties, glucose-regulated protein 78(GRP78) overexpression was found to be a predictive marker for the development of taxane-based therapeutic resistance [74]. Survivin is a member of the family of inhibitor of apoptosis proteins (IAPs), and its expression levels have been demonstrated to be inversely correlated with taxane treatment [66].

Numerous studies have shown that Forkhead box protein M1 (FOXM1), which plays an important role in cell cycle regulation, mediates docetaxel resistance in gastric cancer patients [75, 76]. In addition, docetaxel resistance was shown to be reversed upon inhibition of FOXM1 [77]. Furthermore, genes that play a role in the DNA damage response pathway, including BRCA1, have been shown to also play a critical role in a patient's response to taxane agents. Tumors exhibiting high BRCA1 expression were found to exhibit an increased susceptibility to docetaxel [23]. As discussed earlier in the section regarding platinum, our study found that of 59 patients who received first-line FOLFOX and second-line docetaxel-based chemotherapy, the median overall survival was 25.8 months for patients with high BRCA1 expression levels, 19.1 months for patients with intermediate BRCA1 expression levels, and 9.5 months for those with low BRCA1 expression levels ($p = 0.0062$) [78].

In addition, previous studies have demonstrated that ErbB3 overexpression and AKT/ERK activation can induce gastric cancer cell resistance to paclitaxel treatment [79]. Homomeric α7-nicotinic acetylcholine receptor (A7-nAChR) was found to be a key modulator of smoking-induced gastric cancer metastasis. Interestingly, A7-nAChR knockdown cells were shown to exhibit higher sensitivity to paclitaxel treatment in gastric cancer cells [80].

4.3.4 Irinotecan(CPT-11)

Irinotecan (CPT-11)-based treatment regimens were commonly used for the treatment of gastric cancer. This treatment exhibited a good response rate in patients, varying from 14–70% when used as a single or combination treatment agent [81].

Irinotecan is a semisynthetic, water-soluble derivative of the plant alkaloid camptothecin. This compound belongs to the class of topoisomerase I inhibitors. Addition of irinotecan to the topoisomerase I (Topo I)-DNA complex obstructs the ligation of double-stranded DNA during the process of DNA replication. This causes Topo I to be trapped on a nicked DNA intermediate in replicating cells, resulting in cell death [82]. A variety of DNA repair genes, including aprataxin (APTX), BRCA1, ERCC1, and ATM, are involved in the repair of irinotecan-associated DNA damage. Studies have reported that high gene expression levels of Topo I are associated with irinotecan sensitivity in gastric cancer [83]. Interestingly, significantly lower gene expression levels of APTX, BRCA1, and ERCC1 have been reported to be associated with irinotecan-sensitive gastric cancer samples, compared with that of irinotecan-resistant samples [84]. Furthermore, low expression levels of the DNA repair gene, ATM kinase, were also found to be associated with increased irinotecan drug sensitivity in gastric cancer cell lines [85]. Consistent results were observed in the molecular biomarker study of GC0301/TOP-002 phase III trials in gastric cancer. The results of these trials show that low TS, low ERCC1, and high TP mRNA levels function as biomarkers for irinotecan treatment [83].

Recently, gene hyper-methylation has been demonstrated to be an important epigenetic mechanism of drug response in gastric cancer [86]. Methylation of the oncogene, heparan sulfate 6-O-endosulfatase (SULF2), and methylation of the tumor-suppressor gene, WRN, were both reported to render gastric cancer sensitive to irinotecan treatment [87].

Recent studies regarding cell signaling revealed that irinotecan resistance was accompanied by an activation of EGFR and Src signaling in human cancer models [88]. Furthermore, gene XB130 knockdown demonstrated an improved response to irinotecan treatment in gastric cancer cells [89].

4.3.5 Pemetrexed

Pemetrexed is a new antifolate drug that has been shown to target multiple components within the folate pathway, including thymidylate synthase (TS), dihydrofolate reductase (DHFR), and glycinamide ribonucleotide formyltransferase (GARFT) [90]. Pemetrexed was demonstrated to mediate its antitumor effect by impeding both DNA synthesis and folate metabolism [91]. Clinical antitumor activity of pemetrexed in gastric cancer has also been observed in several clinical trials where it has been used either as a single agent or in combination with another chemotherapy agent. The response rate in these trials was found to range from 23–36% [92–95].

Thymidylate synthase (TS) is a critical enzyme that plays a role in the synthesis of DNA. Research from our group indicates that low expression levels of TS in the plasma and tumor were negatively correlated with pemetrexed sensitivity in gastric cancer patients ($p < 0.001$) [96]. TS levels in plasma and tumor were found to be lower in the pemetrexed-sensitive group compared to the pemetrexed-resistant group. Previous study also confirmed that low DHFR and GARFT gene expression levels exhibited a significant correlation with chemosensitivity to pemetrexed in freshly explanted tumor cells in vitro [97].

4.3.6 Other Regimens

Other regimens, such as doxorubicin, epirubicin, and mitomycin, could also function as effective treatments in gastric cancer patients.

Doxorubicin is a member of the anthracycline group of compounds and is known to exhibit activity against a wide range of tumors. The primary mechanism of action of this compound appears to be through inhibition of topoisomerase II. In addition, it has also been shown to be capable of forming adducts with DNA in order to induce cell death [98]. Studies have shown that high expression levels of the apoptosis repressor with caspase recruitment domain (ARC) in gastric cancer cell lines contribute to doxorubicin chemotherapy resistance [99]. Recent microarray data has enabled researchers to identify novel genes including ADAM22, CYR61, FN1, SPHK1, and GNAI1 as predictive markers of doxorubicin sensitivity in gastric cancer [100].

Epirubicin is another example of an antitumor agent of anthracyclines. This specific compound is thought to enter tumor cells more efficiently in order to exert its antitumor effects though the inhibition of nucleic acid synthesis and mitosis, both leading to cell death [101]. Studies have reported that high expression levels of MDR genes, including MDR1, MRP1, and ABCG2, in gastric cancer patients correlated with the development of resistance to epirubicin [102]. Gastric cancer patients with high expression levels of DNA synthesis-related genes, such as topoisomerase IIA (TOP2A), have been shown to benefit from epirubicin therapy [20]. Furthermore, amplification of human epidermal growth factor receptor-2 (HER-2) or HER-2 overexpression was identified as a potential biomarker to flag those patients who benefited from either perioperative or postoperative epirubicin-based therapy in gastroesophageal adenocarcinoma [103].

Mitomycin is a cell cycle nonspecific agent, an anticancer drug that is commonly used to treat numerous cancer types, including stomach, anal, and lung cancer [104]. Studies investigating the antitumor mechanism of mitomycin revealed that this drug induced DNA damage via DNA alkylation. This was found to result in the production of DNA mono-adducts, intrastrand cross-links, and interstrand cross-links (ICLs) [105, 106]. However, the specific mechanism underlying mitomycin resistance has not been fully understood. In vitro studies have revealed that TCF transcription factor 3 played a role in mitomycin resistance in gastric cancer patients [107]. AKT activation and loss of heterozygosity (LOH) of phosphatase and tensin homolog on chromosome ten (PTEN) were also found to be associated with mitomycin-related chemoresistance in GC patients [108]. Both normal and cancer cells that were found to lack the suppressor gene, FHIT, exhibited mitomycin C resistance [109].

4.3.7 Markers for Toxicity

Common adverse drug events of chemotherapy treatment for gastric cancer include nausea and vomiting, fatigue, diarrhea, liver and kidney dysfunction, blennophlogisma, and hematopoietic disorders such as granulocytopenia, thrombocytopenia, and anemia. Numerous studies have been carried out in an effort to discover the biomarkers that can be used to predict drug toxicity in chemotherapy treatments for gastric cancer [110].

Genetic polymorphisms were found to play a critical role in the pharmacologic activity of commonly utilized medications, which was found to contribute to the different responses observed to chemical agents. Polymorphisms in key components of the nucleotide excision repair (NER) pathway or drug metabolic pathways were found to be significantly associated with a higher drug toxicity incidence with platinum or S-1 treatment [111–114]. Polymorphic abnormalities in the human TS gene was also identified as a risk factor for serious adverse reactions to 5-FU-based therapy [115]. In addition, studies focused on polymorphisms in gene UGT1A1 revealed that patients who carry the UGT1A1*6 A/A allele or UGT1A1*28 variants experienced increased diarrhea and were more prone to developing hematopoietic disorders upon treatment with irinotecan [116–119]. DHFR F/S-TS G52S, which is a fusion gene of both mutant enzymes, dihydrofolate reductase (DHFR F/S) and thymidylate synthase (TS G52S), has recently been shown to possess the ability to confer resistance to pemetrexed-induced toxicity. Retroviral transduction to express this fusion gene in cells was found to result in a significantly higher pemetrexed IC50 and increased survival of CFU-GM colonies compared with those transduced with either of the mutants alone [120].

In addition to the genetic indicators, biochemical indicators in serum or urine could also function as valuable markers for predicting side effects from anticancer drugs. Serum diamine oxidase (DAO) activity, which reflects the integrity and maturity of the small mucosa, has been shown to function as an indicator of gastrointestinal damage prior to symptom onset in patients undergoing chemotherapy treatment [121]. Large clinical studies have shown that elevated baseline concentrations of both homocysteine and methylmalonic acid indicate severe hematological toxicity, as a result of pemetrexed treatment [122]. The presence of neutrophil gelatinase-associated lipocalin (NGAL) in urine is also widely accepted as an assessment of renal injury in patients receiving cisplatin treatment [123].

Conclusions

Biomarkers can be investigated at various levels. These include genetic analyses that identify polymorphisms, DNA sequencing, transcriptional assays such as reverse transcriptional-polymerase chain reaction (RT-PCR) that measure mRNA levels, and transductional tests, such as immunohistochemistry, that measure protein expression levels. However, having such a variety of available tools to identify biomarkers is not always advantageous. While this number of tools is advantageous in that it allows for a wider comprehension of biomarkers, it can also be misleading due to discrepancies obtained between different techniques. With the exception of HER-2 status for trastuzumab-based targeted treatment, no other molecular markers have entered the mainstream of clinical practice. The primary obstacle toward the identification of reliable markers lies in technical difficulties that arise in the ability to quantitatively assess molecular alterations. In addition, the use of a single biomarker allows only limited power toward predicting the prognosis or response to specific chemotherapy treatments. Thus, the most promising approach would entail the evaluation of a combination of variables in order to achieve a more reliable predictive value than using a single biomarker.

References

1. Fujitani K, Yang HK, Mizusawa J, Kim YW, Terashima M, Han SU, et al. Gastrectomy plus chemotherapy versus chemotherapy alone for advanced gastric cancer with a single non-curable factor (REGATTA): a phase 3, randomised controlled trial. Lancet Oncol. 2016;17(3):309–18. doi:10.1016/S1470-2045(15)00553-7.

2. Wagner AD, Unverzagt S, Grothe W, Kleber G, Grothey A, Haerting J, et al. Chemotherapy for advanced gastric cancer. Cochrane Database Syst Rev. 2010;3:CD004064. doi:10.1002/14651858.CD004064.pub3.
3. Al-Batran SE, Atmaca A, Hegewisch-Becker S, Jaeger D, Hahnfeld S, Rummel MJ, et al. Phase II trial of biweekly infusional fluorouracil, folinic acid, and oxaliplatin in patients with advanced gastric cancer. J Clin Oncol. 2004;22(4):658–63.
4. Lordick F, Lorenzen S, Stollfuss J, Vehling-Kaiser U, Kullmann F, Hentrich M, et al. Phase II study of weekly oxaliplatin plus infusional fluorouracil and folinic acid (FUFOX regimen) as first-line treatment in metastatic gastric cancer. Br J Cancer. 2005;93(2):190–4.
5. Chao Y, Yeh KH, Chang CJ, Chen LT, Chao TY, Wu MF, et al. Phase II study of weekly oxaliplatin and 24-h infusion of high-dose 5-fluorouracil and folinic acid in the treatment of advanced gastric cancer. Br J Cancer. 2004;91(3):453–8.
6. De Vita F, Orditura M, Matano E, Bianco R, Carlomagno C, Infusino S, et al. A phase II study of biweekly oxaliplatin plus infusional 5-fluorouracil and folinic acid (FOLFOX-4) as first-line treatment of advanced gastric cancer patients. Br J Cancer. 2005;92(9):1644–9.
7. Al-Batran SE, Hartmann JT, Probst S, Schmalenberg H, Hollerbach S, Hofheinz R, et al. Phase III trial in metastatic gastroesophageal adenocarcinoma with fluorouracil, leucovorin plus either oxaliplatin or cisplatin: a study of the Arbeitsgemeinschaft Internistische Onkologie. J Clin Oncol Off J Am Soc Clin Oncol. 2008;26(9):1435–42. doi:10.1200/JCO.2007.13.9378.
8. Cunningham D, Allum WH, Stenning SP, Thompson JN, Van de Velde CJ, Nicolson M, et al. Perioperative chemotherapy versus surgery alone for resectable gastroesophageal cancer. N Engl J Med. 2006;355(1):11–20. doi:10.1056/NEJMoa055531.
9. Kang YK, Kang WK, Shin DB, Chen J, Xiong J, Wang J, et al. Capecitabine/cisplatin versus 5-fluorouracil/cisplatin as first-line therapy in patients with advanced gastric cancer: a randomised phase III noninferiority trial. Ann Oncol. 2009;20(4):666–73. doi:10.1093/annonc/mdn717.
10. Okines AF, Norman AR, McCloud P, Kang YK, Cunningham D. Meta-analysis of the REAL-2 and ML17032 trials: evaluating capecitabine-based combination chemotherapy and infused 5-fluorouracil-based combination chemotherapy for the treatment of advanced oesophago-gastric cancer. Ann Oncol. 2009;20(9):1529–34. doi:10.1093/annonc/mdp047.
11. Van Cutsem E, Moiseyenko VM, Tjulandin S, Majlis A, Constenla M, Boni C, et al. Phase III study of docetaxel and cisplatin plus fluorouracil compared with cisplatin and fluorouracil as first-line therapy for advanced gastric cancer: a report of the V325 Study Group. J Clin Oncol Off J Am Soc Clin Oncol. 2006;24(31):4991–7. doi:10.1200/JCO.2006.06.8429.
12. Van Cutsem E, Boni C, Tabernero J, Massuti B, Richards DA, Prenen H, et al. Randomized phase II study (GATE study) of docetaxel plus oxaliplatin with or without fluorouracil or capecitabine in metastatic or locally recurrent gastric cancer. J Clin Oncol. 2011;29(S15):abstract 4018!!
13. Koizumi W, Narahara H, Hara T, Takagane A, Akiya T, Takagi M, et al. S-1 plus cisplatin versus S-1 alone for first-line treatment of advanced gastric cancer (SPIRITS trial): a phase III trial. Lancet Oncol. 2008;9(3):215–21. doi:10.1016/S1470-2045(08)70035-4.
14. Ajani JA, Rodriguez W, Bodoky G, Moiseyenko V, Lichinitser M, Gorbunova V, et al. Multicenter phase III comparison of cisplatin/S-1 with cisplatin/infusional fluorouracil in advanced gastric or gastroesophageal adenocarcinoma study: the FLAGS trial. J Clin Oncol Off J Am Soc Clin Oncol. 2010;28(9):1547–53. doi:10.1200/JCO.2009.25.4706.
15. Dank M, Zaluski J, Barone C, Valvere V, Yalcin S, Peschel C, et al. Randomized phase III study comparing irinotecan combined with 5-fluorouracil and folinic acid to cisplatin combined with 5-fluorouracil in chemotherapy naive patients with advanced adenocarcinoma of the stomach or esophagogastric junction. Ann Oncol. 2008;19(8):1450–7. doi:10.1093/annonc/mdn166.
16. Guimbaud R, Louvet C, Ries P, Ychou M, Maillard E, Andre T, et al. Prospective, randomized, multicenter, phase III study of fluorouracil, leucovorin, and irinotecan versus epirubicin, cisplatin, and capecitabine in advanced gastric adenocarcinoma: a French intergroup (Federation Francophone de Cancerologie Digestive, Federation Nationale des Centres de Lutte Contre le Cancer, and Groupe Cooperateur Multidisciplinaire en Oncologie) study. J Clin Oncol Off J Am Soc Clin Oncol. 2014;32(31):3520–6. doi:10.1200/JCO.2013.54.1011.
17. Song P, Yin Q, Lu M, Fu BO, Wang B, Zhao Q. Prognostic value of excision repair cross-complementation group 1 expression in gastric cancer: a meta-analysis. Exp Ther Med. 2015;9(4):1393–400. doi:10.3892/etm.2015.2284.
18. Yamada Y, Boku N, Nishina T, Yamaguchi K, Denda T, Tsuji A, et al. Impact of excision repair cross-complementing gene 1 (ERCC1) on the outcomes of patients with advanced gastric cancer: correlative study in Japan Clinical Oncology Group Trial JCOG9912. Ann Oncol. 2013;24(10):2560–5. doi:10.1093/annonc/mdt238.
19. Wei J, Zou Z, Qian X, Ding Y, Xie L, Sanchez JJ, et al. ERCC1 mRNA levels and survival of advanced gastric cancer patients treated with a modified FOLFOX regimen. Br J Cancer. 2008;98(8):1398–402. doi:10.1038/sj.bjc.6604317.
20. Miura JT, Johnston FM, Thomas J, George B, Eastwood D, Tsai S, et al. Molecular profiling in gastric cancer: examining potential targets for chemotherapy. J Surg Oncol. 2014;110(3):302–6. doi:10.1002/jso.23639.
21. Matsuoka S, Ballif BA, Smogorzewska A, McDonald 3rd ER, Hurov KE, Luo J, et al. ATM and ATR substrate

analysis reveals extensive protein networks responsive to DNA damage. Science. 2007;316(5828):1160–6. doi:10.1126/science.1140321.
22. Harper JW, Elledge SJ. The DNA damage response: ten years after. Mol Cell. 2007;28(5):739–45.
23. Quinn JE, Kennedy RD, Mullan PB, Gilmore PM, Carty M, Johnston PG, et al. BRCA1 functions as a differential modulator of chemotherapy-induced apoptosis. Cancer Res. 2003;63(19):6221–8.
24. Quinn JE, James CR, Stewart GE, Mulligan JM, White P, Chang GK, et al. BRCA1 mRNA expression levels predict for overall survival in ovarian cancer after chemotherapy. Clin Cancer Res. 2007;13(24):7413–20. doi:10.1158/1078-0432.CCR-07-1083.
25. Wang L, Wei J, Qian X, Yin H, Zhao Y, Yu L, et al. ERCC1 and BRCA1 mRNA expression levels in metastatic malignant effusions is associated with chemosensitivity to cisplatin and/or docetaxel. BMC Cancer. 2008;8:97. doi:10.1186/1471-2407-8-97.
26. Stucki M, Clapperton JA, Mohammad D, Yaffe MB, Smerdon SJ, Jackson SP. MDC1 directly binds phosphorylated histone H2AX to regulate cellular responses to DNA double-strand breaks. Cell. 2005;123(7):1213–26. doi:10.1016/j.cell.2005.09.038.
27. Stewart GS, Wang B, Bignell CR, Taylor AM, Elledge SJ. MDC1 is a mediator of the mammalian DNA damage checkpoint. Nature. 2003;421(6926):961–6. doi:10.1038/nature01446.
28. Rauch T, Zhong X, Pfeifer GP, Xu X. 53BP1 is a positive regulator of the BRCA1 promoter. Cell Cycle. 2005;4(8):1078–83.
29. Bunting SF, Callen E, Wong N, Chen HT, Polato F, Gunn A, et al. 53BP1 inhibits homologous recombination in Brca1-deficient cells by blocking resection of DNA breaks. Cell. 2010;141(2):243–54. doi:10.1016/j.cell.2010.03.012.
30. Galanty Y, Belotserkovskaya R, Coates J, Polo S, Miller KM, Jackson SP. Mammalian SUMO E3-ligases PIAS1 and PIAS4 promote responses to DNA double-strand breaks. Nature. 2009;462(7275):935–9. doi:10.1038/nature08657.
31. Qin Y, Xu J, Aysola K, Oprea G, Reddy A, Matthews R, et al. BRCA1 proteins regulate growth of ovarian cancer cells by tethering Ubc9. Am J Cancer Res. 2012;2(5):540–8.
32. Pei H, Zhang L, Luo K, Qin Y, Chesi M, Fei F, et al. MMSET regulates histone H4K20 methylation and 53BP1 accumulation at DNA damage sites. Nature. 2011;470(7332):124–8. doi:10.1038/nature09658.
33. Hudlebusch HR, Santoni-Rugiu E, Simon R, Ralfkiaer E, Rossing HH, Johansen JV, et al. The histone methyltransferase and putative oncoprotein MMSET is overexpressed in a large variety of human tumors. Clin Cancer Res. 2011;17(9):2919–33. doi:10.1158/1078-0432.CCR-10-1302.
34. Kassambara A, Klein B, Moreaux J. MMSET is overexpressed in cancers: link with tumor aggressiveness. Biochem Biophys Res Commun. 2009;379(4):840–5. doi:10.1016/j.bbrc.2008.12.093.
35. Hudlebusch HR, Skotte J, Santoni-Rugiu E, Zimling ZG, Lees MJ, Simon R, et al. MMSET is highly expressed and associated with aggressiveness in neuroblastoma. Cancer Res. 2011;71(12):4226–35. doi:10.1158/0008-5472.CAN-10-3810.
36. Brito JL, Walker B, Jenner M, Dickens NJ, Brown NJ, Ross FM, et al. MMSET deregulation affects cell cycle progression and adhesion regulons in t(4;14) myeloma plasma cells. Haematologica. 2009;94(1):78–86. doi:10.3324/haematol.13426.
37. Pei H, Wu X, Liu T, Yu K, Jelinek DF, Lou Z. The histone methyltransferase MMSET regulates class switch recombination. J Immunol. 2013;190(2):756–63. doi:10.4049/jimmunol.1201811.
38. Morris JR, Boutell C, Keppler M, Densham R, Weekes D, Alamshah A, et al. The SUMO modification pathway is involved in the BRCA1 response to genotoxic stress. Nature. 2009;462(7275):886–90. doi:10.1038/nature08593.
39. Sobhian B, Shao G, Lilli DR, Culhane AC, Moreau LA, Xia B, et al. RAP80 targets BRCA1 to specific ubiquitin structures at DNA damage sites. Science. 2007;316(5828):1198–202. doi:10.1126/science.1139516.
40. Morris JR. SUMO in the mammalian response to DNA damage. Biochem Soc Trans. 2010;38(Pt 1):92–7. doi:10.1042/BST0380092.
41. Wei J, Costa C, Ding Y, Zou Z, Yu L, Sanchez JJ, et al. mRNA expression of BRCA1, PIAS1, and PIAS4 and survival after second-line docetaxel in advanced gastric cancer. J Natl Cancer Inst. 2011; doi:10.1093/jnci/djr326.
42. Wei J, Costa C, Shen J, Yu L, Sanchez JJ, Qian X, et al. Differential effect of MMSET mRNA levels on survival to first-line FOLFOX and second-line docetaxel in gastric cancer. Br J Cancer. 2014;110(11):2662–8. doi:10.1038/bjc.2014.231.
43. Yang SM, Huang C, Li XF, Yu MZ, He Y, Li J. miR-21 confers cisplatin resistance in gastric cancer cells by regulating PTEN. Toxicology. 2013;306:162–8. doi:10.1016/j.tox.2013.02.014.
44. Fang Y, Shen H, Li H, Cao Y, Qin R, Long L, et al. miR-106a confers cisplatin resistance by regulating PTEN/Akt pathway in gastric cancer cells. Acta Biochim Biophys Sin. 2013;45(11):963–72. doi:10.1093/abbs/gmt106.
45. Hu J, Fang Y, Cao Y, Qin R, Chen Q. miR-449a Regulates proliferation and chemosensitivity to cisplatin by targeting cyclin D1 and BCL2 in SGC7901 cells. Dig Dis Sci. 2014;59(2):336–45. doi:10.1007/s10620-013-2923-3.
46. Popa EC, Shah MA. Capecitabine in the treatment of esophageal and gastric cancers. Expert Opin Investig Drugs. 2013;22(12):1645–57. doi:10.1517/13543784.2013.842974.
47. Maehara Y. S-1 in gastric cancer: a comprehensive review. Gastric Cancer. 2003;6(Suppl 1):2–8.
48. Pietrantonio F, De Braud F, Da Prat V, Perrone F, Pierotti MA, Gariboldi M, et al. A review on biomarkers

for prediction of treatment outcome in gastric cancer. Anticancer Res. 2013;33(4):1257–66.
49. Lenz HJ, Leichman CG, Danenberg KD, Danenberg PV, Groshen S, Cohen H, et al. Thymidylate synthase mRNA level in adenocarcinoma of the stomach: a predictor for primary tumor response and overall survival. J Clin Oncol Off J Am Soc Clin Oncol. 1996;14(1):176–82.
50. Langer R, Specht K, Becker K, Ewald P, Bekesch M, Sarbia M, et al. Association of pretherapeutic expression of chemotherapy-related genes with response to neoadjuvant chemotherapy in Barrett carcinoma. Clin Cancer Res. 2005;11(20):7462–9. doi:10.1158/1078-0432.CCR-05-0042.
51. Choi J, Lim H, Nam DK, Kim HS, Cho DY, Yi JW, et al. Expression of thymidylate synthase in gastric cancer patients treated with 5-fluorouracil and doxorubicin-based adjuvant chemotherapy after curative resection. Br J Cancer. 2001;84(2):186–92. doi:10.1054/bjoc.2000.1553.
52. Terashima M, Fujiwara H, Takagane A, Abe K, Irinoda T, Nakaya T, et al. Prediction of sensitivity to fluoropyrimidines by metabolic and target enzyme activities in gastric cancer. Gastric Cancer. 2003;6(Suppl 1):71–81.
53. Wang Z, Chen JQ, Liu JL, Qin XG, Huang Y. Polymorphisms in ERCC1, GSTs, TS and MTHFR predict clinical outcomes of gastric cancer patients treated with platinum/5-Fu-based chemotherapy: a systematic review. BMC Gastroenterol. 2012;12:137. doi:10.1186/1471-230X-12-137.
54. Wang YC, Xue HP, Wang ZH, Fang JY. An integrated analysis of the association between Ts gene polymorphisms and clinical outcome in gastric and colorectal cancer patients treated with 5-FU-based regimens. Mol Biol Rep. 2013;40(7):4637–44. doi:10.1007/s11033-013-2557-8.
55. Koizumi W, Tanabe S, Azuma M, Ishido K, Nishimura K, Sasaki T, et al. Impacts of fluorouracil-metabolizing enzymes on the outcomes of patients treated with S-1 alone or S-1 plus cisplatin for first-line treatment of advanced gastric cancer. Int J Cancer. 2010;126(1): 162–70. doi:10.1002/ijc.24726.
56. Lu M, Gao J, Wang XC, Shen L. Expressions of thymidylate synthase, thymidine phosphorylase, class III beta-tubulin, and excision repair cross-complementing group 1 predict response in advanced gastric cancer patients receiving capecitabine plus paclitaxel or cisplatin. Chin J Cancer Res. 2011;23(4):288–94. doi:10.1007/s11670-011-0288-8.
57. Sekikawa A, Fukui H, Zhang X, Maruo T, Tsumura T, Okabe Y, et al. REG Ialpha is a biomarker for predicting response to chemotherapy with S-1 plus cisplatin in patients with unresectable stage IV gastric cancer. Br J Cancer. 2013;108(2):395–401. doi:10.1038/bjc.2012.572.
58. Mitani Y, Oue N, Matsumura S, Yoshida K, Noguchi T, Ito M, et al. Reg IV is a serum biomarker for gastric cancer patients and predicts response to 5-fluorouracil-based chemotherapy. Oncogene. 2007;26(30):4383–93. doi:10.1038/sj.onc.1210215.
59. Iwao-Koizumi K, Matoba R, Ueno N, Kim SJ, Ando A, Miyoshi Y, et al. Prediction of docetaxel response in human breast cancer by gene expression profiling. J Clin Oncol Off J Am Soc Clin Oncol. 2005;23(3):422–31. doi:10.1200/JCO.2005.09.078.
60. Kavallaris M. Microtubules and resistance to tubulin-binding agents. Nat Rev Cancer. 2010;10(3):194–204. doi:10.1038/nrc2803.
61. Horwitz SB, Lothstein L, Manfredi JJ, Mellado W, Parness J, Roy SN, et al. Taxol: mechanisms of action and resistance. Ann N Y Acad Sci. 1986;466:733–44.
62. Pasquier E, Kavallaris M. Microtubules: a dynamic target in cancer therapy. IUBMB Life. 2008;60(3): 165–70. doi:10.1002/iub.25.
63. Hodgkinson JE, Clark HJ, Kaplan RM, Lake SL, Matthews JB. The role of polymorphisms at beta tubulin isotype 1 codons 167 and 200 in benzimidazole resistance in cyathostomins. Int J Parasitol. 2008;38(10):1149–60. doi:10.1016/j.ijpara.2008.02.001.
64. Sale S, Sung R, Shen P, Yu K, Wang Y, Duran GE, et al. Conservation of the class I beta-tubulin gene in human populations and lack of mutations in lung cancers and paclitaxel-resistant ovarian cancers. Mol Cancer Ther. 2002;1(3):215–25.
65. Mozzetti S, Ferlini C, Concolino P, Filippetti F, Raspaglio G, Prislei S, et al. Class III beta-tubulin overexpression is a prominent mechanism of paclitaxel resistance in ovarian cancer patients. Clin Cancer Res. 2005;11(1):298–305.
66. He W, Zhang D, Jiang J, Liu P, Wu C. The relationships between the chemosensitivity of human gastric cancer to paclitaxel and the expressions of class III beta-tubulin, MAPT, and survivin. Med Oncol. 2014;31(5):950. doi:10.1007/s12032-014-0950-3.
67. Urano N, Fujiwara Y, Doki Y, Kim SJ, Miyoshi Y, Noguchi S, et al. Clinical significance of class III beta-tubulin expression and its predictive value for resistance to docetaxel-based chemotherapy in gastric cancer. Int J Oncol. 2006;28(2):375–81.
68. Gao J, Lu M, Yu JW, Li YY, Shen L. Thymidine Phosphorylase/beta-tubulin III expressions predict the response in Chinese advanced gastric cancer patients receiving first-line capecitabine plus paclitaxel. BMC Cancer. 2011;11:177. doi:10.1186/1471-2407-11-177.
69. Hwang JE, Lee JH, Park MR, Kim DE, Bae WK, Shim HJ, et al. Blockade of VEGFR-1 and VEGFR-2 enhances paclitaxel sensitivity in gastric cancer cells. Yonsei Med J. 2013;54(2):374–80. doi:10.3349/ymj.2013.54.2.374.
70. Wang Q, Wang N, Shao G, Qian J, Shen D, Fei Y, et al. Relationship between gastric cancer tau protein expression and paclitaxel sensitivity. Pathol Oncol Res. 2013;19(3):429–35. doi:10.1007/s12253-012-9598-5.
71. Xie L, Wei J, Qian X, Chen G, Yu L, Ding Y, et al. CXCR4, a potential predictive marker for docetaxel

sensitivity in gastric cancer. Anticancer Res. 2010;30(6):2209–16.
72. Bhalla KN. Microtubule-targeted anticancer agents and apoptosis. Oncogene. 2003;22(56):9075–86.
73. Li R, Moudgil T, Ross HJ, Hu HM. Apoptosis of non-small-cell lung cancer cell lines after paclitaxel treatment involves the BH3-only proapoptotic protein Bim. Cell Death Differ. 2005;12(3):292–303.
74. Yang L, Yang S, Liu J, Wang X, Ji J, Cao Y, et al. Expression of GRP78 predicts taxane-based therapeutic resistance and recurrence of human gastric cancer. Exp Mol Pathol. 2014;96(2):235–41.
75. Li X, Qiu W, Liu B, Yao R, Liu S, Yao Y, et al. Forkhead box transcription factor 1 expression in gastric cancer: FOXM1 is a poor prognostic factor and mediates resistance to docetaxel. J Transl Med. 2013;11:204.
76. Okada K, Fujiwara Y, Takahashi T, Nakamura Y, Takiguchi S, Nakajima K, et al. Overexpression of forkhead box M1 transcription factor (FOXM1) is a potential prognostic marker and enhances chemoresistance for docetaxel in gastric cancer. Ann Surg Oncol. 2013;20(3):1035–43.
77. Li X, Yao R, Yue L, Qiu W, Qi W, Liu S, et al. FOXM1 mediates resistance to docetaxel in gastric cancer via up-regulating Stathmin. J Cell Mol Med. 2014;18(5):811–23.
78. Wei J, Costa C, Ding Y, Zou Z, Yu L, Sanchez JJ, et al. mRNA expression of BRCA1, PIAS1, and PIAS4 and survival after second-line docetaxel in advanced gastric cancer. J Natl Cancer Inst. 2011;103(20):1552–6.
79. Wu G, Qin XQ, Guo JJ, Li TY, Chen JH. AKT/ERK activation is associated with gastric cancer cell resistance to paclitaxel. Int J Clin Exp Pathol. 2014;7(4):1449–58.
80. Tu CC, Huang CY, Cheng WL, Hung CS, Uyanga B, Wei PL, et al. The alpha7-nicotinic acetylcholine receptor mediates the sensitivity of gastric cancer cells to taxanes. Tumour Biol. 2016;37(4):4421–8.
81. Farhat FS. A general review of the role of irinotecan (CPT11) in the treatment of gastric cancer. Med Oncol. 2007;24(2):137–46.
82. Gilbert DC, Chalmers AJ, El-Khamisy SF. Topoisomerase I inhibition in colorectal cancer: biomarkers and therapeutic targets. Br J Cancer. 2012;106(1):18–24.
83. Tsuburaya A, Sugimoto N, Imamura H, Nishikawa K, Imamoto H, Tsujinaka T, et al. Molecular biomarker study in a randomised phase III trial of irinotecan plus S-1 versus S-1 for advanced gastric cancer (GC0301/TOP-002). Clin Oncol (R Coll Radiol). 2016;28(8):e45–51. doi:10.1016/j.clon.2016.04.001.
84. Shen J, Wei J, Wang H, Yue G, Yu L, Yang Y, et al. A three-gene signature as potential predictive biomarker for irinotecan sensitivity in gastric cancer. J Transl Med. 2013;11:73. doi:10.1186/1479-5876-11-73.
85. Subhash VV, Tan SH, Yeo MS, Yan FL, Peethala PC, Liem N, et al. ATM expression predicts Veliparib and Irinotecan sensitivity in gastric cancer by mediating P53 independent regulation of cell cycle and apoptosis. Mol Cancer Ther. 2016; doi:10.1158/1535-7163.MCT-15-1002.
86. Das PM, Singal R. DNA methylation and cancer. J Clin Oncol Off J Am Soc Clin Oncol. 2004;22(22):4632–42. doi:10.1200/JCO.2004.07.151.
87. Wang L, Xie L, Wang J, Shen J, Liu B. Correlation between the methylation of SULF2 and WRN promoter and the irinotecan chemosensitivity in gastric cancer. BMC Gastroenterol. 2013;13:173. doi:10.1186/1471-230X-13-173.
88. Petitprez A, Larsen AK. Irinotecan resistance is accompanied by upregulation of EGFR and Src signaling in human cancer models. Curr Pharm Des. 2013;19(5):958–64.
89. Shi M, Huang W, Lin L, Zheng D, Zuo Q, Wang L, et al. Silencing of XB130 is associated with both the prognosis and chemosensitivity of gastric cancer. PLoS One. 2012;7(8):e41660. doi:10.1371/journal.pone.0041660.
90. Takezawa K, Okamoto I, Okamoto W, Takeda M, Sakai K, Tsukioka S, et al. Thymidylate synthase as a determinant of pemetrexed sensitivity in non-small cell lung cancer. Br J Cancer. 2011;104(10):1594–601. doi:10.1038/bjc.2011.129.
91. Taylor EC, Kuhnt D, Shih C, Rinzel SM, Grindey GB, Barredo J, et al. A dideazatetrahydrofolate analogue lacking a chiral center at C-6, N-[4-[2-(2-amino-3,4-dihydro-4-oxo-7H-pyrrolo[2,3-d]pyrimidin-5- yl) ethyl]benzoyl]-L-glutamic acid, is an inhibitor of thymidylate synthase. J Med Chem. 1992;35(23):4450–4.
92. Kut V, Patel JD, Argiris A. Pemetrexed: a novel antifolate agent enters clinical practice. Expert Rev Anticancer Ther. 2004;4(4):511–22. doi:10.1586/14737140.4.4.511.
93. Chen JS, Chao Y, Bang YJ, Roca E, Chung HC, Palazzo F, et al. A phase I/II and pharmacogenomic study of pemetrexed and cisplatin in patients with unresectable, advanced gastric carcinoma. Anticancer Drugs. 2010;21(8):777–84. doi:10.1097/CAD.0b013e32833cfbca.
94. Zhang DS, Jin Y, Luo HY, Wang ZQ, Qiu MZ, Wang FH, et al. Pemetrexed for previously treated patients with metastatic gastric cancer: a prospective phase II study. Br J Cancer. 2015;112(2):266–70. doi:10.1038/bjc.2014.607.
95. Celio L, Sternberg CN, Labianca R, La Torre I, Amoroso V, Barone C, et al. Pemetrexed in combination with oxaliplatin as a first-line therapy for advanced gastric cancer: a multi-institutional phase II study. Ann Oncol. 2009;20(6):1062–7. doi:10.1093/annonc/mdn766.
96. Shen J, Wei J, Guan W, Wang H, Ding Y, Qian X, et al. Plasma mRNA expression levels of BRCA1 and TS as potential predictive biomarkers for chemotherapy in gastric cancer. J Transl Med. 2014;12:355. doi:10.1186/s12967-014-0355-2.
97. Hanauske AR, Eismann U, Oberschmidt O, Pospisil H, Hoffmann S, Hanauske-Abel H, et al. In vitro chemosensitivity of freshly explanted tumor cells to

pemetrexed is correlated with target gene expression. Invest New Drugs. 2007;25(5):417–23. doi:10.1007/s10637-007-9060-9.
98. Cutts SM, Nudelman A, Rephaeli A, Phillips DR. The power and potential of doxorubicin-DNA adducts. IUBMB Life. 2005;57(2):73–81. doi:10.1080/15216540500079093.
99. Wang JX, Li Q, Li PF. Apoptosis repressor with caspase recruitment domain contributes to chemotherapy resistance by abolishing mitochondrial fission mediated by dynamin-related protein-1. Cancer Res. 2009;69(2):492–500. doi:10.1158/0008-5472.CAN-08-2962.
100. Liu H, Li N, Yao L, Jiang L, Bao G, Li J, et al. Prediction of doxorubicin sensitivity in gastric cancers based on a set of novel markers. Oncol Rep. 2008;20(4):963–9.
101. Ganzina F. 4′-epi-doxorubicin, a new analogue of doxorubicin: a preliminary overview of preclinical and clinical data. Cancer Treat Rev. 1983;10(1):1–22.
102. Yuan SQ, Zhou ZW, Liang YJ, Fu LW, Chen G, Keshari RP, et al. Correlation of chemosensitivity measured by histoculture drug response assay to expression of multidrug resistance genes and proteins in gastric cancer. Ai Zheng. 2009;28(4):337-43.
103. Personeni N, Baretti M, Bozzarelli S, Spaggiari P, Rubino L, Tronconi MC, et al. Assessment of HER2 status in patients with gastroesophageal adenocarcinoma treated with epirubicin-based chemotherapy: heterogeneity-related issues and prognostic implications. Gastric Cancer. 2016; doi:10.1007/s10120-016-0625-1.
104. Bradner WT. Mitomycin C: a clinical update. Cancer Treat Rev. 2001;27(1):35–50. doi:10.1053/ctrv.2000.0202.
105. Weng MW, Zheng Y, Jasti VP, Champeil E, Tomasz M, Wang Y, et al. Repair of mitomycin C mono- and interstrand cross-linked DNA adducts by UvrABC: a new model. Nucleic Acids Res. 2010;38(20):6976–84. doi:10.1093/nar/gkq576.
106. Shinohara K, Bando T, Sasaki S, Sakakibara Y, Minoshima M, Sugiyama H. Antitumor activity of sequence-specific alkylating agents: pyrolle-imidazole CBI conjugates with indole linker. Cancer Sci. 2006;97(3):219–25. doi:10.1111/j.1349-7006.2006.00158.x.
107. Sagara N, Katoh M. Mitomycin C resistance induced by TCF-3 overexpression in gastric cancer cell line MKN28 is associated with DT-diaphorase down-regulation. Cancer Res. 2000;60(21):5959–62.
108. Oki E, Baba H, Tokunaga E, Nakamura T, Ueda N, Futatsugi M, et al. Akt phosphorylation associates with LOH of PTEN and leads to chemoresistance for gastric cancer. Int J Cancer. 2005;117(3):376–80. doi:10.1002/ijc.21170.
109. Ottey M, Han SY, Druck T, Barnoski BL, McCorkell KA, Croce CM, et al. Fhit-deficient normal and cancer cells are mitomycin C and UVC resistant. Br J Cancer. 2004;91(9):1669–77. doi:10.1038/sj.bjc.6602058.
110. Canter RJ. Chemotherapy: does neoadjuvant or adjuvant therapy improve outcomes? Surg Oncol Clin N Am. 2016;25(4):861–72. doi:10.1016/j.soc.2016.05.013.
111. Ruzzo A, Graziano F, Galli F, Giacomini E, Floriani I, Rulli E, et al. Genetic markers for toxicity of adjuvant oxaliplatin and fluoropyrimidines in the phase III TOSCA trial in high-risk colon cancer patients. Sci Rep. 2014;4:6828. doi:10.1038/srep06828.
112. Cortejoso L, Garcia MI, Garcia-Alfonso P, Gonzalez-Haba E, Escolar F, Sanjurjo M, et al. Differential toxicity biomarkers for irinotecan- and oxaliplatin-containing chemotherapy in colorectal cancer. Cancer Chemother Pharmacol. 2013;71(6):1463–72. doi:10.1007/s00280-013-2145-6.
113. Cortejoso L, Lopez-Fernandez LA. Pharmacogenetic markers of toxicity for chemotherapy in colorectal cancer patients. Pharmacogenomics. 2012;13(10):1173–91. doi:10.2217/pgs.12.95.
114. Jeung HC, Rha SY, Park CH, Im CK, Shin SJ, Ahn JB, et al. Copy number changes can be a predictor for hemoglobin reduction after S-1 monotherapy in gastric cancer. Int J Oncol. 2009;34(3):787–96.
115. Shahrokni A, Rajebi MR, Saif MW. Toxicity and efficacy of 5-fluorouracil and capecitabine in a patient with TYMS gene polymorphism: A challenge or a dilemma? Clin Colorectal Cancer. 2009;8(4):231–4. doi:10.3816/CCC.2009.n.039.
116. Onoue M, Terada T, Kobayashi M, Katsura T, Matsumoto S, Yanagihara K, et al. UGT1A1*6 polymorphism is most predictive of severe neutropenia induced by irinotecan in Japanese cancer patients. Int J Clin Oncol. 2009;14(2):136–42. doi:10.1007/s10147-008-0821-z.
117. Takano M, Kato M, Yoshikawa T, Sasaki N, Hirata J, Furuya K, et al. Clinical significance of UDP-glucuronosyltransferase 1A1*6 for toxicities of combination chemotherapy with irinotecan and cisplatin in gynecologic cancers: a prospective multi-institutional study. Oncology. 2009;76(5):315–21. doi:10.1159/000209335.
118. Minami H, Sai K, Saeki M, Saito Y, Ozawa S, Suzuki K, et al. Irinotecan pharmacokinetics/pharmacodynamics and UGT1A genetic polymorphisms in Japanese: roles of UGT1A1*6 and *28. Pharmacogenet Genomics. 2007;17(7):497–504. doi:10.1097/FPC.0b013e328014341f.
119. Han JY, Lim HS, Shin ES, Yoo YK, Park YH, Lee JE, et al. Influence of the organic anion-transporting polypeptide 1B1 (OATP1B1) polymorphisms on irinotecan-pharmacokinetics and clinical outcome of patients with advanced non-small cell lung cancer. Lung Cancer. 2008;59(1):69–75. doi:10.1016/j.lungcan.2007.07.019.
120. Capiaux GM, Budak-Alpdogan T, Alpdogan O, Bornmann W, Takebe N, Banerjee D, et al. Protection of hematopoietic stem cells from pemetrexed toxicity by retroviral gene transfer with a mutant dihydrofolate reductase-mutant thymidylate synthase fusion

gene. Cancer Gene Ther. 2004;11(12):767–73. doi:10.1038/sj.cgt.7700683.

121. Miyoshi J, Miyamoto H, Goji T, Taniguchi T, Tomonari T, Sogabe M, et al. Serum diamine oxidase activity as a predictor of gastrointestinal toxicity and malnutrition due to anticancer drugs. J Gastroenterol Hepatol. 2015;30(11):1582–90. doi:10.1111/jgh.13004.

122. Niyikiza C, Baker SD, Seitz DE, Walling JM, Nelson K, Rusthoven JJ, et al. Homocysteine and methylmalonic acid: markers to predict and avoid toxicity from pemetrexed therapy. Mol Cancer Ther. 2002;1(7):545–52.

123. Maghsoudi O, Mirjalili SH, Dolatabadi M, Joshaghani MF, Zarea M, Yahaghi E, et al. Investigations of renal function using the level of neutrophil gelatinase-associated lipocalin associated with single-dose of cisplatin during chemotherapy. Diagn Pathol. 2015;10:98. doi:10.1186/s13000-015-0338-5.

Targeted Therapy in Advanced Gastric Cancer

5

Li Xie, Jia Wei, Lijing Zhu, and Wenjing Hu

Despite the fact that numerous advances have been made toward the development of new tumor screening methods, as well as surgical skills and systematic chemotherapy regimens, the overall prognosis for advanced gastric cancer patients remains dismal. This is especially true for patients with late-stage disease. The 5-year survival rate for patients with metastatic gastric cancer remains around 10%. Thus, improvements in the management of gastric cancer, specifically through treatment with targeted therapeutic agents, are urgently required. With advances in our understanding of the biology of malignancy and the molecular evolution of gastric cancer, the potential for targeted therapy has begun to emerge [1]. However, only a limited number of molecular-targeted drugs have been approved at this point in time. Tumor cells possess unique characteristics that enable them to drive the disease to the malignancy stage, including immortality, the ability to infiltrate other tissues, and promote changes in the tumor microenvironment. Thus, the molecular targets of gastric cancer should include not only genetic mutations of the tumor cells but also the factors that enable the alteration of the tumor stroma, such as tumor angiogenesis, inflammatory cell infiltration, extracellular matrix, and others [2].

5.1 Novel Comprehensive Classification of Gastric Cancer

Different types of gastric cancer are traditionally subdivided by histologic subtype via the World Health Organization (WHO) or Lauren classifications [3], with each subtype having distinct clinical and epidemiologic features. In the case of Lauren classifications, intestinal gastric cancer tends to be associated with *Helicobacter pylori* infection, tends to occur in the antrum, and is found to often develop from intestinal metaplasia. Diffuse gastric cancers, on the other hand, are more poorly differentiated. These cancers tend to be found in younger patients and are associated with a poorer prognosis. The WHO classification divides gastric cancers based on their resemblance to a metaplastic intestinal tissue [4]. While these classifications are different, both help little in the selection for the most appropriate treatment for advanced gastric cancer patients.

Genetic alterations are the main typical feature of cancer cells, playing crucial roles in carcinogenesis and tumor progression [5]. Current research is still being carried out to understand the detailed mechanisms of tumor development associated with gene

L. Xie (✉) • J. Wei • L. Zhu • W. Hu
The Comprehensive Cancer Centre of Drum Tower Hospital, Medical School of Nanjing University and Clinical Cancer Institute of Nanjing University, Nanjing 210008, China

J. Wei, B. Liu (eds.), *Personalized Management of Gastric Cancer*,
DOI 10.1007/978-981-10-3978-2_5

amplification, mutation, or translocation. However, quite a few aberrant genes have been identified as valid targets for the treatment of cancer in the clinic. Distinguishing driver oncogenes from other coexisting passenger gene alterations and subsequently blocking the activated signaling transduction have been a critical strategy for the development of molecular-targeted therapeutics. In order to facilitate the discovery and validation of "driver" genes, patient-derived specimen-based molecular analysis techniques and in vivo disease models have been widely used. Deng et al. [6] screened 233 gastric cancer patients and identified five distinct gastric cancer patient subgroups. These subgroups were defined by the signature genomic alterations of FGFR2 (9% of tumors), KRAS (9%), EGFR (8%), ERBB2 (7%), and MET (4%). They proposed that at least 37% of gastric cancer patients could be potentially treated with receptor tyrosine kinase-directed therapies. This was considered to be the first detailed molecular map of genomic alterations in gastric cancer, a step bringing the field closer to the development of targeted treatment. The development of high-throughput, multi-platform sequencing has led to increased efficacy and accessibility of genomic sequencing, in turn driving the development of classification systems based not only on histopathology but also on molecular features. Currently, several studies have provided insight into the molecular basis of gastric cancer, enabling improved molecular classification of gastric cancers. In 2014, a comprehensive molecular classification of gastric cancer was carried out by the Cancer Genome Atlas (TCGA) project, and they identified a series of genomic alterations which were expected to provide insight into potentially novel therapeutic targets [7]. This study carried out sequencing of 295 gastric cancer patients and resulted in the patients being clustered into four groups, which included *Epstein-Barr virus* (EBV)-positive tumors (9%), tumors with microsatellite instability (MSI) (22%), genomically stable tumors (20%), and those with chromosomal instability (50%). A similar research study carried out by the Asian Cancer Research Group (ACRG) analyzed a panel of 300 gastric tumor tissues. For each tumor, gene expression profiling, targeted gene sequencing, and genomic copy number microarrays were carried out [8]. Following the profiling of 251 gastric cancer tissues, the authors then further divided gastric cancers into four groups, MSS/EMT (microsatellite stable/epithelial-to-mesenchymal transition), which encompassed the outliers on the EMT distribution, MSI, MSS/TP53+, and MSS/TP53−. TCGA and ACRG classifications showed both similarities and differences. In the two classification systems, a MSI subtype with high mutation frequency shared similar genomic characteristics and the best prognosis. TCGA that is genomically stable, EBV+, and CIN subtypes were enriched in but not identical to ACRG MSS/EMT, MSS/TP53+, and TP53–, respectively. Due to the different frequency of CDH1 and RHOA mutations, the TCGA GS subtype was found to not be equivalent to the ACRG MSS/EMT subtype. Besides, MSS/TP53 was not found to cover TCGA EBV subtype, as only 12/18 EBV+ tumors were present in the MSS/TP53+ group [9]. Once trastuzumab, a drug that targets overexpressed HER2, was approved as the first targeted drug against advanced/metastatic gastric cancer in 2010, research efforts have almost failed on the development of other promising targets, including c-Met, EGFR, IGFR, PI3K, mTOR, and others. Clinical trials were carried out to identify promising therapeutics, while abortive attempts find a number of candidates not so satisfactory (Table 5.1). While the molecular classification of gastric cancer greatly helped to provide insight into the carcinogenesis and progression of gastric cancer and identify patients having different genetic and epigenetic alterations resulting in a different prognosis, few remarkable treatment targets have been identified for molecular-targeted therapy.

The tumor microenvironment, which is comprised of immune cells, tumor cells, stromal cells, and extracellular matrix, is considered to be the primary battleground during the neoplastic process, fostering the proliferation, survival, and migration of tumor cells. Current classification of malignancy relies highly on not only the information of tumor cells but also the tumor microenvironment, including tumor vessels and the tumor immunity status [10]. Following years of research efforts, it was discovered that tumors can not only survive and disseminate but can more importantly mimic certain

Table 5.1 Completed phase III clinical trials of targeted therapies in gastroesophageal adenocarcinoma

Agents	Targets	Type	Chemotherapy	Study	OS	PFS
Trastuzumab	HER2	Recombinant humanized mAb	Capecitabine/ fluorouracil + cisplatin	ToGA	13. 8 vs. 11.1	6.5 vs. 5.5
Lapatinib	EGFR, HER2	Tyrosine kinase inhibitor	Capecitabin e + oxaliplatin	TRIO-013/ LOGIC	12.2 vs. 10.5	6.0 vs. 5.4
Lapatinib	EGFR, HER2	Tyrosine kinase inhibitor	Paclitaxel	TyTAN	11 vs. 8.9	5.4 vs. 4.4
Cetuximab	EFGR	Humanized mAb	Cisplatin + capecitabine	EXPAND	9.4 vs. 10.7	4.4 vs. 5.6
Panitumumab	EFGR	Humanized mAb	Epirubicin + oxaliplatin + capecitabine	REAL-3	8.8 vs. 11.3	6.0 vs. 7.4
Rilotumumab	HGF	Humanized mAb	Epirubicin + cisplatin + capecitabine	RILOMET-1	9.7 vs. 11.1	5.1 vs. 4.2
Onartuzumab	c-Met	Humanized mAb	mFOLFOX6	METGastric	11 vs. 9.7	–
Ramucirumab	VEGFR2	Humanized mAb	Paclitaxel	RAINBOW	9.6 vs. 7.4	4.4 vs. 2.9
Bevacizumab	VEGF	Humanized mAb	Capecitabine + Cisplatin	AVAGAST	12.1 vs. 10.1	5.3 vs. 6.7
Apatinib	VEGFR2	Tyrosine kinase inhibitor	–	Phase III study of apatinib tablets in the treatment of advanced or metastatic gastric cancer	6.5 vs. 4.7	–
Everolimus	mTOR	Inhibitor	–	GRANITE	5.4 vs. 4.3	1.7 vs. 1.4

signaling pathways of the immune system to propagate conditions that favor tumor immune tolerance. In addition, focused anti-angiogenesis was found to fail as a treatment, demonstrating the sustained anticancer effect. Thus, multiple pathways within the tumor microenvironment must be co-targeted in order to release the full effector function of tumor-specific immune cells.

5.2 Targeting the Driver Oncogenes of Tumor Cells

5.2.1 HER2

HER2, also known as ERBB2 (ErbB2 receptor tyrosine kinase 2), is a member of the human epidermal growth factor receptor family, and almost 15–20% of gastric adenocarcinomas have shown HER2 amplification [11]. Clinically, HER2-positive gastric cancer is termed with a score of 3+ using immunohistochemistry (IHC) method or positive fluorescence in situ hybridization (FISH) (HER2 to CEP17 ratio, 2:2). In contrast to breast cancer, using HER2 as a predictor for prognosis in gastroesophageal cancer is contradictory, with some studies showing an association between HER2 overexpression and poor overall survival (OS) and other studies showing no significant relationship with OS [12, 13].

Trastuzumab (Herceptin), a recombinant humanized IgG1 monoclonal antibody, binds to the HER2 receptor, resulting in an elimination or reduction in receptor activity. This weakens subsequent signaling events involving proteins such as protein kinase B (PKB) and signal transducer and activator of transcription 3 (STAT3). In another way, trastuzumab has been shown to induce antibody-dependent cytotoxicity (ADCC) which resulted in cell cycle disorders [14]. Trastuzumab was initially approved in HER2-overexpressing metastatic breast cancer patients and, later, in the postoperation adjuvant treatment of breast cancer. When combined with chemotherapy, it was shown to significantly prolong OS compared with chemotherapy treatment alone. Based on the positive results seen with breast cancer patients and the high prevalence of HER2 amplification and overexpression associated with gastroesophageal cancer, a study using trastuzumab for the treatment of gastric cancer patients was carried out. The ToGA (Trastuzumab for Gastric Cancer) trial was a multicenter, phase III trial which assigned advanced or metastatic gastroesophageal cancer patients with positive HER2 in tumor cells to receive 5-fluorouracil or capecitabine and cisplatin treatments, with or without trastuzumab, randomly as the first-line treatment [15]. After a primary screening, a total of 594 patients were randomly assigned to the two different groups. The patients who received trastuzumab were found to have a higher overall response rate (47% vs. 35%; $p = 0.0017$) and a longer median PFS (6.7 vs. 5.5 months; $p = 0.0002$) and median OS (13.8 vs. 11.1 months; $p = 0.0046$). Based on the results from the above study of ToGA, trastuzumab treatment with fluoropyrimidine and cisplatin was considered as the standard first-line treatment for HER2-positive gastric cancer patients.

Following the established paradigm for HER2-positive breast cancer treatment, small molecule inhibitors of HER2 were subsequently analyzed in advanced gastric cancer. Lapatinib (Tykerb) is known to bind the intracellular tyrosine kinase domains of epidermal growth factor receptor (EGFR) and HER2, subsequently blocking autophosphorylation and downstream signaling. Similar with what was observed with metastatic breast cancer, lapatinib treatment appeared to be less effective than trastuzumab treatment in gastric cancer patients. Based on the preclinical data and a 9% response rate in a phase II trial of single-agent lapatinib in advanced gastroesophageal adenocarcinoma [16], two phase III trials of lapatinib treatment for HER2-positive gastric cancer patents were launched. These two trials differed in the status of the previous treatment. The TRIO-013 (Translational Research in Oncology)/LOGiC (Lapatinib Optimization Study in the HER2-Positive Gastric Cancer) trial was a multicenter, double-blinded, phase III trial which randomly assigned patients with previously untreated HER2-positive advanced gastroesophageal cancers to groups that received Xelox chemotherapy plus either lapatinib treatment or a placebo control [17]. While patients in the lapatinib treatment arm of the study were observed to have a significantly higher response rate compared with the control group (53% vs. 39%; $p = 0.0031$), this study did not reach its primary endpoint, as there was no significant improvement in OS detected (median OS 12.2 vs. 10.5 months; HR = 0.91; $p = 0.3492$). The subgroup analyses revealed an OS improvement of lapatinib treatment in both younger patients (12.9 vs. 9.0 months, HR = 0.69; 95% CI, 0.51–0.94, $p = 0.0141$) and Asian patients (16.5 vs. 10.9 months, HR = 0.68; 95% CI, 0.48–0.96, $p = 0.0261$). It should be noted that there was no correlation observed between the IHC status of HER2 and survival. The TyTAN (Lapatinib [Tykerb] with Paclitaxel [Taxol] in Asian ErbB2+ [HER2+] Gastric Cancer Study) study was a phase III clinical trial where paclitaxel was given as a treatment with or without lapatinib as the second-line treatment of advanced HER2-positive gastric cancer in Asian population [18]. The median OS was not found to be different between the two arms of the study (11.0 vs. 8.9 months; HR = 0.84; $p = 0.1044$). Subgroup analyses identified a significant OS benefit for patients with HER2 IHC 3+ (14 vs. 7.6 months; HR = 0.59; $p = 0.0176$). Specifically, the biomarker for determining enrollment in the two trials was the presence of HER2 amplification, as identified with FISH-positive samples, regardless of HER2 expression levels observed with IHC. Gastric cancer patients exhibiting more amplification of HER2 were found to be more likely to benefit from anti-HER2 treatment. Interestingly, in a recent series of patients with metastatic gastric cancer that were treated with trastuzumab alongside chemotherapy, a higher HER2 to CEP17 ratio ($\geq$ 4.7) in FISH detection was identified to be the optimal cutoff as a prediction response for HER2-directed therapy [19].

Given the successful results observed with trastuzumab, novel HER2-targeted therapeutics are currently being evaluated in both of the first- and second-line settings. Pertuzumab, which is a monoclonal antibody that block the heterodimerization of HER2 and other HER proteins, is currently being investigated in a first-line therapy to be used in conjunction with trastuzumab and chemotherapy in the phase III trial, JACOB (A Study of Perjeta [Pertuzumab] in Combination with Herceptin and Chemotherapy in Patients with HER2-Positive Metastatic Gastroesophageal Junction or Gastric Cancer) trial (ClinicalTrials.gov ID: NCT01774786) [20]. Pertuzumab was shown to inhibit the ligand-induced dimerization of HER2. This suggests that a broader range of individuals would benefit from pertuzumab, which needs further verification. Trastuzumab emtansine (T-DM1) is an antibody drug conjugate that combines trastuzumab with emtansine, a cytotoxic agent similar to taxane. Recently, T-DM1 was evaluated in HER2-positive gastric cancer since it has been approved in the treatment of trastuzumab-refractory metastatic breast cancer. In addition, phase II/III adaptive trial (A Study of Trastuzumab Emtansine Versus Taxane in Patients With Advanced Gastric Cancer) examined the efficacy of T-DM1 compared to taxane treatment as the second-line therapy for advanced HER2-positive gastroesophageal cancer patients (ClinicalTrials.gov ID: NCT01641939) [21]. The final results of this trial indicated a possible benefit from higher dose of T-DM1 (3.6 mg/kg). Afatinib is a second-generation irreversible tyrosine kinase inhibitor, both of EGFR and HER2, and is thought to potentially show greater efficacy over lapatinib. A phase II study of afatinib comparing to paclitaxel monotherapy in patients with trastuzumab-refractory HER2-positive advanced gastric cancer is currently underway (ClinicalTrials.gov ID: NCT01522768).

5.2.2 EGFR

The epidermal growth factor receptor (EGFR) is a receptor tyrosine kinase within the HER family. EGFR has been demonstrated to be amplified in 10–15% of gastric cancer patients. However, a higher proportion (27–55%) of gastric cancer patients have been shown to overexpress EGFR [22]. To date, few trials of EGFR-directed agents of monotherapy or in combination with chemotherapy have shown an improvement in outcomes. A few of phase III studies have focused primarily on the use of monoclonal antibodies targeting EGFR (such as cetuximab and panitumumab), while some smaller phase II trials have focused on studying the activity and efficacy of EGFR tyrosine kinase inhibitors (such as gefitinib).

Cetuximab (C225) is a humanized IgG1 monoclonal antibody that has been shown to bind specifically to the extracellular domain of EGFR and competitively inhibits the binding of natural ligands to EGFR, thereby blocking the ligand-induced phosphorylation of the tyrosine kinase domain of EGFR. Cetuximab has been shown to downregulate the expression of cell surface receptors, weaken receptor-mediated signaling, and kill tumor cells via an ADCC effect. The EXPAND (Erbitux (cetuximab) in combination with Xeloda (capecitabine) and cisplatin in advanced esophagogastric cancer) study was a multicenter, phase III trial which treated subjects with cisplatin and capecitabine, with or without cetuximab among patients with previously untreated advanced or metastatic gastroesophageal adenocarcinomas [23]. This study showed no differences in OS or PFS between the two arms (median OS 9.4 vs. 10.7 months; HR = 1.0; p = 0.95 median PFS 4.4 vs. 5.6 months; HR = 1.09; p = 0.32). Exploratory analysis showed a tendency toward survival benefit for patients that received a combination treatment of both cetuximab and chemotherapy in the EGFR-overexpressing group. Multivariate analysis indicated that mutations in the KRAS and PIK3CA act as poor prognosis factors. Similarly disappointing results were reported from the REAL-3 (Randomized Trial of EOC ± Panitumumab for Advanced and

Locally Advanced Esophagogastric Cancer) trial. This trial randomly assigned patients with previously untreated advanced gastroesophageal cancer to receive a EOC (epirubicin, oxaliplatin and capecitabine) chemotherapy with or without panitumumab, a fully human monoclonal antibody targeted against EGFR. The addition of panitumumab treatment to EOC not only failed to improve outcomes but was also observed to result in a detrimental effect on OS (8.8 vs. 11.3 months; HR = 1.37; 95% CI, 1.07–1.76; $p = 0.013$) [24]. The tendency toward shorter survival could be attributed to inadequate chemotherapy drug dosages and an accelerated cancer progression following drug withdrawal. An additional phase III trial comparing nimotuzumab + irinotecan vs. placebo + irinotecan, ENRICH, is currently ongoing. The aim of this study is to assess the activity of these treatment regimens in advanced gastric cancer patients with EGFR IHC 2+ or 3+(ClinicalTrials.gov ID: NCT01813253).

Trials that have studied the efficacy of EGFR tyrosine kinase inhibitors have also shown modest results. The objective response rates ranged only from 0 to 11% [25]. The fact that these trials failed in the end suggests that EGFR may not be the primary oncogenic driver in advanced gastric cancer. It should be noted that all EGFR-directed trials were performed using unselected patient populations, which could explain some of the disappointing results. Therefore, the identification of predictive markers of anti-EGFR treatment outcomes in order to determine a population that would be the most likely to benefit from this therapy is crucial for understanding the true therapeutic efficacy of these treatments. Further evaluation of EGFR inhibitors should therefore be warranted in a carefully selected patient population, primarily choosing patients with EGFR-amplified gastric cancer.

5.2.3 HGF Pathway

Over activation of the MET oncogene and hepatocyte growth factor (HGF) pathways has been demonstrated to promote tumor growth and metastasis in gastric cancer patients. While MET amplification is identified only in approximately 4–6% of gastric cancer patients, MET expression has been reported in almost more than a half of gastric cancers. Trials evaluating the clinical efficacy of monoclonal antibodies against HGF (rilotumumab) and the MET receptor (onartuzumab) were carried out recently without impressive results.

The phase III trials RILOMET-1 (phase III, randomized, double-blinded, multicenter, placebo-controlled trial of rilotumumab plus epirubicin, cisplatin, and capecitabine as first-line therapy in patients with advanced MET-positive gastric or gastroesophageal junction cancer) and RILOMET-2 for Asian patients only were initiated based on the positive results stemming from a randomized phase II trial of rilotumumab treatment in patients with MET-overexpressing gastroesophageal cancer [26–28]. However, both studies are closed due to toxicity concerns. The RILOMET-1 trial randomly assigned untreated advanced MET-positive gastroesophageal cancer patients to receive ECX with or without rilotumumab treatment. There were 600 patients that were randomly assigned after screening approximately 1500 patients and identifying 1043 patients as MET-positive by IHC methods. Similar to the clinical trial assessing panitumumab, RILOMET-1 identified a detrimental effect on OS at the addition of rilotumumab treatment to chemotherapy (OS 9.6 vs. 11.5 months; HR = 1.37; $p = 0.0016$), resulting in an early termination of the trial. Correlative biomarker studies are currently still underway. However, neither MET overexpression, as determined by IHC, nor MET amplification, as determined by FISH, was associated with more positive outcomes in the rilotumumab arm, surprisingly. The METGastric (A Study of Onartuzumab in Combination With mFOLFOX6 in Participants with Metastatic HER2-Negative and MET-Positive Gastroesophageal Cancer) trial studied the efficacy of onartuzumab, a monoclonal antibody targeted against the MET receptor, in patients with untreated, advanced MET-positive gastroesophageal cancer. The study was designed such that 800 patients would be randomly assigned to receive FOLFOX plus onartuzumab or a placebo treatment. In this trial, the addition of onartuzumab to first-line mFOLFOX6 chemotherapy in the intent to treat or MET 2+/3+ populations did not significantly improve clinical benefits [29]. A total of 562 patients were enrolled prior to the closure of the METGastric study due to the sponsor decision. For the entire study population, onartuzumab was found to fail to improve outcomes (median OS 11.3 vs. 11.0 months; HR = 0.82; p = 0.244). In the case of patients that possessed MET-overexpressing tumors, as determined by IHC (2+ and 3+), there was a trend observed toward improved OS in the onartuzumab arm of the study (11.0 vs. 9.7 months; HR = 0.64; p = 0.062) [30]. Biomarker-based analyses should focus on both the reason underlying these negative results and the method to identify subgroups that may respond to MET inhibition.

Unlike monoclonal antibody treatments, potentially promising results were recently achieved using a highly selective MET small molecule inhibitor, AMG 337. A pilot trial was described that a dramatic response for AMG337 was observed in13 patients with MET-amplified gastroesophageal cancer at the 2015 American Society of Clinical Oncology Gastrointestinal Cancers Symposium. AMG 337 monotherapy made eight patients (62%) achieve either a partial or complete response. Given these encouraging results, a phase II study of AMG 337 in MET-amplified gastroesophageal cancer patients and patients with other solid tumors is currently in process (ClinicalTrials.gov ID: NCT02016534).

5.2.4 FGFR2

Fibroblast growth factor receptor 2 (FGFR2) is a receptor tyrosine kinase that plays pivotal roles in cell proliferation, differentiation, and migration. FGFR2 amplification has been shown to occur in less than 10% of gastric adenocarcinomas and is associated with lymphatic invasion and a poor clinical prognosis [31, 32]. A biomarker-driven clinical trial that investigated the efficacy of FGFR2 inhibition was carried out recently. The SHINE study was a randomized phase II trial that compared the FGFR inhibitor, AZD4547, to paclitaxel in a second-line setting in FGFR2-amplified advanced gastric cancer patients (ClinicalTrials.gov ID: NCT01457846). A total of 71 patients with FGFR2 polysomy or gene amplification were randomized to receive either AZD4547 or paclitaxel treatment. The median PFS was 1.8 months for patients treated with AZD4547 vs. 3.5 months for patients treated with paclitaxel. Subsequently, exploratory biomarker analysis revealed marked intra-tumor heterogeneity of FGFR2 amplification, with four out of seven tumors tested showing amplification in 20% of the tumor section. Furthermore, only 21% of FGFR2-amplified tumors were found to possess high FGFR2 expression levels. While the correlation of heterogeneity and FGFR2 expression with response to AZD4547 were not reported in this study, both of these reasons could explain part of the lack of efficacy observed with FGFR2 inhibition. Another phase II clinical trial to explore the activity of the FGFR2 inhibitor, dovitinib, in the second- and third-line setting is still recruiting patients (ClinicalTrials.gov ID: NCT01719549). Further biomarker studies to identify biomarkers that could better predict the response or resistance to FGFR inhibition will be essential in future studies.

5.2.5 mTOR

mTOR is an important member of the PI3K-related kinase family, which is primarily responsible for the regulation of cell growth, cell proliferation, cell cycle, and other physiological functions via the PI3K/Akt/mTOR signaling pathway. Phosphorylated mTOR expression is a prognosis factor used for gastric cancer, a factor that is found to negatively correlate with cancer prognosis. Everolimus has been shown to prevent the phosphorylation of p70S6K and 4E-BP1, which is mediated by mTOR and results in G0/G1 cell cycle arrest [33]. A phase II trial of everolimus monotherapy showed a disease control rate of 56% in patients who had exhibited failure with previous chemotherapy (without CR and PR cases) [34]. However, an international multicenter, double-blinded, randomized phase III GRANITE-1 study of everolimus demonstrated that there was no significant efficacy of everolimus in the palliative treatment of advanced gastric cancer patients who failed the first line of chemotherapy treatment [35]. The median OS was 5.4 months with everolimus treatment, compared to 4.3 months with placebo (HR = 0.90; 95% CI, 0.75–1.08; $p = 0.124$). The median PFS was 1.7 months in the everolimus arm comparing to and 1.4 months in the placebo treatment arm, respectively (HR = 0.66; 95% CI, 0.56–0.78). A combination of everolimus and chemotherapy was further evaluated in the clinical trial (ClinicalTrials.gov ID:NCT01248403).

5.2.6 Cell Cycle

Disorder of cell cycle regulatory mechanisms is one of the primary hallmarks of cancer. There are three main types of proteins involved in cell cycle regulation: cyclins, CDKs (cyclin-dependent kinase), and CDK inhibitors (CKIs). CDKs bind to cyclins, an initial event that facilitates the crossing of restriction points during cell cycle progression. CDKs also work with CKIs to inhibit cell cycle progression or induce apoptosis. Therefore, CKIs are likely to induce cell cycle arrest at certain phases within the cell cycle. Flavopiridol is a semisynthetic flavonoid CKI and has been evaluated as the first cell cycle inhibitor in a clinical trial. Flavopiridol has been demonstrated to extensively suppress messenger RNA translation by blocking the transport of transcripts to ribosomes, halting the expression of cell proliferation-related proteins [36]. However, flavopiridol was found to fail to exert the desired effect in the case of gastric cancer patients with a serious adverse reaction [37].

5.3 Targeting Angiogenesis

Angiogenesis is a process that results in the generation of new blood vessels as a mechanism to provide oxygen and nutrients to peripheral tissues and maintain appropriate levels of perfusion. However, the uncontrolled formation of new blood vessels is known to dramatically worsen a cancer patients' clinical outcome. Angiogenesis and the vascular endothelial growth factor (VEGF) pathway play key roles in the pathogenesis of gastroesophageal cancer (Fig. 5.1). A meta-analysis published in 2015 reported the benefit of antiangiogenic agents in terms of overall survival of advanced gastric cancer patients (HR = 0.759; 95% CI, 0.655–0.880; $p < 0.001$) [38]. Current available strategies developed to inhibit the VEGF pathway are shown in Fig. 5.1 and include anti-VEGF antibody therapy (e.g., bevacizumab), inhibitors of angiogenic receptor tyrosine kinases (e.g., sunitinib, pazopanib, sorafenib, regorafenib), inhibitors of VEGFR-2 tyrosine kinases (apatinib), and anti-VEGFR antibody therapy (ramucirumab).

5.3.1 Anti-VEGF Antibody (Bevacizumab)

Following the success seen with bevacizumab, a monoclonal antibody targeted against VEGF-A, which was used to treat patients with metastatic colorectal cancer, the AVAGAST (Avastin in Gastric Cancer) study, was initiated. The purpose of this study was to evaluate bevacizumab activity in advanced gastroesophageal cancer patients. In this multicenter, phase III clinical trial, a total of 774 patients were randomly assigned to treatment groups that received cisplatin and capecitabine with or without bevacizumab. In this trial, both of the median PFS (6.7 vs. 5.3 months; HR = 0.8; 95% CI, 0.68–0.93; $p = 0.0037$) and overall response rates (46% vs. 37.4%, $p = 0.0315$) were found to be improved with bevacizumab comparing to placebo treatment. However, the median OS was not found to be significantly different between the two arms of the study (12.1 vs. 10.1 months; HR = 0.87; 95% CI, 0.73–1.03; $p = 0.1002$), preventing the application of bevacizumab in clinic [39]. Patients with high plasma levels of VEGF-A and low neuropilin levels, a co-receptor of VEGF-A, were found to have obtained the greatest benefit from the combination treatment of bevacizumab

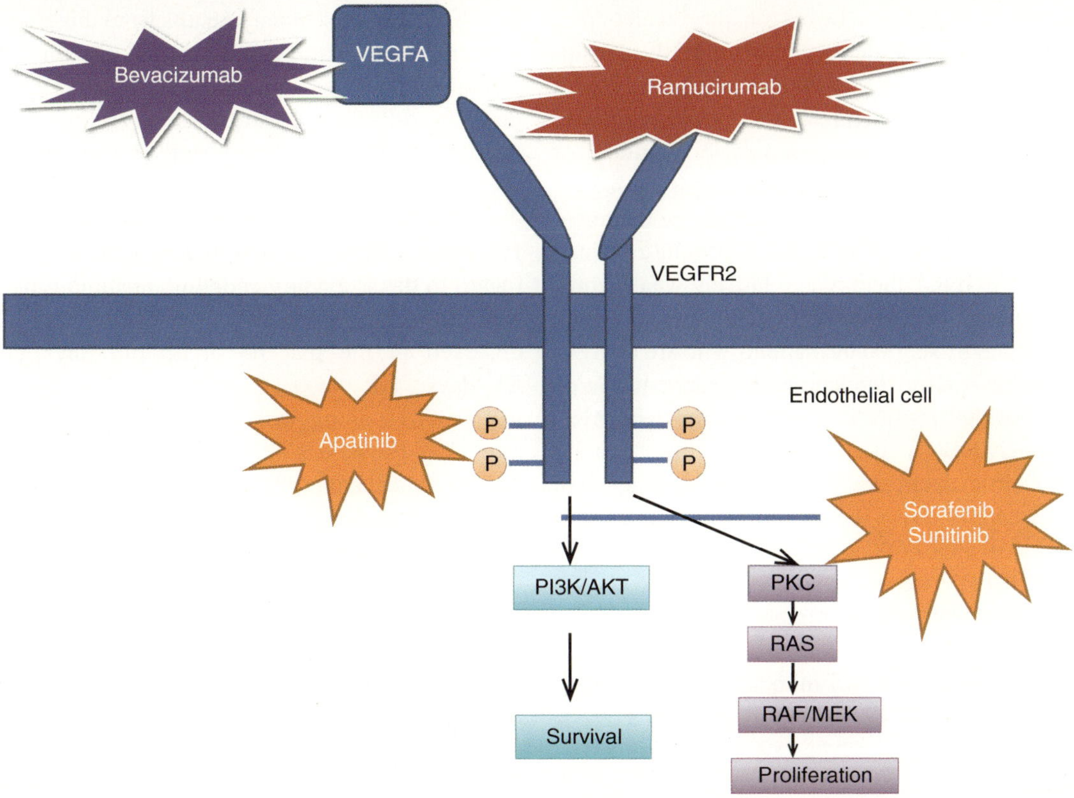

Fig. 5.1 VEGF pathway and the inhibitors

with chemotherapy [40, 41]. However, in the case of both biomarkers, subgroup analyses demonstrated significance only in patients originating from non-Asian regions.

5.3.2 Anti-VEGFR-2 Antibody (Ramucirumab)

VEGFR-2 is typically expressed on circulating bone marrow-derived endothelial progenitor cells and on vascular endothelial cells. This receptor is thought to be one of the primary factors responsible for tumor angiogenesis. The VEGFR-2 antibody, ramucirumab, has been shown to be more effective as a treatment in patients compared to bevacizumab. Two different phase III trials have evaluated the efficacy of ramucirumab in the second-line setting. In the first study, ramucirumab was used as a monotherapy, whereas it was used in combination with paclitaxel in the second study. In the REGARD (ramucirumab monotherapy for previously treated advanced gastric or gastroesophageal junction adenocarcinoma) trial, patients who failed in the first-line chemotherapy for advanced gastroesophageal adenocarcinoma were randomly assigned to treatment groups to receive either ramucirumab or placebo. The median OS was found to be 5.2 months for the ramucirumab treatment group and 3.8 months for the placebo group (HR = 0.776; 95% CI, 0.603–0.998; $p = 0.047$) [42]. A subsequent study went on to compare the combinatorial treatment of ramucirumab + paclitaxel and single agent of paclitaxel as the second-line treatment of advanced gastroesophageal adenocarcinoma. The RAINBOW (A Study of Paclitaxel With or Without Ramucirumab in Metastatic Gastric Adenocarcinoma) study achieved its primary end point, with a median OS of 9.6 months for the ramucirumab arm of the study versus 7.4 months for the control arm (HR = 0.807; 95% CI, 0.678–

0.962; $p = 0.0017$). Based on the results from these studies, ramucirumab is currently considered to be a new standard therapy for patients with advanced gastroesophageal adenocarcinoma who have failed a first-line treatment of platinum or 5-fluorouracil. Though ramucirumab is the second antibody that has been approved for the treatment of gastric cancer, the clinical benefit obtained from VEGFR-2 therapy is relatively weak. Thus, it is critical to identify biomarkers that will enable researchers to enrich the patients who are likely to show respond to ramucirumab treatment. Given the positive results identified in the REGARD and RAINBOW trials, new trials investigating ramucirumab efficacy in the first-line setting were launched. A phase II trial comparing the combination of FOLFOX with ramucirumab treatment to FOLFOX treatment alone in advanced gastroesophageal adenocarcinoma patients as the first-line treatment failed to improve outcomes (median PFS 6.4 vs. 6.7 months; HR = 0.98; 95% CI, 0.69–1.37; $p = 0.89$; and median OS 11.7 vs. 11.5 months; HR = 1.08; 95% CI, 0.73–1.58). It should be paid particular attention that the high discontinuation rate in the ramucirumab arm of 48% could have affected the results of this trial. Additional clinical trials aimed at exploring other combination treatments with ramucirumab are currently underway.

5.3.3 Anti-VEGFR-2 Receptor Tyrosine Kinases (Apatinib)

Apatinib mesylate, a compound derived from valatinib, has been demonstrated to exhibit a particularly intriguing antitumor efficacy. This compound, formerly referred to as YN968D1 (N-[4-(1-cyano-cyclopentyl) phenyl]-2-(4-pyridylmethyl) amino-3-pyridinecarboxamide mesylate), is a novel inhibitor of VEGFR-2 tyrosine kinase which targets the intracellular ATP-binding site of the receptor, preventing phosphorylation and subsequent downstream signaling. Apatinib was shown to elicit suppressed kinase activities of VEGFR-2, c-kit and c-Src. In addition, this compound was found to inhibit the intracellular phosphorylation of VEGFR-2, c-kit, and PDGFRβ. Preliminary results from this study were reported at the ASCO annual meeting in 2014. The authors of the phase III study of apatinib in advanced gastric cancer reported a median OS that was significantly longer in the apatinib group compared with that observed in the placebo group (195 days vs. 140 days; HR = 0.71; 95% CI, 0.54–0.94; $p < 0.016$). In regard to the secondary endpoint, apatinib group exhibited a longer PFS compared with what was observed in the placebo group (78 days vs. 53 days, HR = 0.44, 95% CI, 0.33–0.61; $p < 0.0001$), along with an improved response rate of 2.84% vs. 0.00%, in favor of apatinib [43, 44] (ClinicalTrials.gov ID: NCT01512745). Apatinib was approved by the China Food and Drug Administration in 2014.

The most common adverse events of apatinib were identical to those typical of other antiangiogenic agents. These adverse events include hypertension in approximately 70% of patients, proteinuria in approximately 50% of patients, and hand–foot syndrome in 46% of patients. Both hypertension and the hand–foot syndrome were generally easily managed with the use of corresponding drugs.

5.3.4 Angiogenic Receptor Tyrosine Kinases (Sunitinib, Sorafenib, Etc.)

Both sunitinib and sorafenib are small molecule, multi-targeted, tyrosine kinase inhibitors that have been demonstrated to inhibit VEGFR. In a second-line phase II trial for the treatment of advanced gastric cancer, patients were randomized to groups for treatment with docetaxel, with or without sunitinib treatment. This study showed a higher objective response rate (41.1% vs. 14.3%, $p = 0.002$). However, there were no significant differences observed in the median time to progression (3.9 vs. 2.6 months, $p = 0.206$) and median OS (8.0 vs. 6.6 months, $p = 0.802$) [45]. Sorafenib has been studied as a treatment in combination with docetaxel and cisplatin a first-line, phase II study for advanced gastric cancer patients. In this study, a median survival of

13.6 months was observed, and an objective tumor response was seen in 41% of the patients, with the main grade 3/4 adverse event being neutropenia [46]. However, in another phase II study, where sorafenib was included in the second line of treatment of gastric cancer patients, a median PFS of 3 months (95% CI, 2.3–4.1) and a median OS of 6.5 months (95% CI, 5.2–9.6) was achieved when sorafenib was combined with oxaliplatin treatment following failure of first-line cisplatin and fluoropyrimidine treatment. No further phase III trials were launched [47]. Regorafenib is an orally available, small molecule multikinase inhibitor that targets signaling pathways implicated in tumor angiogenesis (VEGF receptors 1–3 and TIE2), oncogenesis (KIT, RET, RAF1, and BRAF), and tumor microenvironment (platelet-derived growth factor receptor and fibroblast growth factor receptor) [48]. Regorafenib has been shown to exhibit sufficient activity and safety in a randomized, placebo-controlled, phase II trial (INTEGRATE). In this trial, the regorafenib arm had a longer PFS (11.1 vs. 3.9 weeks; HR = 0.41, $p < 0.001$), warranting this drug for consideration for further phase III evaluation [49]. Foretinib (GSK1363089) is also an oral multi-kinase inhibitor, inhibiting multiple targets, including MET, VEGFR-2, RON, and AXL. Preclinical studies demonstrated that foretinib treatment could effectively inhibit the growth of gastric cancer cells through inhibition of the signal transduction pathway of tyrosine kinase [50]. A phase II clinical study showed foretinib, the cMET/VEGFR-2 inhibitor, was insufficient to improve the survival of patients with advanced gastric cancer who had not received previous chemotherapy treatment [51]. Further studies are needed in order to understand the effect of foretinib on gastric cancer patients.

5.4 Immune-Checkpoint Blockade

Immunotherapy holds potential promise for the treatment of two different subgroups, specifically EBV+ and MSI + tumors. This is due to the fact that there are a high number of mutations present in MSI+ tumors, which in turn results in the creation of neoantigens that affect the patients' response to immune-checkpoint inhibitors [52]. In the case of EBV+ patients, both the overexpression of PD-L1and activation of the immune pathway provide strong motive to justify the targeting of these molecules and pathways via immunotherapy, as they are likely to be good candidates of an immune response reactivation [53].

The development of a monoclonal antibody that targets immune-checkpoints has generated great interest in recent years. These antibodies have been shown to be able to induce sustained tumor remission and demonstrated to be effective in the treatment of a variety of tumor types. Immune-checkpoints are inhibitory signaling pathways within the immune system that function to regulate the sustainability and strength of the immune response in the peripheral tissue in order to prevent tissue damage. In addition, immune-checkpoints also play a role in the maintenance of the system's tolerance to self-antigens. The ability to target these inhibitory signaling pathways to result in the improvement of T cell activity is a key mechanism in preventing the escape of tumors from immunologic cytotoxicity. The use of monoclonal antibodies targeted against PD-1, PD-L1, and CTLA-4 has been gradually implemented in clinical research. In addition, the synergistic effects of various immunosuppressors are thought to represent an effective treatment mechanism. In the near future, the development of antibodies targeted against PD-1, PD-L1, and CTLA-4 is expected for the treatment of gastric cancer. A phase Ib trial enrolled 39 patients with either recurrent or metastatic PD-L1-positive adenocarcinoma of the stomach or gastroesophageal junction. Patients were treated with pembrolizumab, with eight (22%, 95% CI 10–39%) patients found to have had an overall response at central review (ClinicalTrials.gov ID: NCT01848834) [54]. Avelumab, a fully human anti-PD-L1 IgG1 antibody (ClinicalTrials.gov ID: NCT01772004), was assessed either as a second-line therapy or a first-line maintenance treatment in patients with advanced gastric cancer or gastroesophageal junction cancer. Disease control rates were found to be 29% and 57.3%, respectively [55]. A phase I/II trial was carried out to determine the safety and activity of nivolumab, an antibody targeted against PD-1, and ipilimumab, an antibody targeted against CTLA-4 (ClinicalTrials.gov ID: NCT01928394). Initial results from this study are encouraging; however, further confirmation is needed. A pilot study did not show any benefit of ipilimumab treatment in advanced or metastatic gastric cancer patients (ClinicalTrials.gov ID: NCT01585987).

5.5 Targeting Extracellular Matrix (ECM)

MMPs (matrix metalloproteinases) comprise a series of proteolytic enzymes that function to degrade and destruct the extracellular matrix and basement membrane. Abnormal expression of MMPs has been shown to promote local tumor invasion and tumor spread. High expression levels of MMPs have been associated with the progression and poor prognosis of gastric cancer. The MMP inhibitor, marimastat (BB-2516, TA-2516), has been demonstrated to exhibit antitumor activity in gastric cancer patients. Advanced gastric cancer patients have also been shown to benefit from marimastat treatment due to its low hematological toxicity, in which the clinical value of marimastat treatment in gastric cancer patients needs further confirming [56].

5.6 Perspectives

Compared to lung cancer, breast cancer, and colorectal cancer, targeted therapy for gastric cancer is still in its infancy. While genomic studies have identified numerous potential therapeutic targets in approximately 20% of gastroesophageal cancer patients, the low frequency of these events gives significant challenges for the design of biomarker-driven trials. Several thousands of patients must be screened in order to select a population with the specific genomic alteration of interest. A potential solution to this problem is to conduct "basket" trials, where the effect of targeted agents would be tested on patients that possess the same genomic alterations but across a variety of cancer types. However, recent data exists which suggest that the disease-specific context of a genomic alteration plays a key role in the patient response to a targeted therapy. For example, in contrast to the dramatic response observed with BRAF inhibition treatment of BRAF-mutant melanoma, BRAF-mutant colorectal cancers were found to be refractory to these same agents. Thus, histology-agnostic is a great limitation of this kind of trial. Another type of trial design that could prove useful for the assessment of targeted therapies in a more efficient manner is an "umbrella" trial. In this type of trial, patients with one particular tumor type are assigned to different targeted agent treatments according to their tumors' specific genomic alterations. This type of trial design allows for the simultaneous testing of a variety of targeted drugs in biomarker-selected patient cohorts. One example of this type of trial for gastroesophageal cancer patients, the PANGEA (Personalized Antibodies for Gastro-Esophageal Adenocarcinoma) trial, has currently been in process (ClinicalTrials.gov ID: NCT02213289) [57]. This study aims to utilize molecular profiling, including both genomic and proteomic information, to assign patients with advanced gastroesophageal cancer with different molecular characteristics to different treatment arms. These treatment arms consist of chemotherapy group plus a targeted agent group. It is important that the clinical trial design also takes into account the genomic complexity and heterogeneity of gastroesophageal cancer.

From the achievements made in the molecular-targeted therapy of gastric cancer, potential companion biomarkers were also studied from a therapeutic perspective. A consecutive series of 438 gastric cancer tissues were analyzed by ten GC panels. These included EBER in situ hybridization, immunohistochemistry to visualize mismatch repair (MMR) proteins (MLH1, PMS2, MSH2, and MSH6), receptor tyrosine kinases (RTKs, HER2, EGFR, and MET), PTEN, and p53 protein. These studies aim to facilitate the development of successful future clinical trials using molecular-targeted agents [58].

Currently, targeted therapy for the treatment of gastric cancer continues to face enormous challenges. (1) While a large number of phase II clinical trials have been carried out, precise phase III clinical trials are lacking. This could potentially be explained by weak activity of drugs observed. However, additional, in-depth phase III clinical studies must be carried out in order to obtain sufficient evidence to support the use of targeted therapy in the treatment of gastric cancer patients. (2) Oncogene addiction promises a good therapeutic effect of molecular-targeted therapy. However, in the area of gastric cancer, there was no similar situation such as EGFR mutation, as demonstrated in lung cancer [59]. The approach of targeting a single molecule is limited for the effective treatment of gastric cancer, due to the complex pathogenesis of this disease. Consequently, drugs that target a single molecule will likely lose efficacy, as a compensatory mechanism will likely be activated soon after treatment. In addition, it is difficult to target the entire tumor, given the fact that subclones of gastric cancer cells exhibit different biological behaviors. This is just one of the primary reasons that explain the failures observed with treatment with a single agent as a broad treatment mechanism for gastric cancer. Thus, the development of multi-targeted drugs or the development of combination therapies utilizing targeted drugs with surgery, radiotherapy, and chemotherapy could result in new, promising opportunities for the treatment of this cancer. On the other hand, efforts should be focused on identifying trunk oncogenes during the clonal evolution of gastric cancer. (3) Tumor heterogeneity creates great challenges in the treatment of cancer in that not all subclones will respond the same from a new treatment. Liquid biopsies could provide insight into the overall molecular makeup of the tumor based on information from the blood of patients. However, such analysis would rely greatly on bioinformatics analysis [60]. (4) In addition, the cost of targeted drugs remains one of the greatest obstacles to their widespread use in clinical practice. The cost of these drugs must decrease in order to make these a viable treatment option. (5) New challenges stem from understanding the tumor microenvironment. Tumor microenvironments could become potential antitumor targets. Despite these current challenges, we strongly believe that an in-depth understanding of the molecular mechanisms promoting clonal evolution of malignancy will lead to essential breakthroughs in the targeted treatment of gastric cancer. Hopefully, a new chapter for the treatment of advanced gastric cancer will be opened in the very recent future.

Unlike in the case of lung adenocarcinoma, no obvious addiction to an oncogene has been confirmed through preclinical studies and clinical trials for gastric cancer. This has limited the discovery of molecular-targeted therapeutics for this type of cancer. This also makes it difficult to imagine that a breakthrough by a single treatment of a molecular-targeted drug would prove efficacious for gastric cancer treatment. However, molecular-targeted therapeutics for the treatment of gastric cancer could enable a mechanism not only to block activated signaling pathways of tumor cells but also to modulate the tumor microenvironment. Such treatment would show great prospect in the ability to prolong patient survival.

References

1. Vogelstein B, Kinzler KW. The path to cancer–three strikes and you're out. New Engl J Med. 2015;373(20):1895–8.
2. Hainaut P, Plymoth A. Targeting the hallmarks of cancer: towards a rational approach to next-generation cancer therapy. Curr Opin Oncol. 2013;25(1):50–1.
3. Polkowski W, van Sandick JW, Offerhaus GJ, ten Kate FJ, Mulder J, Obertop H, et al. Prognostic value of Lauren classification and c-erbB-2 oncogene overexpression in adenocarcinoma of the esophagus and gastroesophageal junction. Ann Surg Oncol. 1999;6(3):290–7.
4. Dicken BJ, Bigam DL, Cass C, Mackey JR, Joy AA, Hamilton SM. Gastric adenocarcinoma: review and considerations for future directions. Ann Surg. 2005;241(1):27–39.
5. Hanahan D, Weinberg RA. Hallmarks of cancer: the next generation. Cell. 2011;144(5):646–74.
6. Deng N, Goh LK, Wang H, Das K, Tao J, Tan IB, et al. A comprehensive survey of genomic alterations in gastric cancer reveals systematic patterns of molecular exclusivity and co-occurrence among distinct therapeutic targets. Gut. 2012;61(5):673–84.

7. Cancer Genome Atlas Research N. Comprehensive molecular characterization of gastric adenocarcinoma. Nature. 2014;513(7517):202–9.
8. Cristescu R, Lee J, Nebozhyn M, Kim KM, Ting JC, Wong SS, et al. Molecular analysis of gastric cancer identifies subtypes associated with distinct clinical outcomes. Nat Med. 2015;21(5):449–56.
9. Corso S, Giordano S. How can gastric cancer molecular profiling guide future therapies? Trends Mol Med. 2016;22(7):534–44.
10. Smyth MJ, Ngiow SF, Ribas A, Teng MW. Combination cancer immunotherapies tailored to the tumour microenvironment. Nat Rev Clin Oncol. 2016;13(3):143–58.
11. Allgayer H, Babic R, Gruetzner KU, Tarabichi A, Schildberg FW, Heiss MM. c-erbB-2 is of independent prognostic relevance in gastric cancer and is associated with the expression of tumor-associated protease systems. J Clin Oncol Off J Am Soc Clin Oncol. 2000;18(11):2201–9.
12. Hsu JT, Chen TC, Tseng JH, Chiu CT, Liu KH, Yeh CN, et al. Impact of HER-2 overexpression/amplification on the prognosis of gastric cancer patients undergoing resection: a single-center study of 1,036 patients. Oncologist. 2011;16(12):1706–13.
13. Janbabai G, Oladi Z, Farazmandfar T, Taghvaei T, Naghshvar F. The prognostic impact of EGFR, ErbB2 and MET gene amplification in human gastric carcinomas as measured by quantitative Real-Time PCR. J Cancer Res Clin Oncol. 2015;141(11):1945–52.
14. Kim SY, Kim HP, Kim YJ, Oh DY, Im SA, Lee D, et al. Trastuzumab inhibits the growth of human gastric cancer cell lines with HER2 amplification synergistically with cisplatin. Int J Oncol. 2008;32(1):89–95.
15. Bang YJ, Van Cutsem E, Feyereislova A, Chung HC, Shen L, Sawaki A, et al. Trastuzumab in combination with chemotherapy versus chemotherapy alone for treatment of HER2-positive advanced gastric or gastro-oesophageal junction cancer (ToGA): a phase 3, open-label, randomised controlled trial. Lancet. 2010;376(9742):687–97.
16. Iqbal S, Goldman B, Fenoglio-Preiser CM, Lenz HJ, Zhang W, Danenberg KD, et al. Southwest Oncology Group study S0413: a phase II trial of lapatinib (GW572016) as first-line therapy in patients with advanced or metastatic gastric cancer. Ann Oncol. 2011;22(12):2610–5.
17. Hecht JR, Bang YJ, Qin SK, Chung HC, Xu JM, Park JO, et al. Lapatinib in combination with capecitabine plus oxaliplatin in human epidermal growth factor receptor 2-positive advanced or metastatic gastric, esophageal, or gastroesophageal adenocarcinoma: TRIO-013/LOGiC–a randomized Phase III trial. J Clin Oncol Off J Am Soc Clin Oncol. 2016;34(5):443–51.
18. Satoh T, Xu RH, Chung HC, Sun GP, Doi T, Xu JM, et al. Lapatinib plus paclitaxel versus paclitaxel alone in the second-line treatment of HER2-amplified advanced gastric cancer in Asian populations: TyTAN–a randomized, Phase III study. J Clin Oncol Off J Am Soc Clin Oncol. 2014;32(19):2039–49.
19. Gomez-Martin C, Plaza JC, Pazo-Cid R, Salud A, Pons F, Fonseca P, et al. Level of HER2 gene amplification predicts response and overall survival in HER2-positive advanced gastric cancer treated with trastuzumab. J Clin Oncol Off J Am Soc Clin Oncol. 2013;31(35):4445–52.
20. Oh DY, Bang YJ. Pertuzumab in gastrointestinal cancer. Expert Opin Biol Ther. 2016;16(2):243–53.
21. Kang Y SMA, Ohtsu A, Van Cutsem E, Ajani J A, van der Horst T, Harle-Yge M, Piao Y, Althaus B, Thuss-Patience P C. A randomized, open-label, multicenter, adaptive phase 2/3 study of trastuzumab emtansine (T-DM1) versus a taxane (TAX) in patients (pts) with previously treated HER2-positive locally advanced or metastatic gastric/gastroesophageal junction adenocarcinoma (LA/MGC/GEJC). J Clin Oncol Off J Am Soc Clin Oncol. 2016;34S(4):5.
22. Birkman EM, Algars A, Lintunen M, Ristamaki R, Sundstrom J, Carpen O. EGFR gene amplification is relatively common and associates with outcome in intestinal adenocarcinoma of the stomach, gastro-oesophageal junction and distal oesophagus. BMC Cancer. 2016;16:406.
23. Lordick F, Kang YK, Chung HC, Salman P, Oh SC, Bodoky G, et al. Capecitabine and cisplatin with or without cetuximab for patients with previously untreated advanced gastric cancer (EXPAND): a randomised, open-label phase 3 trial. Lancet Oncol. 2013;14(6):490–9.
24. Okines AF, Ashley SE, Cunningham D, Oates J, Turner A, Webb J, et al. Epirubicin, oxaliplatin, and capecitabine with or without panitumumab for advanced esophagogastric cancer: dose-finding study for the prospective multicenter, randomized, phase II/III REAL-3 trial. J Clin Oncol Off J Am Soc Clin Oncol. 2010;28(25):3945–50.
25. Dragovich T, McCoy S, Fenoglio-Preiser CM, Wang J, Benedetti JK, Baker AF, et al. Phase II trial of erlotinib in gastroesophageal junction and gastric adenocarcinomas: SWOG 0127. J Clin Oncol Off J Am Soc Clin Oncol. 2006;24(30):4922–7.
26. Doshi S, Gisleskog PO, Zhang Y, Zhu M, Oliner KS, Loh E, et al. Rilotumumab exposure-response relationship in patients with advanced or metastatic gastric cancer. Clin Cancer Res. 2015;21(11):2453–61.
27. Cunningham D N C Tebbutt, Davidenko I, Murad A M, Al-Batran S, Ilson D H, et al. Phase III, randomized, double-blind, multicenter, placebo (P)-controlled trial of rilotumumab (R) plus epirubicin, cisplatin and capecitabine (ECX) as first-line therapy in patients (pts) with advanced MET-positive (pos) gastric or gastroesophageal junction (G/GEJ) cancer: RILOMET-1 study. J Clin Oncol Off J Am Soc Clin Oncol. 2015; 33S(15):4000.
28. Doi T K Y, Muro K, Jiang Y, Jain R K, Lizambri R. A phase 3, multicenter, randomized, double-blind, placebo-controlled study of rilotumumab in combination with cisplatin and capecitabine (CX) as first-line therapy for Asian patients (pts) with advanced MET-positive gastric or gastroesophageal junction (G/GEJ)

adenocarcinoma: The RILOMET-2 trial. J Clin Oncol Off J Am Soc Clin Oncol. 2015;33S(3):226.
29. Shah MA, Cho JY, Tan IB, Tebbutt NC, Yen CJ, Kang A, et al. A randomized Phase II study of FOLFOX with or without the MET inhibitor onartuzumab in advanced adenocarcinoma of the stomach and gastroesophageal junction. Oncologist. 2016;21(9):1085–90.
30. Shah MA, Bang YJ, Lordick F, Alsina M, Chen M, Hack SP, et al. Effect of fluorouracil, leucovorin, and oxaliplatin with or without onartuzumab in HER2-Negative, MET-positive gastroesophageal adenocarcinoma: the METGastric randomized clinical trial. JAMA Oncol. 2016. Epub ahead press.
31. Ahn S, Lee J, Hong M, Kim ST, Park SH, Choi MG, et al. FGFR2 in gastric cancer: protein overexpression predicts gene amplification and high H-index predicts poor survival. Mod Pathol. 2016;29(9):1095–103.
32. Su X, Zhan P, Gavine PR, Morgan S, Womack C, Ni X, et al. FGFR2 amplification has prognostic significance in gastric cancer: results from a large international multicentre study. Br J Cancer. 2014;110(4):967–75.
33. Yu G, Wang J, Chen Y, Wang X, Pan J, Li G, et al. Overexpression of phosphorylated mammalian target of rapamycin predicts lymph node metastasis and prognosis of chinese patients with gastric cancer. Clin Cancer Res. 2009;15(5):1821–9.
34. Doi T, Muro K, Boku N, Yamada Y, Nishina T, Takiuchi H, et al. Multicenter phase II study of everolimus in patients with previously treated metastatic gastric cancer. J Clin Oncol Off J Am Soc Clin Oncol. 2010;28(11):1904–10.
35. Ohtsu A, Ajani JA, Bai YX, Bang YJ, Chung HC, Pan HM, et al. Everolimus for previously treated advanced gastric cancer: results of the randomized, double-blind, phase III GRANITE-1 study. J Clin Oncol Off J Am Soc Clin Oncol. 2013;31(31):3935–43.
36. Holkova B, Supko JG, Ames MM, Reid JM, Shapiro GI, Perkins EB, et al. A phase I trial of vorinostat and alvocidib in patients with relapsed, refractory, or poor prognosis acute leukemia, or refractory anemia with excess blasts-2. Clin Cancer Res. 2013;19(7):1873–83.
37. Schwartz GK, Ilson D, Saltz L, O'Reilly E, Tong W, Maslak P, et al. Phase II study of the cyclin-dependent kinase inhibitor flavopiridol administered to patients with advanced gastric carcinoma. J Clin Oncol Off J Am Soc Clin Oncol. 2001;19(7):1985–92.
38. Ciliberto D, Staropoli N, Caglioti F, Gualtieri S, Fiorillo L, Chiellino S, et al. A systematic review and meta-analysis of randomized trials on the role of targeted therapy in the management of advanced gastric cancer: evidence does not translate? Cancer Biol Ther. 2015;16(8):1148–59.
39. Ohtsu A, Shah MA, Van Cutsem E, Rha SY, Sawaki A, Park SR, et al. Bevacizumab in combination with chemotherapy as first-line therapy in advanced gastric cancer: a randomized, double-blind, placebo-controlled phase III study. J Clin Oncol Off J Am Soc Clin Oncol. 2011;29(30):3968–76.
40. Hacker UT, Escalona-Espinosa L, Consalvo N, Goede V, Schiffmann L, Scherer SJ, et al. Evaluation of Angiopoietin-2 as a biomarker in gastric cancer: results from the randomised phase III AVAGAST trial. Br J Cancer. 2016;114(8):855–62.
41. Van Cutsem E, de Haas S, Kang YK, Ohtsu A, Tebbutt NC, Ming Xu J, et al. Bevacizumab in combination with chemotherapy as first-line therapy in advanced gastric cancer: a biomarker evaluation from the AVAGAST randomized phase III trial. J Clin Oncol Off J Am Soc Clin Oncol. 2012;30(17):2119–27.
42. Fuchs CS, Tomasek J, Yong CJ, Dumitru F, Passalacqua R, Goswami C, et al. Ramucirumab monotherapy for previously treated advanced gastric or gastro-oesophageal junction adenocarcinoma (REGARD): an international, randomised, multicentre, placebo-controlled, phase 3 trial. Lancet. 2014;383(9911):31–9.
43. S Qin. Phase III study of apatinib in advanced gastric cancer: A randomized, double-blind, placebo-controlled trial. J Clin Oncol Off J Am Soc Clin Oncol. 2014;32S(15):4003.
44. Li J, Qin S, Xu J, Xiong J, Wu C, Bai Y, et al. Randomized, double-blind, placebo-controlled phase III trial of apatinib in patients with chemotherapy-refractory advanced or metastatic adenocarcinoma of the stomach or gastroesophageal junction. J Clin Oncol Off J Am Soc Clin Oncol. 2016;34(13):1448.
45. Yi JH, Lee J, Lee J, Park SH, Park JO, Yim DS, et al. Randomised phase II trial of docetaxel and sunitinib in patients with metastatic gastric cancer who were previously treated with fluoropyrimidine and platinum. Br J Cancer. 2012;106(9):1469–74.
46. Sun W, Powell M, O'Dwyer PJ, Catalano P, Ansari RH, Benson 3rd AB. Phase II study of sorafenib in combination with docetaxel and cisplatin in the treatment of metastatic or advanced gastric and gastroesophageal junction adenocarcinoma: ECOG 5203. J Clin Oncol Off J Am Soc Clin Oncol. 2010;28(18):2947–51.
47. Martin-Richard M, Gallego R, Pericay C, Garcia Foncillas J, Queralt B, Casado E, et al. Multicenter phase II study of oxaliplatin and sorafenib in advanced gastric adenocarcinoma after failure of cisplatin and fluoropyrimidine treatment. Invest New Drugs. 2013;31(6):1573–9.
48. Wilhelm SM, Dumas J, Adnane L, Lynch M, Carter CA, Schutz G, et al. Regorafenib (BAY 73-4506): a new oral multikinase inhibitor of angiogenic, stromal and oncogenic receptor tyrosine kinases with potent preclinical antitumor activity. Int J Cancer. 2011;129(1):245–55.
49. Pavlakis N, Sjoquist KM, Martin AJ, Tsobanis E, Yip S, Kang YK, et al. Regorafenib for the treatment of advanced gastric cancer (INTEGRATE): a multinational placebo-controlled phase II trial. J Clin Oncol Off J Am Soc Clin Oncol. 2016;34(23):2728–35.
50. Kataoka Y, Mukohara T, Tomioka H, Funakoshi Y, Kiyota N, Fujiwara Y, et al. Foretinib (GSK1363089), a multi-kinase inhibitor of MET and VEGFRs, inhibits growth of gastric cancer cell lines by blocking

inter-receptor tyrosine kinase networks. Invest New Drugs. 2012;30(4):1352–60.
51. Shah MA, Wainberg ZA, Catenacci DV, Hochster HS, Ford J, Kunz P, et al. Phase II study evaluating 2 dosing schedules of oral foretinib (GSK1363089), cMET/VEGFR2 inhibitor, in patients with metastatic gastric cancer. PLoS One. 2013;8(3):e54014.
52. Desrichard A, Snyder A, Chan TA. Cancer neoantigens and applications for immunotherapy. Clin Cancer Res. 2016;22(4):807–12.
53. Cohen JI, Fauci AS, Varmus H, Nabel GJ. Epstein-Barr virus: an important vaccine target for cancer prevention. Sci Transl Med. 2011;3(107):107fs7.
54. Muro K, Chung HC, Shankaran V, Geva R, Catenacci D, Gupta S, et al. Pembrolizumab for patients with PD-L1-positive advanced gastric cancer (KEYNOTE-012): a multicentre, open-label, phase 1b trial. Lancet Oncol. 2016;17(6):717–26.
55. Chung H C, Arkenau H Wyrwicz L, Oh D, Lee K, Infante J R, Chin K M, von Heydebreck A, Kang Y, Safran H. Safety, PD-L1 expression, and clinical activity of avelumab (MSB0010718C), an anti-PD-L1 antibody, in patients with advanced gastric or gastroesophageal junction cancer. J Clin Oncol Off J Am Soc Clin Oncol. 2016;34S(4):168.
56. Bramhall SR, Hallissey MT, Whiting J, Scholefield J, Tierney G, Stuart RC, et al. Marimastat as maintenance therapy for patients with advanced gastric cancer: a randomised trial. Br J Cancer. 2002;86(12):1864–70.
57. Catenacci DV. Next-generation clinical trials: novel strategies to address the challenge of tumor molecular heterogeneity. Mol Oncol. 2015;9(5):967–96.
58. Kim HS, Shin SJ, Beom SH, Jung M, Choi YY, Son T, et al. Comprehensive expression profiles of gastric cancer molecular subtypes by immunohistochemistry: implications for individualized therapy. Oncotarget. 2016;7(28):44608–20.
59. Sharma SV, Bell DW, Settleman J, Haber DA. Epidermal growth factor receptor mutations in lung cancer. Nat Rev Cancer. 2007;7(3):169–81.
60. Meador CB, Lovly CM. Liquid biopsies reveal the dynamic nature of resistance mechanisms in solid tumors. Nat Med. 2015;21(7):663–5.

Part II

Precision Regional Therapy in Gastric Cancer

Laparoscopic Surgery and Robotic Surgery

6

Meng Wang and Wenxian Guan

6.1 Laparoscopic Surgery for Gastric Cancer

6.1.1 Introduction

Laparoscopic surgery has become a standard treatment for early-stage gastric cancer. Many studies have demonstrated its safety, efficacy, and the significant advantages resulting from its minimally invasive nature [1, 2]. As the technique developed, laparoscopic surgery has also begun to be widely used in local, advanced gastric cancer treatment [3]. In recent years, the type and resection area in laparoscopic surgery have changed significantly. Moreover, standard procedures have developed from D2 lymph node dissection to digestive tract reconstruction [3].

6.1.2 Indications for Laparoscopic Surgery in Gastric Cancer

The current Japanese gastric cancer treatment guidelines confirm that distal laparoscopic gastrectomy is the standard procedure for Ic stage gastric cancer patients (level B) [4]. However, the current guidelines do not accept laparoscopic surgery as a valid approach for local, advanced gastric cancer. Despite this, several recent studies have reported promising outcomes when laparoscopic surgery was used in the treatment of advanced gastric cancer [5, 6].

Thus, current guideline indications for the use of laparoscopic surgery have been limited to Stage I gastric cancer patients. Further studies in using this approach in advanced gastric cancer will need to be performed in some experienced centers.

6.1.3 Standard Laparoscopic Surgical Procedure

Presently, standard gastrectomy with D2 lymphadenectomy is performed following both Japanese and NCCN gastric cancer treatment guidelines. To this end, D2 lymphadenectomy is a key feature for laparoscopic radical gastrectomy [7, 8]. The procedure for D2 lymphadenectomy in laparoscopic distal gastrectomy is as follows:

(a) A 12-mm trocar is inserted below the navel to allow for laparoscope access. Three 5-mm trocars are also inserted into the middle right, upper right, and left abdomen. Finally, one 12-mm trocar is inserted into the middle left abdomen. A total of five trocars are used in this procedure (Fig. 6.1).

M. Wang • W. Guan (✉)
Department of General Surgery of Drum Tower Hospital, Medical School of Nanjing University, Nanjing 210008, China
e-mail: guan_wx@163.com

J. Wei, B. Liu (eds.), *Personalized Management of Gastric Cancer*, DOI 10.1007/978-981-10-3978-2_6

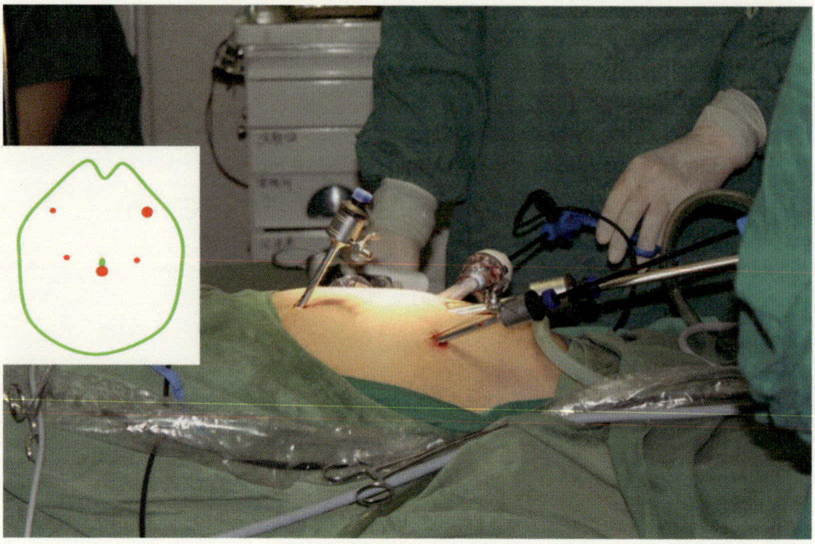

Fig. 6.1 Trocar locations for laparoscopic gastrectomy

(b) A monitor is located over the patient's head, and the surgeon sits between patient's legs for the procedure. First, the greater omentum is cut under a laparoscopic view. The right gastroepiploic vessels were clipped and cut, and the inflapyloric lymph nodes (No. 6) were dissected. The ligament of spleen and stomach was cut, and the No. 4 lymph nodes were dissected. After lymph node dissection, the duodenum is cut with a laparoscopic linear stapler.

(c) The lesser omentum is then cut, the right crus of the diaphragm is exposed, and the inflapyloric lymph nodes are dissected. The lymph nodes beside the proper hepatic artery (No. 8) are dissected. The left gastric artery, common hepatic artery, and the splenic artery are exposed. The left gastric vein is clipped and cut. The left gastric artery is divided after double clipping (Fig. 6.2). The lymph nodes along these vessels (No. 7, No. 8, and No. 9) are confirmed under excellent surgical view and then removed. Finally, the stomach is cut by the laparoscopic linear stapler.

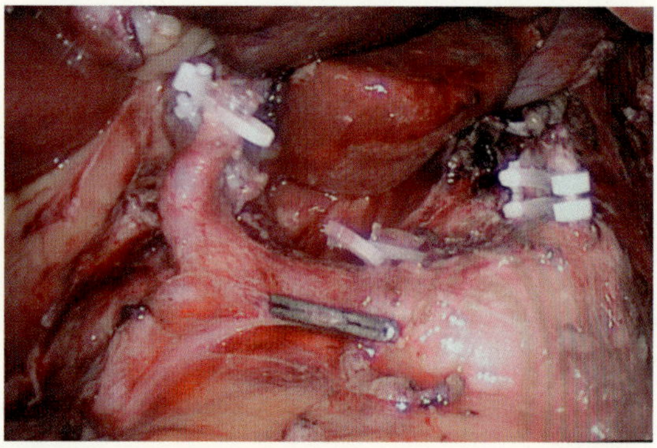

Fig. 6.2 The left gastric artery is divided after double clipping

Safe and effective digestive tract reconstruction is a crucial goal for laparoscopic radical gastrectomy. The basic principles for proper digestive tract reconstruction after laparoscopic gastric surgery include:

- To improve the quality of life for patients with gastric cancer
- To maintain the continuity of the digestive tract while simultaneously preserving its physiological function
- To have reduced surgical complications
- To allow for safe, quick, and easy operating procedures

At present, digestive tract reconstruction procedures for laparoscopic gastrectomy are divided into three types: total laparoscopic surgery, laparoscopic-assisted surgery, and hand-assisted laparoscopic surgery.

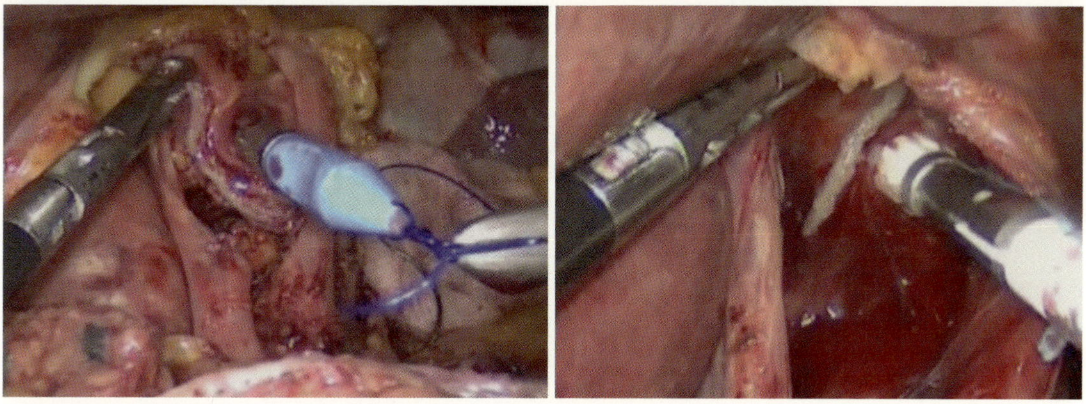

Fig. 6.3 (*Left*) End-end esophago-jejunal anastomosis using an EST device. (*Right*) End-lateral esophago-jejunal anastomosis using an OrVil device

Laparoscopic distal gastrectomy for digestive tract reconstructive methods includes Billroth I, Billroth II, and Roux-en-Y anastomosis. Billroth I anastomosis is close to the normal physiological state: food goes through the duodenal, where mixing of duodenal juice, bile, and pancreatic juice occurs, and there is a reduction or complete avoidance of bile and/or pancreatic juice reflux into the gastric remnant. This approach reduces the occurrence of inflammation and/or cancer of the gastric remnant. On the other hand, Billroth I anastomosis can effectively stimulate cholecystokinin secretion as well as reduce the incidence of postoperative cholecystitis and cholelithiasis. Therefore, Billroth I anastomosis is the recommended method for the reconstruction of digestive tract after laparoscopic distal gastrectomy [9]. However, if the tumor is involved in the duodenum, Billroth II or Roux-en-Y anastomosis should be performed in order to ensure the radical resection of the tumor.

According to the current literature, the gastric digestive tract reconstruction after total gastrectomy amounts to more than 70 methods [10]. Despite this vast amount of work, the best way for digestive tract reconstruction is still unclear. However, according to the principle of "simple, safe, and effective," more and more scholars recommend no pouch esophageal jejunal Roux-en-Y anastomosis after total gastrectomy [11–14]. Common laparoscopic anastomosis techniques for this approach include end-end esophago-jejunal anastomosis using an EST device and termino-lateral esophago-jejunal anastomosis using an OrVil device (Fig. 6.3). To this end, a continuous single-layer hand-sewn esophago-jejunal anastomosis (3.0 Vycril intracorporeal) could be performed.

6.1.4 Laparoscopic Surgery Outcomes

Laparoscopic surgery has been a known technique for more than 40 years. Within the past 20 years, laparoscopic surgery has revolutionized the field of gastric cancer surgery. It has shown to have significant advantages when compared to more traditional approaches, including lower trauma, reduced blood loss, quicker gut function recovery, shorter hospital stay length, and reduced incisional hernia rates [15–17].

Postoperative complications from laparoscopic surgery are similar to open gastrectomy surgery [16]. Exceptions include pneumoperitoneum-related complications, such as incision infection, intra-abdominal bleeding, duodenal stump leakage, and anastomosis leakage. Of these, the most common are duodenal leakage, anastomosis bleeding, and anastomosis leakage [18].

To evaluate long-term outcomes, a multicenter study comprised of 491 patients in 25 units was performed. Resulting statistical analyses showed that

93% were in Stage IA, 5% were in Stage IB, and 2% were in Stage II of the disease [18]. There were only six cancer recurrences (median follow-up time, 23 months), and the 5-year survival rate was 99.4%. In addition, the 5-year disease-free survival rates were 99.6% for Stage IA and 100% for Stage IB, which were the same as open gastrectomy.

In a separate study, Sato and colleagues studied 332 patients from January 2001 through December 2010 [19]. Of these, 47.6% (158) underwent laparoscopic surgery, while the remaining 52.4% (174) underwent open gastrectomy [19]. When comparing laparoscopic surgery to open gastrectomy with D1 and D1+ lymph node dissection, the mean operation time was significantly longer for the former. The rate of postoperative complications, morbidity, and recurrence was not significantly different between the two methods. However, the mean blood loss was significantly smaller with the laparoscopic surgery, and the average number of lymph nodes was significantly greater. Thus, laparoscopic surgery with D1 and D1+ lymph node dissection is as safe as open gastrectomy. To this end, Lee et al. studied 211 patients, of whom 106 underwent laparoscopic surgery and the remaining 105 underwent open gastrectomy [15]. Their report showed that the rate of postoperative complications with laparoscopic surgery was smaller than that of open gastrectomy. Additionally, postoperative recovery was significantly faster for patients who underwent laparoscopic surgery. To this end, they started a liquid diet sooner, and their postoperative hospital stays were shorter. Concerning long-term outcomes, the 5-year survival rate for laparoscopic surgery versus open gastrectomy was 95.9% and 94.9%, with no significant difference between the two. Collectively, these data suggest that laparoscopic surgery for EGC is feasible and safe. As a result, laparoscopic surgery has been included as one of the standard procedures in the Third edition of the Japanese gastric cancer treatment guidelines for the treatment of Stage I of the disease. Similarly, NCCN guidelines also recommend that patients with early gastric cancer undergo laparoscopic gastrectomy.

To further validate the laparoscopic approach, Korean-funded and Japanese-funded researches (KLASS and JCOG0912, respectively) have performed random control trials (RCTs) at multiple centers to compare the outcomes of laparoscopic and open surgery in early-stage gastric cancer patients [20, 21]. KLASS research demonstrated that there were no significant differences in complication rate and mortality of distal radical operation between the two groups. However, they were unable to draw any conclusions regarding long-term outcomes. Similarly, Korean-funded and Chinese-funded researches (KLASS II and CLASS, respectively) are currently underway to compare the outcomes of laparoscopic and open surgery in advanced gastric cancer patients [22, 23]. We eagerly look forward to the final results when they become available.

6.1.4.1 Limitations of Laparoscopic Surgery

Despite its many advantages, laparoscopic gastrectomy for gastric cancer has some major disadvantages compared with the open gastrectomy. First is the missing haptic perception, which is important in some fields of gastrointestinal surgery. Since neither the liver nor the small bowel can be palpated during laparoscopy without haptic perception. The second disadvantage is the limited field of surgical vision. Some procedures especially in the handling of intraoperative complications (bleeding, hurting small bowel, and so on) are more difficult in laparoscopic surgery when compared to open surgery due to the limited intra-abdominal space [24].

6.1.4.2 Laparoscopic Sentinel Lymph Node Navigation Surgery

Recently, large-scale prospective studies demonstrated that laparoscopic sentinel lymph node mapping and biopsy was safe and beneficial for early-stage gastric cancer patients [25, 26]. The author also performed the sentinel lymph node biopsy in early gastric cancer patients using ICG (Fig. 6.4). This kind of surgery uses either ICG or nanoparticles to assess the lymphatic drainage from lymph channels to sentinel lymph node. The sentinel lymph node navigation surgery (SNNS) diagnostically identifies the sentinel lymph nodes and resects them using a laparoscopic surgical approach. A recent study reported that the detection

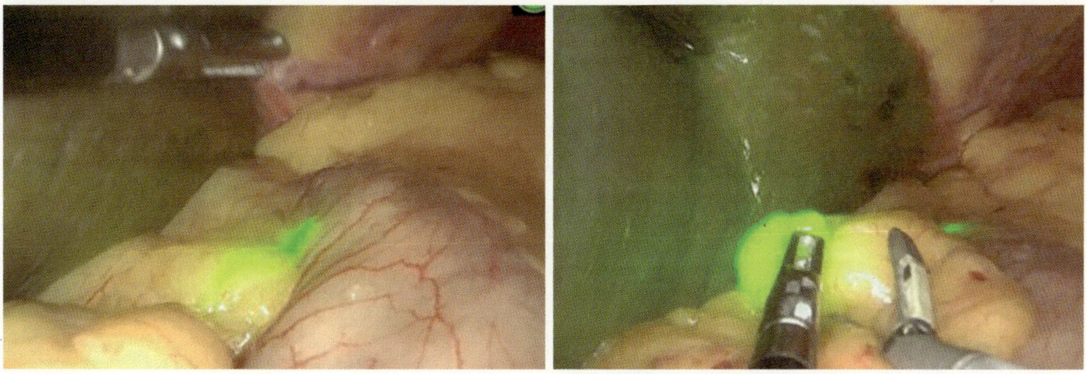

Fig. 6.4 Application of ICG in a gastric cancer patient to assess lymphatic drainage from lymphatic vessels to sentinel lymph nodes (*left*, ICG accumulated in lymphatic vessels; *right*, ICG accumulated in sentinel lymph nodes)

rate, sensitivity, and accuracy for Stage I gastric cancer was 97.5%, 93%, and 99%, respectively. The false negative rate was only 1% [27].

However, some studies have reported that the benefits of SLN navigation are limited [28, 29]. These studies reported that laparoscopic lymphadenectomy may not improve the patients' postoperative quality of life (QOL).

Some researchers have undertaken studies related to sentinel lymph node tracing [25–27]. Although the Japan Clinical Oncology Group trial (JCOG0302) was terminated due to high rates of false negatives, another clinical Phase II trial in Japan initially confirmed the feasibility of sentinel lymph node tracing as applied to gastric cancer [30, 31]. The Korea Phase III SENORITA trial sought to determine the presence of lymph node metastasis by endoscopic injection of 99TCm and subsequent ICG around the tumor [32]. The results of this study will further aid in determining whether sentinel lymph node tracing is applicable for treatment of gastric cancer, thus making surgical resection of early gastric cancer more plausible, accurate, and individualized.

6.2 Robotic Surgery for Gastric Cancer

6.2.1 Introduction

Robotic surgery has rapidly become one of the standard treatments for early-stage gastric cancer. Since robot-assisted gastrectomy was first reported in 2003, many studies have demonstrated its safety, efficacy, and significantly reduced invasiveness when compared to other approaches [33–35]. Robotic gastric cancer surgery including total gastrectomy with D2 lymph node dissection and radical subtotal gastrectomy is technically feasible and safe [35]. The indication for robotic surgery for gastric cancer is similar to that for laparoscopic surgery for Stage I gastric cancer.

6.2.2 Potential Advantages of Robotic Surgery

Robotic surgery for gastric cancer has shown increasing applications in experienced surgical centers [36]. Robotic surgery offers the surgeon the benefit of the freedom of free wrist function, the superior 3D visualization, and the easy control of robotic arms. When compared to laparoscopic surgery, the results of short-term outcomes have been shown to be similar [37]. Due to the technical advantages, the robotic surgical device may facilitate the expansion of minimally invasive surgery over laparoscopy. The potential advantages of robotic surgery include performing an extended lymphadenectomy to the lymph node (itself a difficult dissection) and performing an anastomosis under excellent surgical view [36].

The da Vinci robot-assisted surgical system is the most widely used robotic surgical platform

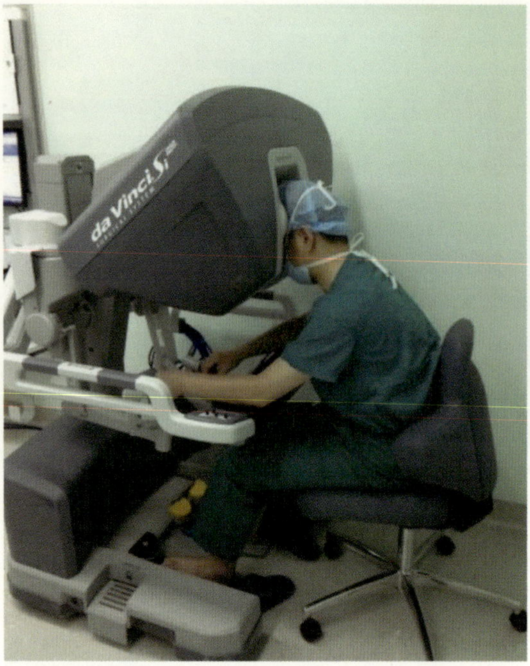

Fig. 6.5 Da Vinci robot-assisted surgical system

(Fig. 6.5). Its technical advantages include eliminating hand tremor, setting the action scaling, and indexing actions. The high-definition, 3D stereo-images transferred by the system are high resolution and have achieved real three-dimensional depth of field. Three emulated mechanical wrists have different types of free activities, and the range of motion of each joint exceeds 90°, making them more interactive than human hands (Fig. 6.5). Therefore, this system has greatly improved surgical stability, accuracy, and safety. Currently, da Vinci robot-assisted surgery within the realm of gastric cancer operations is still confined to just a few countries.

To this end, Song et al. has performed 100 robot-assisted gastrectomy for early-stage gastric cancer patients [38]. Of these, 33 were cases of total gastrectomy, and 67 were partial gastrectomy together with D1+ and D2 lymph node dissection. Operating times averaged from 231 min to 150 min, respectively. On average, patients were eating after 4.2 days and left the hospital 7.8 days post-op. Currently, da Vinci robot-assisted surgeries have been applied in advanced-stage gastric cancer patients in Japan, South Korea, and China [39, 40]. For instance, Köckerling et al. investigated and analyzed robotic gastrectomy surgeries performed in recent years. They found that robot-assisted surgery is safer with a lower converting rate, reduced rate of complications, and mortality rates comparable with those found in traditional laparoscopic surgery [41]. The aforementioned results revealed that the da Vinci robot-assisted total gastrectomy surgery is safe and effective, as measured by short-time outcomes. However, its outcomes over the long term remain to be seen.

A final potential benefit of robot-assisted surgery deals with surgeon fatigue, which has been a historically neglected measure. Surgeon fatigue appears to be reduced in robotic pelvic procedures when compared with standard laparoscopy or open procedures. However, definitive data do not currently exist.

6.2.3 Limitations of Robotic Surgery

Despite its benefits, there are several limitations of robotic surgery for gastric cancer. They are as follows:

The high cost of robotic surgery is one of the key limitations that must be overcome in the future. The costs for patients are significantly higher than for either laparoscopic or traditional open surgical approaches. Some costs are difficult to calculate, including the cost of training surgical staff and the time consumed in the docking process. As such, it is critical to consider the balance of costs and benefits to this approach.

In some studies, there is a selection bias in generating the comparative groups when compared the outcomes of robotic with laparoscopic surgeries [42]. Most studies do not clearly indicate the specific method of anastomotic technique (e.g., intracorporeal versus extracorporeal reconstruction). In some centers, the data of intracorporeal anastomosis are often mixed with those of extracorporeal anastomosis.

Some analyses of complications have revealed that the anastomotic leak rate was twice higher in laparoscopic and robotic group than open surgery group. However, the methods of digestive tract reconstruction in these studies are not clear [43]. Almost all of the studies comparing laparoscopic and robotic surgery reported little about digestive tract reconstruction. More random case-control clinical trials are needed to evaluate the safety and potential advantages of robotic surgery for gastric cancer patients.

6.3 Summary

Laparoscopic and robotic surgery provides us a unique opportunity for gastric cancer treatment, as they present a range of advantages including vision expansion and precision operating and are minimally invasive. We hope to promote the application of laparoscopic and robotic surgery both in the treatment of early- and advanced-stage gastric cancers. Furthermore, the sentinel lymph node navigation surgery (SNNS) is a key feature for precise surgery in gastric cancer. Through the development of laparoscopic and robotic techniques as well as sentinel lymph node tracing technology, it is extremely likely that we will be able to improve the quality of life quality for our patients in addition to achieving better future outcomes for them.

References

1. Kim BS, Yook JH, Choi YB, et al. Comparison of early outcomes of intracorporeal and extracorporeal gastroduodenostomy after laparoscopic distal gastrectomy for gastric cancer. J Laparoendosc Adv Surg Tech A. 2011;21(5):387–91.
2. Varela JE, Hiyashi M, Nguyen T, et al. Comparison of laparoscopic and open gastrectomy for gastric cancer. Am J Surg. 2006;192(6):837–42.
3. Son T, Hyung WJ. Laparoscopic gastric cancer surgery: current evidence and future perspectives. World J Gastroenterol. 2016;22(2):727–35.
4. Japanese Gastric Cancer Association. Japanese gastric cancer treatment guidelines 2010 (ver. 3). Gastric Cancer. 2011;14(2):113–23.
5. Aurello P, Sagnotta A, Terrenato I, et al. Oncologic value of laparoscopy-assisted distal gastrectomy for advanced gastric cancer: A systematic review and meta-analysis. J Minim Access Surg. 2016;12(3):199–208.
6. Haverkamp L, Ruurda JP, Offerhaus GJ, et al. Laparoscopic gastrectomy in Western European patients with advanced gastric cancer. Eur J Surg Oncol. 2016;1:110–5.
7. Lee JH, Ahn SH, Park DJ, et al. Laparoscopic total gastrectomy with D2 lymphadenectomy for advanced gastric cancer. World J Surg. 2012;36(10):2394–9.
8. Martinez-Ramos D, Miralles-Tena JM, Cuesta MA, et al. Laparoscopy versus open surgery for advanced and resectable gastric cancer: a meta-analysis. Rev Esp Enferm Dig. 2011;103(3):133–41.
9. Adachi Y, Suematsu T, Shiraishi N, et al. Quality of life after laparoscopy-assisted Billroth I gastrectomy. Ann Surg. 1999;229(1):49–54.
10. Lehnert T, Buhl K. Techniques of reconstruction after total gastrectomy for cancer. Br J Surg. 2004;91(5):528–39.
11. Zou Z, Mou T, Deng Z, et al. Exploration of digestive tract reconstruction with totally laparoscopic total gastrectomy for gastric cancer. Zhonghua Wei Chang Wai Ke Za Zhi. 2014;17(8):844–7.
12. Smolarek S, Salih A, Kazanowski M, et al. Laparoscopic assisted total gastrectomy for gastric cancer—operative technique. Wideochir Inne Tech Maloinwazyjne. 2015;10(1):133–7.
13. Ishigami S, Natsugoe S, Hokita S, et al. Postoperative long-term evaluation of interposition reconstruction compared with Roux-en-Y after total gastrectomy in gastric cancer: prospective randomized controlled trial. Am J Surg. 2011;202(3):247–53.
14. Kitagami H, Morimoto M, Nakamura K, et al. Technique of Roux-en-Y reconstruction using overlap method after laparoscopic total gastrectomy for gastric cancer: 100 consecutively successful cases. Surg Endosc. 2016;30(9):4086–91.
15. Lee JH, Yom CK, Han HS. Comparison of long-term outcomes of laparoscopy-assisted and open distal gastrectomy for early gastric cancer. Surg Endosc. 2009;23(8):1759–63.
16. Viñuela EF, Gonen M, Brennan MF, et al. Laparoscopic versus open distal gastrectomy for gastric cancer: a meta-analysis of randomized controlled trials and high-quality nonrandomized studies. Ann Surg. 2012;255(3):446–56.
17. Pak KH, Hyung WJ, Son T, et al. Long-term oncologic outcomes of 714 consecutive laparoscopic gastrectomies for gastric cancer: results from the 7-year experience of a single institute. Surg Endosc. 2012;26(1):130–6.
18. Kitano S, Shiraishi N, Uyama I, et al. A multicenter study on oncologic outcome of laparoscopic gastrectomy for early cancer in Japan. Ann Surg. 2007;245(1):68–72.
19. Sato H, Shimada M, Kurita N, et al. Comparison of long-term prognosis of laparoscopy-assisted gastrectomy and conventional open gastrectomy with special reference to D2 lymph node dissection. Surg Endosc. 2012;26(8):2240–6.
20. Nakamura K, Katai H, Mizusawa J, et al. A phase III study of laparoscopy-assisted versus open distal gastrectomy with nodal dissection for clinical stage IA/IB gastric Cancer (JCOG0912). Jpn J Clin Oncol. 2013;43(3):324–7.

21. Kim HH, Han SU, Kim MC, et al. Prospective randomized controlled trial (phase III) to comparing laparoscopic distal gastrectomy with open distal gastrectomy for gastric adenocarcinoma (KLASS 01). J Korean Surg Soc. 2013;84(2):123–30.
22. Hu Y, Ying M, Huang C, et al. Oncologic outcomes of laparoscopy-assisted gastrectomy for advanced gastric cancer: a large-scale multicenter retrospective cohort study from China. Surg Endosc. 2014;28(7):2048–56.
23. Kim HI, Hur H, Kim YN, et al. Standardization of D2 lymphadenectomy and surgical quality control (KLASS-02-QC): a prospective, observational, multicenter study [NCT01283893]. BMC Cancer. 2014;14:209. doi:10.1186/1471-2407-14-209.
24. Küper MA, Eisner F, Königsrainer A, et al. Laparoscopic surgery for benign and malign diseases of the digestive system: indications, limitations, and evidence. World J Gastroenterol. 2014;20(17):4883–91.
25. Lee JH, Park DJ, Kim YH, et al. Clinical implementations of preoperative computed tomography lymphography in gastric cancer: a comparison with dual tracer methods in sentinel node navigation surgery. Ann Surg Oncol. 2013;20(7):2296–303.
26. Kitagawa Y, Takeuchi H, Takagi Y, et al. Sentinel node mapping for gastric cancer: a prospective multicenter trial in Japan. J Clin Oncol. 2013;31(29):3704–10.
27. Tangoku A, Seike J, Nakano K, et al. Current status of sentinel lymph node navigation surgery in breast and gastrointestinal tract. J Med Invest. 2007;54(1–2):1–18.
28. Mitsumori N, Nimura H, Takahashi N, et al. Sentinel lymph node navigation surgery for early stage gastric cancer. World J Gastroenterol. 2014;20(19):5685–93.
29. Tani T, Sonoda H, Tani M. Sentinel lymph node navigation surgery for gastric cancer: does it really benefit the patient. World J Gastroenterol. 2016;22(10):2894–9.
30. Miyashiro I, Hiratsuka M, Sasako M, et al. High false-negative proportion of intraoperative histological examination as a serious problem for clinical application of sentinel node biopsy for early gastric cancer: final results of the Japan Clinical Oncology Group multicenter trial JCOG0302. Gastric Cancer. 2014;17(2):316–23.
31. Park JY, Ryu KW, Eom BW, et al. Proposal of the surgical options for primary tumor control during sentinel node navigation surgery based on the discrepancy between preoperative and postoperative early gastric cancer diagnoses. Ann Surg Oncol. 2014;21(4):1123–9.
32. Park JY, Kim YW, Ryu KW, et al. Assessment of laparoscopic stomach preserving surgery with sentinel basin dissection versus standard gastrectomy with lymphadenectomy in early gastric cancer-A multicenter randomized phase III clinical trial (SENORITA trial) protocol. BMC Cancer. 2016;16(1):1–8.
33. Shen WS, Xi HQ, Chen L, et al. A meta-analysis of robotic versus laparoscopic gastrectomy for gastric cancer. Surg Endosc. 2014;28(10):2795–802.
34. Maeso S, Reza M, Mayol JA, et al. Efficacy of the Da Vinci surgical system in abdominal surgery compared with that of laparoscopy: a systematic review and meta-analysis. Ann Surg. 2010;252(2):254–62.
35. Marano A, Choi YY, Hyung WJ, et al. Robotic versus Laparoscopic versus Open Gastrectomy: A Meta-Analysis. J Gastric Cancer. 2013;13(3):136–48.
36. Hur H, Kim JY, Cho YK, et al. Technical feasibility of robot-sewn anastomosis in robotic surgery for gastric cancer. J Laparoendosc Adv Surg Tech A. 2010;20(8):693–7.
37. Kim MC, Heo GU, Jung GJ. Robotic gastrectomy for gastric cancer: surgical techniques and clinical merits. Surg Endosc. 2010;24(3):610–5.
38. Song J, Oh SJ, Kang WH, et al. Robot-assisted gastrectomy with lymph node dissection for gastric cancer: lessons learned from an initial 100 consecutive procedures. Ann Surg. 2009;249(6):927–32.
39. Liu XX, Jiang ZW, Chen P, et al. Full robot-assisted gastrectomy with intracorporeal robot-sewn anastomosis produces satisfying outcomes. World J Gastroenterol. 2013;19(38):6427–37.
40. Suda K, Man-I M, Ishida Y, et al. Potential advantages of robotic radical gastrectomy for gastric adenocarcinoma in comparison with conventional laparoscopic approach: a single institutional retrospective comparative cohort study. Surg Endosc. 2015;29(3):673–85.
41. Köckerling F. Robotic vs. standard laparoscopic technique—what is better. Front Surg. 2014;1(15):1–4.
42. Hyun MH, Lee CH, Kim HJ, et al. Systematic review and meta-analysis of robotic surgery compared with conventional laparoscopic and open resections for gastric carcinoma. Br J Surg. 2013;100(12):1566–78.
43. Parisi A, Trastulli S, Ricci F, et al. Robotic double-loop reconstruction method following total gastrectomy. Endoscopy. 2016;48(1):55–6.

7 Radiotherapy in Gastric Cancer with Peritoneal Carcinomatosis

Yang Yang, Ju Yang, and Jing Yan

7.1 Introduction

Peritoneal dissemination is one of the most common metastatic methods of advanced gastric cancer. Radiotherapy has a positive effect for the prevention or treatment of peritoneal metastasis of gastric cancer. Preoperative neoadjuvant radiochemotherapy and postoperative adjuvant radiochemotherapy can effectively reduce the risk of peritoneal metastasis for patients with locally advanced gastric cancer. For patients who already have peritoneal dissemination, local palliative radiotherapy can effectively relieve the symptoms of local compression and reduce pain. Over the past decade, there are many developments for radiotherapy. Helical tomography, proton radiotherapy, intraoperative radiotherapy, and other new technologies have been used in clinical practice. These clinical applications improved the response rate and reduced adverse reactions for radiotherapy and finally bring benefit to patients.

Y. Yang • J. Yang • J. Yan (✉)
The Comprehensive Cancer Centre of Drum Tower Hospital, Medical School of Nanjing University and Clinical Cancer Institute of Nanjing University, 321 Zhongshan Road, Nanjing 210008, China
e-mail: yj20030610@126.com

7.2 Roles of Radiotherapy in Gastric Cancer with Peritoneal Carcinomatosis

7.2.1 Symptoms of Gastric Cancer with Peritoneal Carcinomatosis

Dissemination to the peritoneal cavity—also known as peritoneal carcinomatosis (PC)—is the most frequent metastasis for gastric cancer. Data gathered by our institute from 2006 to 2013 showed that 81.1% of 349 patients with locally advanced or metastatic gastric cancer (stages III–IV) developed PC (including metastases in the peritoneum, ovary, liver, or retroperitoneal adenopathy). A retrospective Korean study looking at 382 patients with stage III gastric cancer that underwent D2 resection yielded similar results. The total incidence rates of local failure, peritoneal failure (including the peritoneum, colorectal, ovary, and ureter), and distant failure as any component of first recurrence were 7.3%, 33.2%, and 19.9%, respectively, indicating that peritoneal recurrence and metastasis are the most common cause of treatment failure in gastric cancer [1].

Metastatic gastric cancer symptoms vary according to the affected body part as well as the size and location of the metastases. For

J. Wei, B. Liu (eds.), *Personalized Management of Gastric Cancer*,
DOI 10.1007/978-981-10-3978-2_7

instance, metastatic adenopathy around the porta hepatis is associated with obstructive jaundice, while peritoneal metastasis causes abdominal pain, bloating, ascites, and intestinal obstruction. In contrast, retroperitoneal adenopathy presents with back pain. Regional metastases are rarely completely resected, and patients with extensive metastases are always too weak to tolerate the chemo-/radiotherapy. The diagnosis for patients with PC is poor. These are difficulties oncologists strive to overcome.

7.2.2 Crucial Roles of Radiotherapy for Gastric Cancer with PC

Platinum and fluorouracil are the most common agents and have been in use for 30 years in patients with gastric cancer undergoing chemotherapy. Although the new generations of platinum and oral fluorouracil compounds are effective and well tolerated, they do not significantly improve the overall survival of gastric cancer patients. However, targeted agents also have limitations. For example, the total expression rate of HER2 is less than 25%, and half of them cannot benefit from trastuzumab. Crucially, in 2014 a phase III trial found that ramucirumab, a monoclonal antibody VEGFR-2 antagonist, improved the median survival of patients with previously treated advanced gastric cancer from 3.8 months to 5.2 months [2]. In 2016, another phase III study found that apatinib prolonged overall survival (OS) of patients with chemotherapy-refractory advanced or metastatic gastric cancer by 1.8 months [3]. These results highlight that local therapy is critical for those types of gastric cancer characterized by a high incidence of regional metastases. On the other hand, radiotherapy improves the radical resection rate for pre-therapeutic patients with regional metastases, decreases the risk of local recurrence in patients with high-risk factors of PC after surgery, and controls symptoms in patients with extensive peritoneal spread.

7.2.2.1 Neoadjuvant Chemoradiotherapy (NACRT)

Neoadjuvant chemoradiotherapy (NACRT) is recommended in pre-therapeutic patients with perigastric or other regional lymph node metastases and without distant metastasis to decrease the tumor size and facilitate surgical resection.

In their study, Kim et al. retrospectively analyzed 29 patients with locally advanced gastric disease (clinically T3 with distal esophagus invasion/T4 or bulky regional node metastasis) which received NACRT. Following NACRT intervention, 20 patients (69%) had a resectable tumor, and 18 patients (62.1%) underwent a D2 gastrectomy. The R0 resection rate was 94.4%, and two patients (2/18, 11.1%) showed a complete response. The 1-year PFS and OS rates were 48.9% and 72.4%, respectively, and no grade 3–4 late treatment-related toxicities or postoperative mortalities were observed [4].

In another study, Orditura et al. evaluated the effect of NACRT on outcome of patients with locally advanced esophagogastric junction adenocarcinoma. A total of total 41 patients received Folfox4 (leucovorin 5, fluorouracil, and oxaliplatin) for four cycles while concurrent three-dimensional conformal radiotherapy was delivered using five daily fractions of 1.8 Gy per week for a total dose of 45 Gy. Following treatment, resection surgery was performed. Following NACRT treatment, 78% of the patients showed a partial clinical response, 17% were stable, and 5% experienced disease progression. Pathological examination of surgical specimens demonstrated a 10% complete response rate [5].

Sun et al. retrospectively analyzed 2764 patients with gastric cancer, of which 55 patients received neoadjuvant radiotherapy (RT). At the time of surgery, total (vs. partial) gastrectomy was more common among patients who underwent neoadjuvant RT (70.9% vs. 46.7%, $p < 0.01$). No differences in overall complications (23.6% vs. 29.7%, $p = 0.49$) or 30-day mortality (3.6% vs. 3.6%, $p = 0.99$) were recorded [6].

RTOG 9904, released in 2006, was a phase II trial to study preoperative chemoradiation in patients with localized gastric adenocarcinoma.

Among the 43 assessed patients, the pathCR and R0 resection rates were 26% and 77%, respectively. After 1 year, the survival rate was higher in patients with pathCR (82%) than in those with less than pathCR (69%). The pathCR rate was much higher than the estimated rate. A D2 dissection was performed in 50% of patients [7]. These findings were encouraging for the subsequent phase III trial.

Oppedijk et al. investigated the patterns of recurrence in 422 patients with cancer of the esophagus or gastroesophageal junction from the CROSS trials after surgery alone compared to combined preoperative chemoradiotherapy and surgery. Preoperative CRT reduced locoregional recurrence (LRR) from 34% to 14% ($p < 0.001$) and peritoneal carcinomatosis from 14% to 4% ($p < 0.001$). LRR occurred in 5% within the target volume [8]. These data indicate that NACRT decreases the risk of local recurrence.

A phase III clinical trial undertaken in Germany compared preoperative chemotherapy with chemoradiotherapy in patients with locally advanced adenocarcinoma of the esophagogastric junction. Patients in arm A received 15 weeks of cisplatin/leucovorin/5-fluorouracil (PLF) induction chemotherapy followed by surgery, while patients in arm B received 12 weeks of chemotherapy (PLF) followed by 3 weeks of chemoradiotherapy (Dt: 30 Gy/15f/3w) followed by surgery. In total, 119 eligible patients were evaluated. Patients in arm B were significantly more likely to show a pathologic complete response (15.6% vs. 2.0%) at resection. Preoperative radiotherapy also improved the 3-year survival rate from 27.7% to 47.4% (log-rank $p = 0.07$). Postoperative mortality was not significantly increased in the chemoradiotherapy group (10.2% vs. 3.8%, $p = 0.26$). Although statistical significance was not achieved, results suggested a survival advantage for preoperative chemoradiotherapy compared with preoperative chemotherapy [9].

In summary, preoperative NACRT showed superior results in patients with locally advanced gastric cancer, with acceptable tolerance and without an increased risk of postoperative mortality or complications, compared to chemotherapy or surgery alone. TOPGEAR, an ongoing multicenter trial sponsored by the Australasian Gastro-Intestinal Trials Group (AGITG) and conducted in collaboration by the Trans-Tasman Radiation Oncology Group (TROG), the European Organization for Research and Treatment of Cancer (EORTC), and the NCIC Clinical Trials Group (NCIC CTG), was started to investigate whether the addition of chemoradiotherapy to chemotherapy is superior to chemotherapy alone in the neoadjuvant setting by improving pathological complete response rates in the first instance and, subsequently overall survival, in patients with resectable gastric cancer.

7.2.2.2 Postoperative Adjuvant Radiotherapy

Definitive surgery for gastric cancer includes D1 lymphadenectomy and D2 lymphadenectomy. The choice of adjuvant therapy depends on the different dissections. Compared to D1 lymphadenectomy, D2 lymphadenectomy does not show superior results in the survival of patients with resectable gastric cancer. A prospective randomized phase III trial published in Lancet in 1996 analyzed postoperative morbidity and mortality after D1 and D2 resections in gastric cancer, with 200 patients enrolled in each arm. Both postoperative hospital mortality (13% vs. 6.5%; $p = 0.04$ [95% CI 9–18% for D2, 4–11% for D1]) and overall postoperative morbidity (46% vs. 28%, $p < 0.001$) were significantly increased in the D2 group. The increased postoperative morbidity and mortality in the D2 group were linked to distal pancreaticosplenectomy and splenectomy. In the whole group of 400 patients, survival beyond 3 years was only 30% in patients whose gastrectomy included en bloc pancreatico-splenic resection versus 50% in the remainder. Therefore, D2 resection was not superior to D1 resection [10]. The study also found that the 5-year survival rates were not significantly different between the two arms, with 35% for the D1 resection group and 33% for the D2 resection group (HR = 1.10, 95% CI 0.87–1.39). Similarly, survival based on death from gastric cancer as the event was similar in the D1 and D2 groups (HR = 1.05, 95% CI 0.79–1.39), as was recurrence-free survival (HR = 1.03, 95% CI 0.82–1.29) [11]. A prospective study published in the Journal of Clinical Oncology in 2004 observed the similar results. After 11 years of follow-up, there was no overall difference in survival (30% vs. 35%, $p = 0.53$) between the D1 and D2 dissection groups. Subgroup analysis showed that only patients with N2 disease might benefit from a D2 dissection, while the relative risk ratio for morbidity and mortality is significantly higher in D1 than in D2 dissections [12].

Following the results of the INT0116 study, adjuvant radiochemotherapy has become the standard treatment after complete resection of gastric adenocarcinoma. In the INT0116 study, patients with stage Ib–IV (M0) were enrolled and randomly assigned to surgery alone versus postoperative radiochemotherapy. Radiochemotherapy consisted of bolus fluorouracil (FU) and leucovorin (LV) before, during, and after radiotherapy. FU and LV on days 1 through 5 began on day 1, and radiation to a total of 45 Gy (1.8 Gy/d 5 days/week for 5 weeks) started on day 28. FU and LV were administered for the first four and the last 3 days of radiotherapy. One month after radiotherapy, two additional cycles of FU+LV were given once every 28 days. Radiotherapy targeted common LRF sites such as the tumor bed, regional nodes, and anastomoses. Of the enrolled patients, more than 2/3 had stage T3 or T4 disease, and 85% had lymph node metastases. Of the patients receiving chemoradiotherapy, 182 (65%) completed the treatment course, 49 (17%) stopped treatment because of toxicity (23 of these 49 received ≥ 40 Gy), 5% progressed during treatment, 1% died during therapy, and 4% discontinued treatment for other reasons. Twelve percent (8% assigned to treatment, 4% assigned to observation) declined to continue the assigned therapy. Compared to the surgery-alone group, the 3-year survival rate in the postoperative radiochemotherapy group was increased from 30% to 41%, and the median survival was prolonged by 9 months (36 vs. 27 months). The median follow-up was 10.3 years. The OS and RFS data demonstrated a continued strong benefit from postoperative radiochemotherapy. HRs were virtually unchanged since the original report. HR for OS was 1.32 (95% CI, 1.10–1.60; $p = 0.0046$), and the HR for RFS was 1.51 (95% CI, 1.25–1.83; $p = 0.001$). These results showed the highly significant benefit of radiochemotherapy. No treatment-related late toxicities were observed during the follow-up. In conclusion, postoperative adjuvant chemoradiotherapy is superior to surgery alone for patients with locally advanced gastric cancer [13, 14]. In this trial, most patients (54%) received D0 dissection, 35% D1 dissection, and only 10% received D2 dissection. Thus, postoperative chemoradiotherapy could improve the survival of patients with gastric cancer receiving D0 or D1 dissection.

However, the benefits of postoperative radiotherapy in D2 dissection still remain unclear.

Kim et al. retrospectively analyzed the role of adjuvant chemoradiotherapy (CRT) in D2-resected gastric cancer patients from 1995 to 2001. In total, 544 patients received postoperative CRT after curative D2 resection, while 446 patients received surgery without further adjuvant treatment. The median follow-up period was 66 months (range 37–108 months). Overall survival was significantly longer in the CRT group than in the comparison group (95.3 months vs. 62.6 months). The 5-year survival rate was 57.1% in the CRT group and 51.0% in the comparison group ($p = 0.0198$). The 5-year survival rates were consistently higher in the CRT group at stages II, IIIA, IIIB, and IV than those in the comparison group. In conclusion, patients receiving D2 dissection might benefit from postoperative chemoradiotherapy [15].

The first study to investigating the role of postoperative chemoradiotherapy in patients with curatively resected gastric cancer with D2 lymph node dissection was ARTIST (Adjuvant Chemoradiation Therapy in Stomach Cancer), a Korean phase III trial. ARTIST was designed to compare two postoperative treatment regimens, capecitabine plus cisplatin (XP) versus XP plus radiotherapy with capecitabine (XP/XRT/XP). The XP group received six cycles of XP (2000 mg/m^2 capecitabine per day on days 1–14 and 60 mg/m^2 cisplatin on day 1, repeated every 3 weeks) chemotherapy, while the XP/XRT/XP group received two cycles of XP followed by 45 Gy XRT (1650 mg/m^2 capecitabine per day

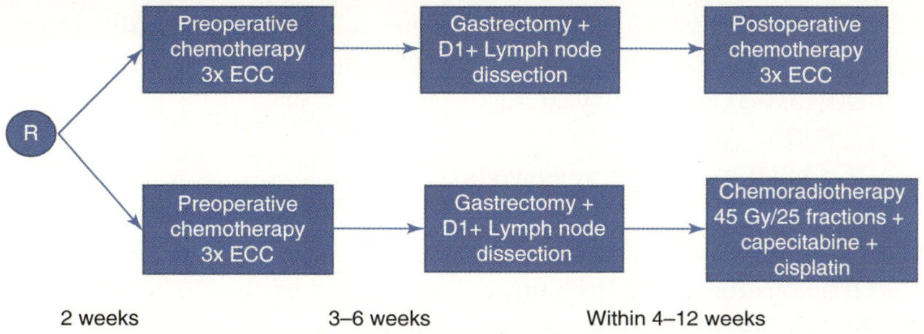

Fig. 7.1 Randomization scheme. *R* randomization, *ECC* epirubicin, cisplatin, capecitabine (Adapted from Neoadjuvant chemotherapy followed by surgery and chemotherapy or by surgery and chemoradiotherapy for patients with resectable gastric cancer (CRITICS). (2011), Dikken JL et al. [18])

for 5 weeks) and two cycles of XP. RT was targeted to the tumor bed, regional lymph nodes, duodenal stump, and anastomosis site and 2 cm beyond the proximal and distal margins of resection. The RT dose was 45 Gy, with 1.8 Gy daily fractions administered over the course of 5 weeks. The median follow-up was 53.2 months. The 3-year DFS rates were not significantly different between treatments, with 78.2% in the XP/XRT/XP arm compared to 74.2% in the XP arm ($p = 0.0862$). In a subgroup analysis of 396 patients with positive pathologic lymph nodes, DFS was significantly prolonged in the XP/XRT/XP arm (estimated 3-year DFS rate of 77.5%) compared to the XP-alone arm (3-year DFS, 72.3%; $p = 0.0365$) [16]. With 7 years of follow-up, DFS remained similar between treatment arms (hazard ratio [HR], 0.740; 95% CI, 0.520–1.050; $p = 0.0922$). OS also was similar (HR, 1.130; 95% CI, 0.775–1.647; $p = 0.5272$). Subgroup analysis demonstrated that patients with lymph node metastatic or intestinal-type gastric cancer would benefit from adjuvant chemoradiotherapy [17].

The ongoing ARTIST II trial was started in 2013 to further investigate adjuvant chemotherapy with S-1 versus S-1/oxaliplatin ± radiotherapy for completely resected gastric adenocarcinoma.

The CRITICS trial, a phase III multicenter prospective study led by a Dutch group, sought to investigate the impact of neoadjuvant chemotherapy followed either by surgery and chemotherapy or by surgery and chemoradiotherapy in patients with resectable gastric cancer. The enrollment started in December 2006 and ended in August 2011, and follow-up is still undergoing. In the CRITICS trial, patients with resectable gastric cancer were treated with three cycles of preoperative ECC (epirubicin, cisplatin, capecitabine) prior to surgery with adequate lymph node dissection. Following surgery, patients are further treated with three additional cycles of ECC alone or with concurrent chemoradiation (45 Gy, cisplatin and capecitabine) (Fig. 7.1). The primary end point is overall survival, while secondary end points are disease-free survival (DFS), toxicity, and health-related quality of life (HRQL) [18]. The results of this study have yet to be released.

In conclusion, postoperative adjuvant chemoradiotherapy should be selectively recommended for patients with resectable locally advanced gastric cancer.

7.2.2.3 Palliative Radiotherapy

Patients with late-stage gastric cancer always develop peritoneal carcinomatosis with symptoms of bleeding, pain, and intestinal obstruction, severely affecting the quality of life. Systemic chemotherapy is associated with low efficacy, higher incidence of toxicities, and poor tolerance. In contrast, local radiotherapy could alleviate symptoms and improve quality of life.

Chaw et al. evaluated the outcomes of 52 patients with gastric cancer bleeding who had been treated with palliative radiotherapy with hemostatic intent. Thirty-nine patients (75%) received single 8 Gy fraction, while 13 patients (25%) received 20 Gy in five daily fractions. The need for transfusion was evaluable in 44 patients, and the response rate was 50%, with fewer requirements for blood transfusions within

4 weeks of radiotherapy. The overall median survival (from treatment end to death) was 160 days (95% CI of 119–201 days), and the 1-year survival rate was 15% [19].

In a retrospective study, Tey et al. reviewed 115 patients that underwent palliative RT for index symptoms of gastric bleeding, obstruction, and pain. Dose fractionation regimens ranged from an 8 Gy single fraction to 40 Gy in 16 fractions. Response rates for bleeding, obstruction, and pain were 80.6% (83/103), 52.9% (9/17), and 45.5% (5/11), respectively. Median survival was significantly longer in patients who responded to RT compared with patients who did not (113.5 vs. 47 days, $p < 0.001$) [20].

7.3 The Technology of Radiotherapy for Gastric Cancer

Many abdominal organs such as the small intestine, liver, and kidneys are highly susceptible to radiotherapy-induced damage. Moreover, gastric cancer is associated with poor radiation sensitivity. Thus, it is necessary to take precautions to reduce radiation damage and to improve radiotherapy response.

7.3.1 The Range of Radiotherapy

According to the 2016 version of the NCCN Guidelines, the range of radiotherapy should be determined based on the location of tumor lesions both for neoadjuvant radiotherapy and postoperative adjuvant radiotherapy (Table 7.1).

Surgery may change the original anatomy, making it more difficult to sketch the postoperative lymphatic drainage area. Haijun et al. performed a phase II clinical study to determine CTV of adjuvant radiotherapy after radical surgery. The study demonstrated that the target area should include residual stomach, anastomosis, tumor bed, as well as the lymphatic drainage area. As lymph nodes are often associated with crucial blood vessels, the radiation target of the regional lymphatic drainage area can be determined based on remaining gastric and perigastric blood vessels. The most common grade 3–4

Table 7.1 The range of radiotherapy for gastric cancer

Tumor site	Radiotherapy mode	CTV primary	CTV node
Esophagogastric junction and upper 1/3 gastric	Neoadjuvant	Primary tumor and 3–5 cm range of proximal esophageal	Perigastric, peritoneal, splenic, hepatic portal lymph node area
	Adjuvant	Tumor bed and 3–5 cm range of proximal esophageal	Perigastric, peritoneal, splenic, hepatic portal lymph node area
Middle 1/3 gastric	Neoadjuvant	Primary tumor and peripheral subclinical lesions	Perigastric, pancreatic, peritoneal, splenic, hepatic portal, and pancreaticoduodenal lymph node area
	Adjuvant	Tumor bed (according to preoperative imaging scan or placement of the peptide clip), residual stomach would be in the CTV if the patient tolerate	Perigastric, pancreatic, peritoneal, splenic, hepatic portal, and pancreaticoduodenal lymph node area
Lower 1/3 gastric	Neoadjuvant	Primary tumor and peripheral subclinical lesions (if the tumor invasion of the stomach—duodenum—should include the first and second part of the duodenum)	Perigastric, pancreatic, peritoneal, hepatic portal, and pancreaticoduodenal lymph node area
	Adjuvant	Tumor bed and 3–5 cm range of duodenum	Perigastric, pancreatic, peritoneal, hepatic portal, and pancreaticoduodenal lymph node area

adverse event observed after adjuvant radiotherapy for gastric cancer was neutropenia (14.8%), while common grade 1–2 toxicities included neutropenia, nausea, and anemia. No treatment-related deaths occurred during the treatment period. The 3-year local recurrence-free survival rate was 91.1%, while the 3-year disease-free survival and overall survival rates were 70.2% and 81.6%, respectively. Eight patients developed peritoneal or distant metastasis [21].

7.3.2 The Dose of Radiotherapy

Due to the tolerable dose limit of abdominal organs such as the small intestine, liver, and kidneys, the maximum dose of neoadjuvant and postoperative adjuvant radiotherapy for gastric cancer is limited to approximately 50 Gy. The recommended dose is 1.8 Gy per fraction, with a total dose of 45–50.4 Gy. In case of positive margins or significant residual lesions after surgery, the radiation dose can be increased depending on the tolerable dose of the organ at risk near the target. Therefore, a radical effect of radiation therapy is difficult to achieve in patients with significant residual or intra-abdominal metastases.

7.3.3 The Tolerable Dose of Normal Tissue (Table 7.2)

Table 7.2 The tolerable dose of intra-abdominal organs

Organ	Tolerable dose
Spinal cord	≤40 Gy
Liver	60% of the liver volume ≤30 Gy
Kidney	33% of one side kidney volume ≤22.5 Gy, 33% of the other side kidney volume ≤45 Gy
Small intestine	≤54 Gy

7.3.4 The Technique of Radiotherapy

7.3.4.1 Three-Dimensional Conformal Intensity-Modulated Radiotherapy

Radiation therapy has developed from two-dimensional to three-dimensional or even four-dimensional. In a retrospective study, Lee et al. investigated the dosimetric and clinical influence of three-dimensional (3D, CT-based) simulation versus conventional two-dimensional (2D)-based simulation in postoperative chemoradiotherapy in patients suffering from advanced gastric cancer. The 3D group showed better dose-volume histogram profiles compared to the 2D group for all dosimetric parameters, including the spinal cord, liver, duodenum, kidneys, and bowel [22].

Three-dimensional conformal radiotherapy (3DCRT) and intensity-modulated radiotherapy (IMRT) were performed using multi-field irradiation. The shape of each field was consistent with tumor shape. Additionally, the radiation dose was adjusted based on tumor cell density. For organs with a limited tolerable dose of radiation such as the spinal cord as well as abdominal organs including the liver, kidneys, and small intestine, the use of three-dimensional conformal intensity-modulated radiotherapy, the cornerstone of radiotherapy technology, is superior to two-dimensional radiotherapy, with better protection of normal abdominal tissue, a reduced frequency of adverse reactions, and improvement of the radiation dose accuracy. Tey's study used three-dimensional conformal radiotherapy techniques to protect the normal tissue. The grade 3 adverse reaction rate was a mere 2.6%, and the therapy was well tolerated [20].

Intensity-modulated radiation therapy is based on reverse dose calculation. The target dose optimization is more reasonable, and the dose conformability is better resulting in improved protection of healthy tissue. In another study, Hawrylewicz et al. compared three-dimensional conformal radiotherapy with intensity-modulated radiotherapy in 25 patients with gastric cancer (adenocarcinoma T1–T4, N0–N3, and GI–GIII, according to AJCC). The area of clinical target volume (CTV) included a gastric tumor and 5 cm surrounding margins as well as the regional lymph nodes: perigastric, celiac trunk, pancreaticoduodenal, splenic, supra-pancreatic, portal vein, and para-aortic.

Table 7.3 Comparison of conformity index and homogeneity index between IMRT and CRT

	Two-field CRT	Three-field CRT	Four-field CRT	IMRT
Homogeneity index	1.118	1.117	1.089	1.087
Conformity index	1.115	1.118	1.088	1.082

CI: conformity index, $CI_{RTOG} = V_{RI}/TV$, where the volume of the reference isodose (V_{RI}) is the volume of the PTV receiving a 95% reference/planned dose, and the target volume (TV) is the volume of the PTV
HI: homogeneity index, $HI = I_{max}/RI$, where I_{max} is the maximum dose to the target, and RI is the reference dose in the PTV

Planning target volume (PTV) was determined by adding a 1 cm margin around the CTV. The planned total preoperative radiotherapy dose was 45 Gy administered in 25 fractions. During chemotherapy, 325 mg/m^2 5-fluorouracil was applied (days 1–5). IMRT technology was used for treatment, and multiple CRT plans were made for comparison. The results of the study showed that the IMRT plan in the CTV conformity and homogeneity is better than the CRT plan (Table 7.3) [23].

7.3.4.2 Volumetric Intensity-Modulated Arc Therapy

Volumetric intensity-modulated arc therapy (VMAT) is one of the most advanced radiotherapy techniques. In VMAT, a computer controls the speed of the linear accelerator multi-leaf collimator velocity movement, the speed of frame rotation, and the dose rate. As a result, the tumor area is more accurately irradiated, while the surrounding healthy tissue only receives minimal radiation. This technique meets the goal of killing the tumor effectively and protecting the surrounding normal tissue.

VMAT technology incorporates various features: (1) a more even dose distribution within the target site through the use of rotating arc irradiation technology. This technology decreases the duration of treatment and improves treatment efficiency. (2) Rotating irradiation allows not only multi-leaf grating but also a dynamic dose rate change, making it easier to adjust the radiation field dose. (3) The current VMAT technology is equipped with image guidance function, making radiation therapy more accurate.

Currently, only two devices of this kind are in existence: the US Varian's RapidArc and Sweden's Elekta VMAT. Zhang et al. compared dose distributions of RapidArc (RA), static gantry intensity-modulated radiotherapy (IMRT), and three-dimensional conformal radiotherapy (3DCRT) as adjuvant radiotherapy modalities for the treatment of gastric cancer. The study included 15 patients with gastric cancer that underwent limited lymphadenectomy of perigastric lymph nodes. The CTV included the anastomosis, tumor bed, and regional lymph nodes. The PTV was defined as a uniform 5 mm expansion of the CTV. The liver, both kidneys, spinal cord, small intestine, heart, and other OAR were delineated. Dosimetric values for a total dose of 45 Gy/25f were calculated for each of the three modalities: the RapidArc, IMRT, and 3DCRT. The results demonstrated the following:

(1) PTV dose uniformity: IMRT and RapidArc were superior to 3DCRT, with RapidArc exhibiting the best dose uniformity.
(2) Dose of OAR: RapidArc excelled at liver and kidney protection compared to IMRT or 3DCRT.
(3) RapidArc significantly reduced the accelerator output dose, with a reduction of 42.5% compared with IMRT.

Furthermore, the dose rate of RapidArc can total 600 MU/min, which significantly decreases treatment time to half the time required for IMRT treatment. In conclusion, RapidArc has a significant advantage over both IMRT and 3DCRT [24].

7.3.4.3 Helical Tomotherapy

Helical tomotherapy (TOMO), the latest generation of radiation therapy equipment, was developed by the University of Wisconsin-Madison and TomoTherapy company. Known for its more precise, larger scope, and more complex treatment, it is a perfect fusion of CT and linear accelerator. TOMO uses the same X-ray source for both treatment and image guidance, thus avoiding the mechanical error of two sources of X-ray and improving the accuracy of the image guidance function. Like a CT scan, TOMO can complete a 160 cm range of irradiation in one session, without requiring multiple isocenter and repetition. TOMO uses the rotating irradiation approach to ensure even dose distribution. The first helical tomotherapy machine received FDA certification in 2002. Today, TOMO has become the mainstream equipment for radiotherapy.

In one study, Dahele et al. compared different types of radiotherapy in postoperative adjuvant radiotherapy in gastric cancer patients. Results showed that TOMO treatment was superior to 2F-CRT, 5F-CRT, and IMRT in the homogeneity of PTV. For the protection of normal tissues such as the kidneys and liver, TOMO was shown to perform comparably to IMRT and much better than CRT for its really lower V20 or V30, giving in an obvious advantage over traditional radiotherapy technology.

TOMO treatment was shown to be superior to CRT or IMRT not only in cases of extensive peritoneal metastasis, a common occurrence in patients with gastric cancer, but also in cases of ovarian cancer (Table 7.4) [25–27]. In this treatment regimen, the whole abdominal area was irradiated using TOMO. CTV included the whole peritoneal cavity, extending from the diaphragm to the Douglas cavity, and the pelvic and para-aortic node regions. These studies indicate an alternative treatment for patients with extensive peritoneal metastasis.

7.3.4.4 Pulsed Reduced-Dose Rate Radiotherapy

Pulsed low-dose-rate radiotherapy (PRDR) refers to a low-dose pulse radiation therapy mode in which the total daily dose is divided into a single small dose and administered at a specific time interval between doses. During these time intervals, irradiation damage is repaired both in tumor and healthy tissue [28–30]. Results of a PRDR study showed that low dose of radiation (<0.3 Gy) significantly increased the cell survival fraction, indicating radiation hypersensitivity (HRS). Conversely, high doses of radiation (0.3–1.0 Gy) decreased the survival fraction of cells, indicating relative radioresistance (IRR).

Low-dose radiation hypersensitivity phenomena can be detected in many different types of cancer including gastric cancer, colorectal cancer, lung adenocarcinoma, and glioma, but also in normal tissue cells such as lung epithelial cells and fibroblasts [31]. PRDR is a new form of clinical radiotherapy based on the principle of low-dose radiation hypersensitivity (HRS) and sublethal injury repair theory. In PRDR, while normal tissue cells are being repaired following irradiation with

Table 7.4 Studies for whole abdominal irradiation using TOMO

Author	Year	Number of cases	Treatment purposes	Irradiation method	Radiation dose	Results	Adverse events
Rochet N	2015	16	Adjuvant radiotherapy	TOMO or step-and-shoot IMRT	30 Gy/20f	Median RFS was 27.6 months, median OS was 42.1 months	Grade 3 toxicities were diarrhea (25%), leucopenia (19%), nausea/vomiting (6%), and thrombocytopenia (6%)
Shetty UM	2013	8	Palliative radiotherapy	TOMO	Whole abdominal: 25 Gy/25f. Tumor: 45 Gy/25f	RFS: 62.5% (5/8)	One grade 3 leukopenia (12.5%) One grade 4 thrombocytopenia (12.5%) Three grade 2 gastrointestinal (37.5%) Two grade 2 liver functions deranged (25%)

small doses, tumor cells remain damaged. By using the difference of the speed of tissue reparation between tumor cells and normal cells, PRDR reduces the normal tissue irradiation reaction around the target area of radiotherapy, completes the effective radiotherapy dose of tumor lesion, improves sensitivity to radiotherapy, and reduces the side effects. The technique was first developed by a research group at the University of Wisconsin and was used in patients who had recurrent tumor growth in the irradiated target area. This re-radiotherapy improved the curative effect while causing no significant side effects in most patients [28, 32, 33]. In one study, Richards et al. [32] re-irradiated 17 patients with breast cancer locoregional recurrence (LRR) using the setting of prior postmastectomy radiation. A median PRDR dose of 54 Gy (range 40–66 Gy) with 1.8–2.0 Gy per fraction was used, with a cumulative dose of 110 Gy (80–236 Gy). The 2-year local control rate was over 90%. Irradiation was well tolerated by all patients. In a series of studies, Marples et al. focused on brain glioma cells [31, 33, 34], concluding that pulsed reduced-dose rate radiotherapy doses of 0.2 Gy × 10 times per day was better than the conventional dose of 2 Gy per day.

Pulsed reduced-dose rate radiotherapy can be applied to several groups of patients: (1) patients who had radiotherapy before but suffered from short-term radiation field relapse, (2) patients that cannot afford conventional three-dimensional conformal due to poor physical fitness, and (3) patients with systemic drug resistance with recurrence of large local tumors. The following case from our hospital exemplifies the use of PRDR. A 36-year-old female was diagnosed with poorly differentiated gastric adenocarcinoma, histologically shown to be partially signet ring cell carcinoma. Her medical history indicated that she initially underwent surgeries and palliative chemotherapy after recurrence. The patient suffered from abdominal pain and back pain caused by abdominal pelvic lymph nodes. The wide range of lesions precluded the use of conventional radiotherapy due to the expected significant radiation-related side effects. The patient was given palliative radiotherapy targeted to the involved abdominal lymph node. Considering the extensive target area, we chose PRDR to reduce the side effects on the normal tissue. A total dose of 50.0 Gy of PRDR was given to the patient. After 20 fractions of (40 Gy) irradiation, the patient's clinical symptoms improved significantly, and a CT scan revealed a >90% reduction in the size of the metastatic tumor lesion, indicating a significant partial remission. The side effects of radiotherapy were only mild (Fig. 7.2).

There are still many unresolved issues for PRDR—(1) the best clinical parameters for PRDR in the treatment of gastric cancer have not yet established, and the following questions remain: what is the optimal pulsed dose for gastric

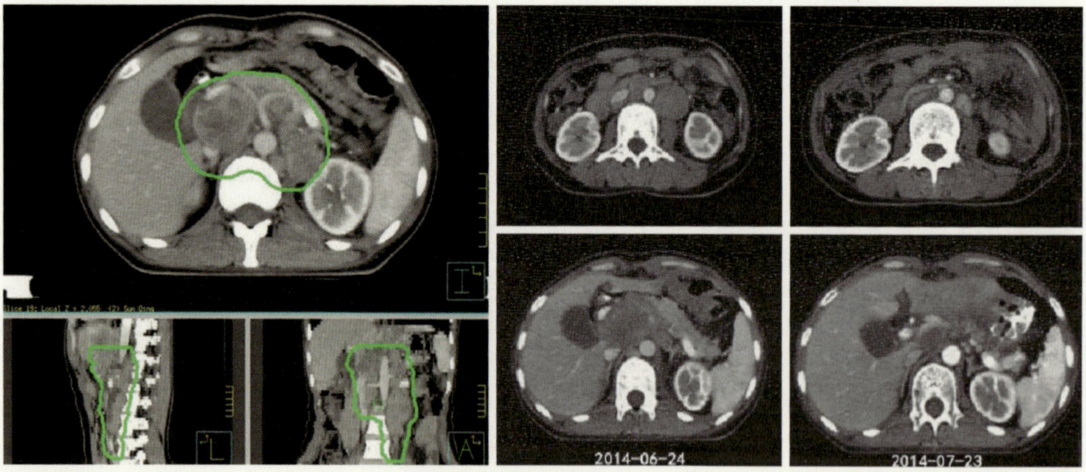

Fig. 7.2 A case of gastric cancer receiving PRDR. *XA* the PTV of radiotherapy, *XB* target lesion before and after radiotherapy

cancer and the interval time of irradiation? Is it possible to exceed the maximum tolerated dose prescribed by conventional radiotherapy? Are the side effects of PRDR different to the ones observed in conventional radiotherapy? (2) Does PRDR combined with chemotherapeutic drugs, i.e., targeted drugs, have synergistic antitumor effects? To this end, further studies are required to further explore and study the transformation of medical-related issues and to lay the foundation for future clinical research.

7.3.4.5 Proton Radiotherapy

Proton therapy is a global trend for radiotherapy, with research into this technique stretching back to the 1950s. In 1954, the Lawrence Berkeley laboratory in the USA used the world's first proton radiotherapy in a patient with advanced breast cancer. From 1961, proton radiotherapy was used to treat pituitary-related diseases such as acromegaly and Cushing syndrome at Harvard University. Soon after, proton technology was used to treat certain diseases in Sweden, the former Soviet Union, France, Canada, Japan, and several other countries. The world's first medical proton therapy center was built in Loma Linda University Medical Center, USA, in 1990. According to reports from the International Proton Therapy Cooperative (PTCOG), by 2013, there were 69 proton therapy centers in existence, and more than 90,000 patients had received proton therapy. In 2003, the Italian Society for Radiation Oncology reported that 12–15% of patients treated with conventional radiotherapy could achieve better outcomes with proton therapy.

Compared with a conventional linear accelerator, proton radiotherapy has several advantages. Radiotherapy harnesses radiation to shrink and destroy tumor tissue. Photons, including X-ray, γ-ray, and electronic lines, are a commonly used medical radiation source. A major feature of photon radiation is that the maximum dose point is reached soon after entering the body, while the energy of radiation gradually decays as the radiation distance increases. However, before and after reaching the tumor, the photons pass through and irradiate normal tissue to a certain degree.

The greatest advantage of proton therapy is its superior dose distribution, which releases the vast majority of destructive energy only at specific depths, known as the Bragg peak. The position of the peak can be calculated from the initial energy. By superimposing the proton Bragg peaks of different energies, an extended Bragg peak can be obtained as shown in Fig. 7.3. The width of the extended Bragg peak can be adjusted

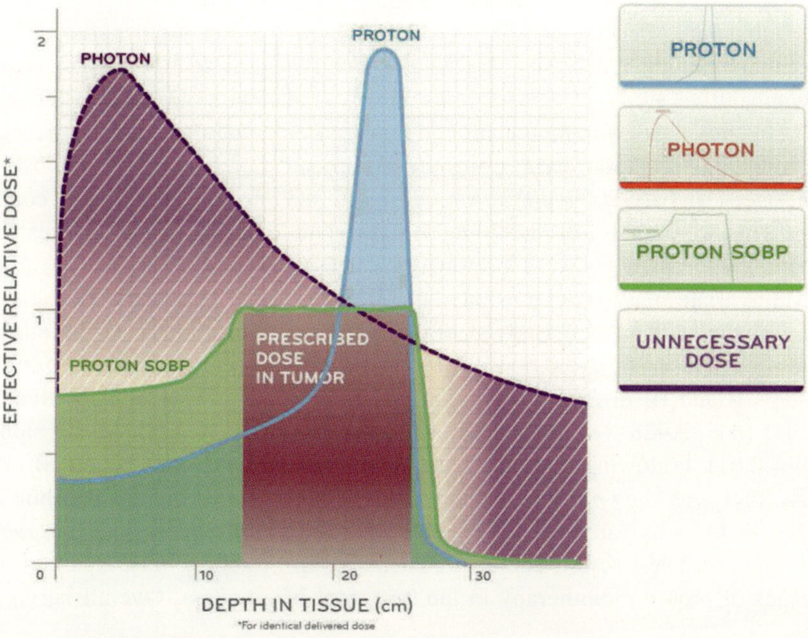

Fig 7.3 The dose comparison between proton beam and photon beam

depending on the thickness of the tumor, thereby maximizing the energy directed at the tumor. Compared to photon therapy, a proton beam can significantly reduce the dose before and after the tumor, thus greatly reducing the damage of the normal tissue surrounding the tumor. In summary, the advantages of proton radiotherapy include (1) a significant improvement of the tumor control rate, (2) a reduction of the side effects caused by radiation, and (3) a reduced risk of secondary tumors.

In one study, Dionisi et al. compared the differences between proton therapy (PT) and intensity-modulated X-ray therapy (IMXT) in postoperative adjuvant chemoradiotherapy of resectable gastric cancer in 13 patients. IMXT provided slightly higher homogeneity indices (median values 0.04 ± 0.01 vs. 0.07 ± 0.01, $p = 0.03$), while PT resulted in significantly ($p < 0.05$) lower intermediate-low doses for all the normal tissues examined (small bowel V15 82 ml vs. 133 ml, liver mean doses 11.9 Gy vs. 14.4 Gy, left/right kidney mean doses 5/0.9 Gy vs. 7.8/3.1 Gy, heart mean doses 7.4 Gy vs. 9.5 Gy). The study demonstrated that PT protects healthy tissue in the adjuvant treatment of gastric cancer, with a potential benefit in terms of treatment compliance as well as acute and late toxicities [35].

At the 2016 ASCO annual meeting, Prof. Madhusmita Behera of the Winship Cancer Center, Emory University, USA, presented a comparative study of proton radiotherapy and X-ray radiotherapy in non-small cell lung cancer (NSCLC) based on data from the American Cancer Database 2004–2012. A total of 140,383 patients were analyzed, including 140,035 photon (PHT) cases and 348 proton (PRT) cases. Multivariate analysis demonstrated that PHT was associated with an increased risk of death relative to PRT (HR 1.46, $p < 0.001$). For patients with stage II and III disease, 5-year OS was 15% in PHT ($n = 78.428$) versus 22.3% in PRT ($n = 193$, $p = 0.01$). Following propensity-matched analysis, PRT was shown to be associated with better 5-year OS compared to PHT (23% vs. 14%, $p = 0.024$). These results demonstrated the advantages of proton radiotherapy in the treatment of NSCLC. While proton radiotherapy has not been extensively studied in gastric cancer, these studies indicate its potential for future treatment options.

7.3.4.6 Intraoperative Radiation Therapy

Intraoperative radiation therapy (IORT) is a type of brachytherapy that can directly administer a single dose of radiation to the tumor or tumor bed during surgery using a small linear accelerator that can be placed in the operating room. The first case of intraoperative radiotherapy was reported in 1955. However, as a result of the special requirements of the operating room as well as other restrictions, this technology has not been widely promoted.

Intraoperative radiotherapy is mainly used in the treatment of abdominal digestive tract tumors. Ogata et al. carried out a study of 183 patients with gastric cancer who underwent radical gastrectomy with or without IORT. One group consisted of 58 patients who underwent radical surgery plus IORT. A single dose of 28–30 Gy was delivered around the celiac axis with an electron beam of 12 MeV. Using the combined treatment modality of radical surgical surgery plus IORT, improved overall survival rates were obtained for patients with stage II and III gastric cancer.

In another study, Zhang et al. analyzed 97 gastric adenocarcinoma patients (T3/4 or N+) treated with adjuvant CRT combined with (47%) or without (53%) intraoperative electron radiation therapy (IOERT; dose range, 12–15 Gy). Five-year locoregional control rates were 50% and 35% for patients treated with or without IOERT, respectively ($p = 0.04$) [36].

The results of a long-term follow-up study of intraoperative radiotherapy in 32 patients with locally advanced gastric cancer were published by Calvo et al. With a median follow-up time of 40 months (2–60 months), locoregional recurrence was observed in five patients (16%, four nodal in hepatic hilum and one anastomotic). No recurrence was observed in the IORT-treated target volume (celiac trunk and peripancreatic nodes). Overall survival at 5 years was 54.6%

(95% CI: 48.57–60.58%). Postoperative mortality was 6% ($n = 2$) and postoperative complications 19% ($n = 6$) [37].

7.4 The Synergistic Effect of Radiation Therapy and Other Treatment Modalities

In recent years, studies found that radiation therapy does not only control local recurrence of tumors but can also stimulate tumor cells to release more antigenic peptides, thus converting immune cells into tumor tissues. Therefore, radiotherapy combined with immunotherapy is an option to consider for the prevention and treatment of tumor metastasis.

Conclusion

Radiation therapy has a crucial role in the comprehensive treatment of gastric cancer. With the continuous progress of radiotherapy and the deeper understanding of tumor biology, radiation therapy and additional treatment methods can be combined to continuously improve the overall efficacy of gastric cancer treatment.

References

1. Chang JS, Lim JS, Noh SH, Hyung WJ, An JY, Lee YC, Rha SY, Lee CG, Koom WS. Patterns of regional recurrence after curative D2 resection for stage III (N3) gastric cancer: implications for postoperative radiotherapy. Radiother Oncol. 2012;104(3):367–73.
2. Fuchs CS, Tomasek J, Yong CJ, Dumitru F, Passalacqua R, Goswami C, Safran H, dos Santos LV, Aprile G, Ferry DR, Melichar B, Tehfe M, Topuzov E, Zalcberg JR, Chau I, Campbell W, Sivanandan C, Pikiel J, Koshiji M, Hsu Y, Liepa AM, Gao L, Schwartz JD, Tabernero J, REGARD Trial Investigators. Ramucirumab monotherapy for previously treated advanced gastric or gastro-oesophageal junction adenocarcinoma (REGARD): an international, randomised, multicentre, placebo-controlled, phase 3 trial. Lancet. 2014;383(9911):31–9.
3. Li J, Qin S, Xu J, Xiong J, Wu C, Bai Y, Liu W, Tong J, Liu Y, Xu R, Wang Z, Wang Q, Ouyang X, Yang Y, Ba Y, Liang J, Lin X, Luo D, Zheng R, Wang X, Sun G, Wang L, Zheng L, Guo H, Wu J, Xu N, Yang J, Zhang H, Cheng Y, Wang N, Chen L, Fan Z, Sun P, Yu H. Randomized, double-blind, placebo-controlled phase III trial of apatinib in patients with chemotherapy-refractory advanced or metastatic adenocarcinoma of the stomach or gastroesophageal junction. J Clin Oncol. 2016;34(13):1448–54.
4. Kim MS, Lim JS, Hyung WJ, Lee YC, Rha SY, Keum KC, Koom WS. Neoadjuvant chemoradiotherapy followed by D2 gastrectomy in locally advanced gastric cancer. World J Gastroenterol. 2015;21(9):2711–8.
5. Orditura M, Galizia G, Di Martino N, Ancona E, Castoro C, Pacelli R, Morgillo F, Rossetti S, Gambardella V, Farella A, Laterza MM, Ruol A, Fabozzi A, Napolitano V, Iovino F, Lieto E, Fei L, Conzo G, Ciardiello F, De Vita F. Effect of preoperative chemoradiotherapy on outcome of patients with locally advanced esophagogastric junction adenocarcinoma-a pilot study. Curr Oncol. 2014;21(3):125–33.
6. Sun Z, Nussbaum DP, Speicher PJ, Czito BG, Tyler DS, Blazer 3rd DG. Neoadjuvant radiation therapy does not increase perioperative morbidity among patients undergoing gastrectomy for gastric cancer. J Surg Oncol. 2015;112(1):46–50.
7. Ajani JA, Winter K, Okawara GS, Donohue JH, Pisters PW, Crane CH, Greskovich JF, Anne PR, Bradley JD, Willett C, Rich TA. Phase II trial of preoperative chemoradiation in patients with localized gastric adenocarcinoma (RTOG 9904): quality of combined modality therapy and pathologic response. J Clin Oncol. 2006;24(24):3953–8.
8. Oppedijk V, van der Gaast A, van Lanschot JJ, van Hagen P, van Os R, van Rij CM, van der Sangen MJ, Beukema JC, Rutten H, Spruit PH, Reinders JG, Richel DJ, van Berge Henegouwen MI, Hulshof MC. Patterns of recurrence after surgery alone versus preoperative chemoradiotherapy and surgery in the CROSS trials. J Clin Oncol. 2014;32(5):385–91.
9. Stahl M, Walz MK, Stuschke M, Lehmann N, Meyer HJ, Riera-Knorrenschild J, Langer P, Engenhart-Cabillic R, Bitzer M, Konigsrainer A, Budach W, Wilke H. Phase III comparison of preoperative chemotherapy compared with chemoradiotherapy in patients with locally advanced adenocarcinoma of the esophagogastric junction. J Clin Oncol. 2009;27(6):851–6.
10. Cuschieri A, Fayers P, Fielding J, Craven J, Bancewicz J, Joypaul V, Cook P. Postoperative morbidity and mortality after D1 and D2 resections for gastric cancer: preliminary results of the MRC randomised controlled surgical trial. The Surgical Cooperative Group. Lancet. 1996;347(9007):995–9.
11. Cuschieri A, Weeden S, Fielding J, Bancewicz J, Craven J, Joypaul V, Sydes M, Fayers P. Patient survival after D1 and D2 resections for gastric cancer: long-term results of the MRC randomized surgical trial. Surgical Co-operative Group. Br J Cancer. 1999;79(9–10):1522–30.
12. Hartgrink HH, van de Velde CJ, Putter H, Bonenkamp JJ, Klein Kranenbarg E, Songun I, Welvaart K, van Krieken JH, Meijer S, Plukker JT, van Elk PJ, Obertop H, Gouma DJ, van Lanschot JJ, Taat CW, de Graaf PW,

von Meyenfeldt MF, Tilanus H, Sasako M. Extended lymph node dissection for gastric cancer: who may benefit? Final results of the randomized Dutch gastric cancer group trial. J Clin Oncol. 2004;22(11):2069–77.
13. Smalley SR, Benedetti JK, Haller DG, Hundahl SA, Estes NC, Ajani JA, Gunderson LL, Goldman B, Martenson JA, Jessup JM, Stemmermann GN, Blanke CD, Macdonald JS. Updated analysis of SWOG-directed intergroup study 0116: a phase III trial of adjuvant radiochemotherapy versus observation after curative gastric cancer resection. J Clin Oncol. 2012;30(19):2327–33.
14. Macdonald JS, Smalley SR, Benedetti J, Hundahl SA, Estes NC, Stemmermann GN, Haller DG, Ajani JA, Gunderson LL, Jessup JM, Martenson JA. Chemoradiotherapy after surgery compared with surgery alone for adenocarcinoma of the stomach or gastroesophageal junction. N Engl J Med. 2001;345(10):725–30.
15. Kim S, Lim DH, Lee J, Kang WK, MacDonald JS, Park CH, Park SH, Lee SH, Kim K, Park JO, Kim WS, Jung CW, Park YS, Im YH, Sohn TS, Noh JH, Heo JS, Kim YI, Park CK, Park K. An observational study suggesting clinical benefit for adjuvant postoperative chemoradiation in a population of over 500 cases after gastric resection with D2 nodal dissection for adenocarcinoma of the stomach. Int J Radiat Oncol Biol Phys. 2005;63(5):1279–85.
16. Lee J, Lim DH, Kim S, Park SH, Park JO, Park YS, Lim HY, Choi MG, Sohn TS, Noh JH, Bae JM, Ahn YC, Sohn I, Jung SH, Park CK, Kim KM, Kang WK. Phase III trial comparing capecitabine plus cisplatin versus capecitabine plus cisplatin with concurrent capecitabine radiotherapy in completely resected gastric cancer with D2 lymph node dissection: the ARTIST trial. J Clin Oncol. 2012;30(3):268–73.
17. Park SH, Sohn TS, Lee J, Lim do H, Hong ME, Kim KM, Sohn I, Jung SH, Choi MG, Lee JH, Bae JM, Kim S, Kim ST, Park JO, Park YS, Lim HY, Kang WK. Phase III trial to compare adjuvant chemotherapy with capecitabine and cisplatin versus concurrent chemoradiotherapy in gastric cancer: final report of the adjuvant chemoradiotherapy in stomach tumors trial, including survival and subset analyses. J Clin Oncol. 2015;33(28):3130–6.
18. Dikken JL, van Sandick JW, Maurits Swellengrebel HA, Lind PA, Putter H, Jansen EP, Boot H, van Grieken NC, van de Velde CJ, Verheij M, Cats A. Neo-adjuvant chemotherapy followed by surgery and chemotherapy or by surgery and chemoradiotherapy for patients with resectable gastric cancer (CRITICS). BMC Cancer. 2011;11:329.
19. Chaw CL, Niblock PG, Chaw CS, Adamson DJ. The role of palliative radiotherapy for haemostasis in unresectable gastric cancer: a single-institution experience. Ecancermedicalscience. 2014;8:384.
20. Tey J, Choo BA, Leong CN, Loy EY, Wong LC, Lim K, Lu JJ, Koh WY. Clinical outcome of palliative radiotherapy for locally advanced symptomatic gastric cancer in the modern era. Medicine (Baltimore). 2014;93(22):e118.
21. Haijun Y, Qiuji W, Zhenming F, Yong H, Zhengkai L, Conghua X, Yunfeng Z, Yahua Z. A new approach to delineating lymph node target volumes for post-operative radiotherapy in gastric cancer: a phase II trial. Radiother Oncol. 2015;116(2):245–51.
22. Lee JA, Ahn YC, Lim do H, Park HC, Asranbaeva MS. Dosimetric and Clinical Influence of 3D Versus 2D Planning in Postoperative Radiation Therapy for Gastric Cancer. Cancer Res Treat. 2015;47(4):727–37.
23. Hawrylewicz L, Leszczynski W, Namysl-Kaletka A, Bronclik I, Wydmanski J. Protection of organs at risk during neoadjuvant chemoradiotherapy for gastric cancer based on a comparison between conformal and intensity-modulated radiation therapy. Oncol Lett. 2016;12(1):692–8.
24. Zhang T, Liang ZW, Han J, Bi JP, Yang ZY, Ma H. Double-arc volumetric modulated therapy improves dose distribution compared to static gantry IMRT and 3D conformal radiotherapy for adjuvant therapy of gastric cancer. Radiat Oncol. 2015;10:114.
25. Rochet N, Jensen AD, Sterzing F, Munter MW, Eichbaum MH, Schneeweiss A, Sohn C, Debus J, Harms W. Adjuvant whole abdominal intensity modulated radiotherapy (IMRT) for high risk stage FIGO III patients with ovarian cancer (OVAR-IMRT-01)—pilot trial of a phase I/II study: study protocol. BMC Cancer. 2007;7:227.
26. Shetty UM, Shankar S, Engineer R, Chopra S, Gupta S, Maheshwari A, Kerkar R, Shrivastava SK. Image-guided intensity-modulated whole abdominal radiation therapy in relapsed epithelial ovarian cancers: a feasibility study. J Cancer Res Ther. 2013;9(1):17–21.
27. Rochet N, Lindel K, Katayama S, Schubert K, Herfarth K, Schneeweiss A, Sohn C, Harms W, Debus J. Intensity-modulated whole abdomen irradiation following adjuvant carboplatin/taxane chemotherapy for FIGO stage III ovarian cancer: four-year outcomes. Strahlenther Onkol. 2015;191(7):582–9.
28. Adkison JB, Tome W, Seo S, Richards GM, Robins HI, Rassmussen K, Welsh JS, Mahler PA, Howard SP. Reirradiation of large-volume recurrent glioma with pulsed reduced-dose-rate radiotherapy. Int J Radiat Oncol Biol Phys. 2011;79(3):835–41.
29. Tome WA, Howard SP. On the possible increase in local tumour control probability for gliomas exhibiting low dose hyper-radiosensitivity using a pulsed schedule. Br J Radiol. 2007;80(949):32–7.
30. Ma CM, Lin MH, Dai XF, Koren S, Klayton T, Wang L, Li JS, Chen L, Price RA. Investigation of pulsed low dose rate radiotherapy using dynamic arc delivery techniques. Phys Med Biol. 2012;57(14):4613–26.
31. Martin LM, Marples B, Lynch TH, Hollywood D, Marignol L. Exposure to low dose ionising radiation: molecular and clinical consequences. Cancer Lett. 2014;349(1):98–106.
32. Richards GM, Tome WA, Robins HI, Stewart JA, Welsh JS, Mahler PA, Howard SP. Pulsed reduced dose-rate radiotherapy: a novel locoregional retreat-

ment strategy for breast cancer recurrence in the previously irradiated chest wall, axilla, or supraclavicular region. Breast Cancer Res Treat. 2009;114(2):307–13.
33. Dilworth JT, Krueger SA, Dabjan M, Grills IS, Torma J, Wilson GD, Marples B. Pulsed low-dose irradiation of orthotopic glioblastoma multiforme (GBM) in a pre-clinical model: effects on vascularization and tumor control. Radiother Oncol. 2013;108(1):149–54.
34. Lee DY, Chunta JL, Park SS, Huang J, Martinez AA, Grills IS, Krueger SA, Wilson GD, Marples B. Pulsed versus conventional radiation therapy in combination with temozolomide in a murine orthotopic model of glioblastoma multiforme. Int J Radiat Oncol Biol Phys. 2013;86(5):978–85.
35. Dionisi F, Avery S, Lukens JN, Ding X, Kralik J, Kirk M, Roses RE, Amichetti M, Metz JM, Plastaras JP. Proton therapy in adjuvant treatment of gastric cancer: planning comparison with advanced x-ray therapy and feasibility report. Acta Oncol. 2014;53(10):1312–20.
36. Zhang Q, Tey J, Peng L, Yang Z, Xiong F, Jiang R, Liu T, Fu S, Lu JJ. Adjuvant chemoradiotherapy with or without intraoperative radiotherapy for the treatment of resectable locally advanced gastric adenocarcinoma. Radiother Oncol. 2012;102(1):51–5.
37. Calvo FA, Sole CV, Obregon R, Gomez-Espi M, Gonzalez-San Segundo C, Gonzalez-Bayon L, Alvarez E, Garcia-Sabrido JL. Intraoperative radiotherapy for the treatment of resectable locally advanced gastric adenocarcinoma: topography of locoregional recurrences and long-term outcomes. Clin Transl Oncol. 2013;15(6):443–9.

8 Personalized Intraperitoneal Strategies in Gastric Cancer

Yang Yang, Nandie Wu, and Jia Wei

8.1 Introduction

Gastric cancer is the fourth most common cancer and the second leading cause of cancer deaths worldwide [1]. Except countries such as Korea and Japan that have routine national screening programs, most patients with gastric cancer are in advanced stages of the disease as early-stage gastric cancers are usually without symptoms and often develop advanced stage even after radical surgery. Despite developments in the surgical treatment of gastric cancer, there is a relatively high recurrence rate. Specifically, the 5-year overall survival rate for all diagnosed patients averages 24.5% in Europe [2] and 40–60% in Asia [3, 4]. The main reason for post-surgery treatment failure for gastric cancer is peritoneal dissemination, which is caused by the seeding of free cancer cells from the primary gastric cancer. This is one of the most common types of metastasis for gastric cancer. Gastric cancer patients with macroscopic peritoneal metastasis have very poor prognoses, with a median overall survival of 3–6 months [5, 6]. In this chapter, we try to describe the influence of peritoneal metastasis on survival in patients with gastric cancer, the possible mechanism of peritoneal metastasis, and individualized treatment strategy of gastric cancer patients at high risk for developing peritoneal metastasis.

Y. Yang (✉) • N. Wu • J. Wei
The Comprehensive Cancer Centre of Drum Tower Hospital, Medical School of Nanjing University and Clinical Cancer Institute of Nanjing University, 321 Zhongshan Road, Nanjing 210008, China

8.2 Peritoneal Metastasis in Gastric Cancer

The recurrence rate for gastric cancer remains high, especially in patients with advanced stages of the disease. In patients receiving radical surgery, 79% have recurrence within 2 years, and the median survival time from the time of recurrence is 6 months [7]. Many patients with gastric cancer (particularly those with Stage III disease) develop locoregional recurrence, peritoneal metastasis, or distant metastasis [8]. Although extensive research has analyzed recurrence patterns of gastric cancer after radical surgery, the data have yielded conflicting results. Schwarz et al. [9] found that most recurrences appeared diffusely at distant or peritoneal sites, and most locoregional recurrences occurred in conjunction with relapse at extraregional sites. Eom et al. [10] reported hematogenous metastasis as the most common pattern in patients with early recurrence, while locoregional and peritoneal recurrence occurred in patients with late recurrence 1 year after radical resection. This divergence was attributed to many

J. Wei, B. Liu (eds.), *Personalized Management of Gastric Cancer*,
DOI 10.1007/978-981-10-3978-2_8

reasons, such as differences in patient cohorts undergoing evaluation, methods for determining recurrence patterns, and the cutoff at which recurrence was determined. In addition, these results as well as those obtained from autopsy studies revealed only end-stage disease rather than early recurrences. Reoperation series likely display early locoregional and peritoneal recurrences. Peritoneal cytology and laparoscopy have been used to detect peritoneal metastatic disease not found in conventional imaging examinations [1].

A recent study of 1178 Korean patients with recurrent or metastatic gastric cancer demonstrated that about 46% of the patients had peritoneal metastases, while 30% had liver metastases [11]. Some clinical studies have found recurrence patterns in patients with early to advanced stages of gastric cancer, showing that 30–54% of patients had peritoneal recurrence alone or in combination with other site recurrence [7, 9, 12–14]. Our investigation with 349 patients with either Stage III or IV gastric cancer found that peritoneal metastasis was part of the metastasis or recurrence pattern in 62.8% of the patients. Of our total patient pool, 81.1% developed metastasis in the peritoneal cavity (peritoneal, liver, lymph node, ascites, or ovary) at the time of diagnosis or recurrence. Furthermore, our analysis showed that peritoneal metastasis was associated with poorer prognosis and poorer quality of life when compared with metastasis to other organs. Finally, patients with peritoneal metastasis had shorter survival time (7.5 vs. 14 months) and a higher risk of mortality (adjusted HR = 2.025, $p = 0.004$).

8.3 Mechanism of Peritoneal Metastasis

A recent comparative study proposed the following sequential steps for cancer cells to form peritoneal metastases: (1) penetration of cancerous tissues into the visceral serosa, (2) exfoliation of the cancer cells from the primary tumor site, (3) dissemination and survival of the cancer cells within the abdominal cavity, (4) adhesion of cancer cells to the peritoneum, (5) invasion of cancer cells through the peritoneal membrane, and (6) formation of the peritoneal metastasis [15]. However, the mechanisms dominating the formation of peritoneal metastasis remain relatively understudied. A global analysis was performed to find the differential gene expression of a gastric cancer cell line established from a primary main tumor and of other cell lines established from the metastasis to the peritoneal cavity. The expression patterns of approximately 21,168 genes were analyzed. Besides expression sequence tags, the investigators found that 24 genes were upregulated and 17 were downregulated [16].

Hiraki et al. [17] used a mouse model to demonstrate that loss of hypoxia inducible factor-1 alpha (HIF-1α) accelerated the development of aggressive peritoneal dissemination in gastric cancer cells by upregulating matrix metalloproteinases-1 (MMP-1) [17]. Matrix metalloproteinases-7 (MMP-7) tissue status in the primary tumor has also been validated as a good indicator for peritoneal metastasis. Patients with MMP-7-positive tumors had significantly shorter overall survival time and more frequently died of peritoneal recurrence than those with MMP-7-negative tumors [18].

Another broad analysis of differential gene expression between the parental cell line GC9811 and its highly metastatic peritoneal counterpart, cell line GC9811-P, confirmed that recombinant human S100 calcium-binding protein A4 (S100A4) and cadherin-associated protein beta 1 (CTNNB1) were upregulated. Moreover, tensin homolog deleted on chromosome ten (PTEN) and phosphatase was downregulated in GC9811-P cells. Identification of these differentially expressed genes could help uncover the underlying mechanisms and provide new targets for therapeutic intervention to avoid peritoneal dissemination of gastric cancer [19]. A recent comparative study demonstrated that advanced gastric cancer patients with a large amount of intraoperative hemorrhage were more likely to develop peritoneal recurrence, maybe due to the increased ability of cancer and mesothelial cells to adhere to each other in the presence of plasma factors [15]. Iroquois homeobox protein (IRX1) [20] and zinc protoporphyrin IX (ZnPPIX) [21] were also confirmed to inhibit peritoneal metastasis via neovascularization. Ultimately, identification of these differentially expressed genes will lead to a better understanding of the molecular mechanisms for peritoneal metastasis and provide new targets for therapeutic agents to avoid peritoneal dissemination of gastric cancer.

To date, P38-mitogen-activated protein kinase (MAKP) inhibition by a targeted small molecule inhibitor has been shown to be effective in preventing the peritoneal dissemination of poorly differentiated gastric cancer. It does so by acting at multiple checkpoints in the process of attachment and diffusion of tumor cells in the peritoneum [22]. Chemokine receptor 5 (CCR5) antagonism can reduce the potential risks of gastric cancer cell dissemination [23]. Nevertheless, the mechanisms of peritoneal dissemination for gastric cancer need to be further examined to lend more insights for peritoneal metastasis therapy.

8.4 Selected Patients for Intraperitoneal Chemotherapy

Positive peritoneal cytology has been classified as M1, metastatic disease in the Seventh Edition of the American Joint Committee on Cancer (AJCC) Staging System for gastric cancer [24]. Free intraperitoneal cancer cells isolated during peritoneal washing in patients with gastric cancer have been reported to be independently and significantly correlated to prognosis, influencing both recurrence-free survival time and overall survival time. It is, therefore, imperative to prevent peritoneal recurrence after radical surgery to improve the prognosis of patients with gastric cancer. The recent progress in treatment is the administration of intraperitoneal adjuvant chemotherapy soon after resection in patients with high risk of peritoneal recurrence [25, 26]. Then the question becomes: What kind of patients may benefit from this therapy, and what kind of patients are at high risk of peritoneal recurrence?

Although the exact mechanism promoting peritoneal recurrence remains controversial, the presence of malignant cells in the peritoneum at the time of surgery leads to peritoneal recurrence [27, 28]. Therefore, tests of peritoneal fluid may be used to identify patients with a high risk of peritoneal recurrence after radical surgery.

The standard and reliable method for detecting free cancer cells in the peritoneal washing fluid and for predicting peritoneal metastasis is conventional peritoneal cytology. However, large-sample studies have revealed that about 4–11% of patients will have positive peritoneal cytology. Therefore, it is neither practical nor cost-effective to perform this test on all patients [29]. Therefore, the sensitivity for the detection of residual cancer cells and prediction of peritoneal spread is not high enough [30, 31]. A recent prospective clinical study suggested that conventional peritoneal cytology test was not very reliable in predicting peritoneal recurrence after radical surgery for patients with gastric cancer, as peritoneal washing cytology was predictive of both peritoneal recurrence and survival time in patients with gastric cancer [32].

Another recent study involving 655 patients examined intraoperatively assessments of macroscopic serosal changes, which were defined as changes in color or nodular texture of the serosal surface on inspection and palpation. Their results showed that such examination led to a poorer prognosis and increased peritoneal recurrence risk for patients with curatively resected gastric cancer. Macroscopic assessment of serosal changes may be a useful indicator that allows for better risk stratification of patients with resected gastric cancer considering both peritoneal recurrence and prognosis [14].

In the last few years, genetic detection using reverse transcriptase polymerase chain reaction (RT-PCR) analysis has been observed to be more sensitive than conventional cytology. The target genes included carcinoembryonic antigen (CEA), zinc finger E-box-binding homeobox 1 (ZEB1), melanoma-associated gene (MAGE), cytokeratin 20, MMP-7, telomerase, and heparanase, and alone or in combination was used as potent molecular markers for the detection of peritoneal metastasis [33–35]. We also detected CEA mRNA in peritoneal washing fluid of gastric cancer patients after radical surgery and found that CEA mRNA was a more sensitive measure to detect peritoneal metastatic disease than peritoneal cytology. The positive rate of CEA mRNA was correlated with either T stage or N stage in patients with gastric cancer.

However, the amplified mRNA may derive from phagocytes or dead cells that engulfed tumor cells and later released it from hematopoietic cells in an inflammatory context [36]. Therefore, the issue of clinical false-positive cases has yet to be addressed. Using DNA methylation or flow cytometry to identify intraperitoneal tumor cells is other valuable alternative for selecting patients who might have a high risk for peritoneal metastasis [37, 38].

8.5 Effective Treatments for Patients with Peritoneal Metastasis

Of patients with gastric cancer, 20–50% who underwent curative surgery will develop postoperative peritoneal recurrence [39]. Intraperitoneal spread of tumor cells is also observed in 54% of gastric cancer patients who died of recurrence after radical surgery [40]. Gastric cancer patients with peritoneal metastasis have a very poor prognosis. Systemic chemotherapy may improve median overall survival time in metastatic gastric cancer by 7–10 months. However, patients with peritoneal carcinomatosis do not show similar improvements [41].

Until now, hyperthermic intraperitoneal chemotherapy (HIPEC) has been the most widely accepted strategy for the treatment of peritoneal metastasis, which is the most frequent metastatic pattern in patients with gastric cancer [42]. The theoretical advantage of HIPEC is to add the direct cytotoxic effects of heat in high concentrations of the cytostatic drug [43, 44]. In addition to the mechanical washing effect, HIPEC also has a theoretical superiority in delivering a higher concentration of anticancer drug into abdominal cavity with reduced systemic toxicity. There are many molecular explanations for these HIPEC effects, such as alterations of cell membrane properties, induction of apoptosis, changes to intracellular proteins and their synthesis, and inhibition of DNA repair enhanced by inhibitors of the cellular heat-shock response [45, 46].

In gastric cancer patients with peritoneal metastasis, surgical treatments that directly remove the primary lesion of peritoneal dissemination are a palliative approach. The combination of cytoreductive surgery (CRS) and HIPEC was first proposed in 1980 by Spratt [47]. After that, Sugarbaker and his team extensively applied this innovative technique for peritoneal carcinomatosis [48]. Some Phase II–III clinical trials revealed that patients with peritoneal metastasis who received CRS and HIPEC had better survival results only if complete cytoreduction (CCR-0) resection was achieved. However, the survival benefit of HIPEC remains low when cytoreductive surgery cannot accomplish sufficient down staging of the carcinomatosis burden [36, 49]. A retrospective study in France that involved 159 patients confirmed the combinatorial advantage in selected CCR-0 groups of patients [50]. The unsatisfactory effect of HIPEC in patients with extensive peritoneal carcinomatosis who were not amenable to down staging to CCR-0 may be explained by a more limited drug penetration ability. This would lead to negligible antitumor effects on the deeply invasive microfoci [51]. Therefore, drug delivery systems with high permeability have a promising, future role in the treatment of extensive peritoneal carcinomatosis patients [52].

8.6 Optional Drugs for Intraperitoneal Treatment

Multimodal treatment strategies have been used to improve the prognosis of gastric cancer patients with peritoneal metastasis. However, the results remain unsatisfactory [53]. The oral chemotherapeutics S1 is a polypharmaceutic, fluoropyrimidine derivative that combines tegafur with two modulators, gimeracil, and oteracil. A recent meta-analysis demonstrated that the use of S1 monotherapy was associated with a significant survival benefit for patients with gastric cancer [54]. The advantage of S1 over other chemotherapeutic agents is in its ability to achieve higher intraperitoneal concentrations. This is due to the higher concentrations of 5-fluorouracil (5-FU) and CDHP achieved in peritoneal tumors relative to plasma [55, 56].

In addition to S1, both docetaxel and paclitaxel also have high sensitivity against diffuse-type adenocarcinoma, which is the most common type of peritoneal tumor. This is due to their ability to bind to tubulin and lead to microtubule stabilization and mitotic arrest. Importantly, some of these compounds can be transported into the peritoneal cavity when administered intravenously [57].

Numerous studies have evaluated intraperitoneal drug delivery in gastric cancer patients, especially in patients with peritoneal metastasis. Intraperitoneal administration of chemotherapeutic agents makes it possible for an extremely high concentration of drugs to directly contact the target cancer lesions in the peritoneal cavity. However, intraperitoneal administration of cisplatin or mitomycin C has not shown significant therapeutic effects against peritoneal metastasis of gastric cancer due to its immediate absorption through the peritoneum [58]. In contrast, intraperitoneal administration of paclitaxel has been demonstrated to enhance antitumor activity against peritoneal metastasis by maintaining a high concentration of the drug in the peritoneal cavity over a long period. A number of convincing clinical trials have confirmed its clinical effects in ovarian cancer with peritoneal metastasis. These superior results were due to the pharmacokinetic advantage of taxanes after regional delivery [59]. Taxanes are absorbed through the openings of the lymphatic system, such as the stomata and the milky spots. These are important sites for the formation of peritoneal dissemination [60], due to their large molecular weight and fat solubility [61]. A Phase I/II study of intraperitoneal docetaxel plus oral S-1 for gastric cancer patients with peritoneal carcinomatosis showed a superior 1-year overall survival rate of 70%. Moreover, peritoneal cytology was negative in 81% of patients [62]. Along similar lines, Fujiwara et al. reported a median survival of 23.6 months in Japanese gastric cancer patients with peritoneal carcinomatosis who had been treated with intraperitoneal docetaxel combined with oral S-1 [63].

Intraperitoneal paclitaxel has shown a profound pharmacokinetic advantage of increased intraperitoneal concentration of the anticancer agent 1000 times higher than intravenous administration of paclitaxel at the same dose. However, the main problem of intraperitoneal chemotherapy is the limited penetration depth of anticancer drugs directly into the tumor. Therefore, the optimum use of paclitaxel may consist of both intraperitoneal and intravenous administrations, since intraperitoneal paclitaxel reaches systemic circulation only in small amounts [64]. In fact, Ishigami et al. established intraperitoneal paclitaxel with oral S-1 plus intravenous paclitaxel as an advantageous means of systemic chemotherapy. Furthermore, a Phase II study reported an overall response rate of 56% among patients with target lesions and a decrease or disappearance of malignant ascites in 62% of these patients [61].

Another recent Phase II clinical trial in serosa-positive gastric cancer patients showed a similar response rate of 71.4%, with 3- and 5-year overall survival rates of 78 and 74.9%, respectively [57].

Also, the efficacy of intraperitoneal irinotecan has been demonstrated in several animal studies. The AUC ratio of SN-38, the bioactive metabolite of irinotecan, varied between 3.7 and 14.8. This depended on the concentration of the administered irinotecan [65]. Moreover, pemetrexed has been considered a viable option when used intraperitoneally in a Phase I trial in both ovarian cancer and diffuse malignant peritoneal mesothelioma [66, 67].

In addition to chemotherapeutic agents, catumaxomab, a rat-mouse hybrid monoclonal antibody, was registered for the treatment of malignant ascites of various epithelial cell adhesion molecule (EpCAM)-positive malignancies, including ovarian, gastric, breast, and colorectal cancer. Two studies have shown that this drug improved progression-free survival in patients with gastric cancer (median 71 vs. 44 days,

$p = 0.03$). Moreover, that it improved survival in gastrointestinal anti-EpCAM-positive tumors when administered intraperitoneally [68, 69].

Conclusion

Gastric cancer is the second leading cause of cancer death worldwide, and more than half of the patients with gastric cancer are found disease progression of peritoneal carcinomatosis and die from it. Proper selection of intraperitoneal chemotherapy in patients with peritoneal metastasis or a potential risk of peritoneal recurrence may be a promising approach to improve the prognosis of advanced gastric cancer cases. Chemotherapeutic agents with high concentration and high permeability in the peritoneal cavity are optimal choices for intraperitoneal chemotherapy and cooperate with systemic chemotherapy. Moreover, future research on potential biomarkers from peritoneal washing could provide valuable information in selecting subsequent treatment combinations.

References

1. Leake PA, Cardoso R, Seevaratnam R, Lourenco L, Helyer L, Mahar A, Rowsell C, Coburn NG. A systematic review of the accuracy and utility of peritoneal cytology in patients with gastric cancer. Gastric Cancer. 2012;15(Suppl 1):S27–37.
2. De Angelis R, Sant M, Coleman MP, Francisci S, Baili P, Pierannunzio D, Trama A, Visser O, Brenner H, Ardanaz E, Bielska-Lasota M, Engholm G, Nennecke A, Siesling S, Berrino F, Capocaccia R. Cancer survival in Europe 1999–2007 by country and age: results of EUROCARE—5-a population-based study. Lancet Oncol. 2014;15(1):23–34.
3. Zeng WJ, Hu WQ, Wang LW, Yan SG, Li JD, Zhao HL, Peng CW, Yang GF, Li Y. Long term follow up and retrospective study on 533 gastric cancer cases. BMC Surg. 2014;14:29.
4. Matsuda T, Saika K. The 5-year relative survival rate of stomach cancer in the USA, Europe and Japan. Jpn J Clin Oncol. 2013;43(11):1157–8.
5. Yonemura Y, Elnemr A, Endou Y, Hirano M, Mizumoto A, Takao N, Ichinose M, Miura M, Li Y. Multidisciplinary therapy for treatment of patients with peritoneal carcinomatosis from gastric cancer. World J Gastrointest Oncol. 2010;2(2):85–97.
6. Yonemura Y, Endou Y, Sasaki T, Hirano M, Mizumoto A, Matsuda T, Takao N, Ichinose M, Miura M, Li Y. Surgical treatment for peritoneal carcinomatosis from gastric cancer. Eur J Surg Oncol. 2010;36(12):1131–8.
7. D'Angelica M, Gonen M, Brennan MF, Turnbull AD, Bains M, Karpeh MS. Patterns of initial recurrence in completely resected gastric adenocarcinoma. Ann Surg. 2004;240(5):808–16.
8. Chang JS, Lim JS, Noh SH, Hyung WJ, An JY, Lee YC, Rha SY, Lee CG, Koom WS. Patterns of regional recurrence after curative D2 resection for stage III (N3) gastric cancer: implications for postoperative radiotherapy. Radiother Oncol. 2012;104(3):367–73.
9. Schwarz RE, Zagala-Nevarez K. Recurrence patterns after radical gastrectomy for gastric cancer: prognostic factors and implications for postoperative adjuvant therapy. Ann Surg Oncol. 2002;9(4):394–400.
10. Eom BW, Yoon H, Ryu KW, Lee JH, Cho SJ, Lee JY, Kim CG, Choi IJ, Lee JS, Kook MC, Park SR, Nam BH, Kim YW. Predictors of timing and patterns of recurrence after curative resection for gastric cancer. Dig Surg. 2010;27(6):481–6.
11. Jo JC, Ryu MH, Koo DH, Ryoo BY, Kim HJ, Kim TW, Choi KD, Lee GH, Jung HY, Yook JH, Oh ST, Kim BS, Kim JH, Kang YK. Serum CA 19-9 as a prognostic factor in patients with metastatic gastric cancer. Asia Pac J Clin Oncol. 2013;9(4):324–30.
12. Deng J, Liang H, Wang D, Sun D, Pan Y, Liu Y. Investigation of the recurrence patterns of gastric cancer following a curative resection. Surg Today. 2011;41(2):210–5.
13. Yoo CH, Noh SH, Shin DW, Choi SH, Min JS. Recurrence following curative resection for gastric carcinoma. Br J Surg. 2000;87(2):236–42.
14. Yoo C, Ryu MH, Park YS, Yoo MW, Park SR, Ryoo BY, Jang SJ, Yook JH, Kim BS, Kang YK. Intraoperatively assessed macroscopic serosal changes in patients with curatively resected advanced gastric cancer: clinical implications for prognosis and peritoneal recurrence. Ann Surg Oncol. 2015;22(9):2940–7.
15. Arita T, Ichikawa D, Konishi H, Komatsu S, Shiozaki A, Hiramoto H, Hamada J, Shoda K, Kawaguchi T, Hirajima S, Nagata H, Fujiwara H, Okamoto K, Otsuji E. Increase in peritoneal recurrence induced by intraoperative hemorrhage in gastrectomy. Ann Surg Oncol. 2015;22(3):758–64.
16. Sakakura C, Hagiwara A, Nakanishi M, Shimomura K, Takagi T, Yasuoka R, Fujita Y, Abe T, Ichikawa Y, Takahashi S, Ishikawa T, Nishizuka I, Morita T, Shimada H, Okazaki Y, Hayashizaki Y, Yamagishi H. Differential gene expression profiles of gastric cancer cells established from primary tumour and malignant ascites. Br J Cancer. 2002;87(10):1153–61.
17. Hiraki M, Kitajima Y, Kai K, Nakamura J, Hashiguchi K, Noshiro H, Miyazaki K. Knockdown of hypoxia-inducible factor-1alpha accelerates peritoneal dissemination via the upregulation of MMP-1 expression in gastric cancer cell lines. Exp Ther Med. 2012;4(3):355–62.
18. Yonemura Y, Endou Y, Fujita H, Fushida S, Bandou E, Taniguchi K, Miwa K, Sugiyama K, Sasaki T. Role of

MMP-7 in the formation of peritoneal dissemination in gastric cancer. Gastric Cancer. 2000;3(2):63–70.
19. Bai FH, Wang NJ, Wang J, Yang L, Zhang FM, Yin F, Liang J, Wu KC, Fan DM. Screening and identification of peritoneal metastasis-related genes of gastric adenocarcinoma using a cDNA microarray. Genet Mol Res. 2012;11(2):1682–9.
20. Jiang J, Liu W, Guo X, Zhang R, Zhi Q, Ji J, Zhang J, Chen X, Li J, Gu Q, Liu B, Zhu Z, Yu Y. IRX1 influences peritoneal spreading and metastasis via inhibiting BDKRB2-dependent neovascularization on gastric cancer. Oncogene. 2011;30(44):4498–508.
21. Shang FT, Hui LL, An XS, Zhang XC, Guo SG, Kui Z. ZnPPIX inhibits peritoneal metastasis of gastric cancer via its antiangiogenic activity. Biomed Pharmacother. 2015;71:240–6.
22. Graziosi L, Mencarelli A, Santorelli C, Renga B, Cipriani S, Cavazzoni E, Palladino G, Laufer S, Burnet M, Donini A, Fiorucci S. Mechanistic role of p38 MAPK in gastric cancer dissemination in a rodent model peritoneal metastasis. Eur J Pharmacol. 2012;674(2-3):143–52.
23. Mencarelli A, Graziosi L, Renga B, Cipriani S, D'Amore C, Francisci D, Bruno A, Baldelli F, Donini A, Fiorucci S. CCR5 Antagonism by Maraviroc Reduces the Potential for Gastric Cancer Cell Dissemination. Transl Oncol. 2013;6(6):784–93.
24. Washington K. 7th edition of the AJCC cancer staging manual: stomach. Ann Surg Oncol. 2010;17(12):3077–9.
25. Matharu G, Tucker O, Alderson D. Systematic review of intraperitoneal chemotherapy for gastric cancer. Br J Surg. 2011;98(9):1225–35.
26. Yan TD, Black D, Sugarbaker PH, Zhu J, Yonemura Y, Petrou G, Morris DL. A systematic review and meta-analysis of the randomized controlled trials on adjuvant intraperitoneal chemotherapy for resectable gastric cancer. Ann Surg Oncol. 2007;14(10):2702–13.
27. Kojima N, Kunieda K, Matsui K, Kato H, Saji S. Evaluation of carcinoembryonic antigen mRNA in living, necrotic, and apoptotic gastric cancer cells by reverse transcriptase-polymerase chain reaction. Surg Today. 2003;33(11):839–46.
28. To EM, Chan WY, Chow C, Ng EK, Chung SC. Gastric cancer cell detection in peritoneal washing: cytology versus RT-PCR for CEA transcripts. Diagn Mol Pathol. 2003;12(2):88–95.
29. De Andrade JP, Mezhir JJ. The critical role of peritoneal cytology in the staging of gastric cancer: an evidence-based review. J Surg Oncol. 2014;110(3):291–7.
30. Bentrem D, Wilton A, Mazumdar M, Brennan M, Coit D. The value of peritoneal cytology as a preoperative predictor in patients with gastric carcinoma undergoing a curative resection. Ann Surg Oncol. 2005;12 (5):347–53.
31. Kodera Y, Nakanishi H, Ito S, Mochizuki Y, Ohashi N, Yamamura Y, Fujiwara M, Koike M, Tatematsu M, Nakao A. Prognostic significance of intraperitoneal cancer cells in gastric carcinoma: analysis of real time reverse transcriptase-polymerase chain reaction after 5 years of followup. J Am Coll Surg. 2006;202(2):231–6.
32. Kang KK, Hur H, Byun CS, Kim YB, Han SU, Cho YK. Conventional cytology is not beneficial for predicting peritoneal recurrence after curative surgery for gastric cancer: results of a prospective clinical study. J Gastric Cancer. 2014;14(1):23–31.
33. Fujiwara Y, Doki Y, Taniguchi H, Sohma I, Takiguchi S, Miyata H, Yamasaki M, Monden M. Genetic detection of free cancer cells in the peritoneal cavity of the patient with gastric cancer: present status and future perspectives. Gastric Cancer. 2007;10(4):197–204.
34. Yabusaki N, Yamada S, Murai T, Kanda M, Kobayashi D, Tanaka C, Fujii T, Nakayama G, Sugimoto H, Koike M, Nomoto S, Fujiwara M, Kodera Y. Clinical significance of zinc-finger E-box binding homeobox 1 mRNA levels in peritoneal washing for gastric cancer. Mol Clin Oncol. 2015;3(2):435–41.
35. Jeon CH, Kim IH, Chae HD. Prognostic value of genetic detection using CEA and MAGE in peritoneal washes with gastric carcinoma after curative resection: result of a 3-year follow-up. Medicine (Baltimore). 2014;93(11):e83.
36. Kowalewska M, Chechlinska M, Nowak R. Carcinoembryonic antigen and cytokeratin 20 in peritoneal cells of cancer patients: are we aware of what we are detecting by mRNA examination? Br J Cancer. 2008;98(2):512–3. author reply 4
37. Kitayama J, Emoto S, Yamaguchi H, Ishigami H, Onoyama H, Yamashita H, Seto Y, Matsuzaki K, Watanabe T. Flow cytometric quantification of intraperitoneal free tumor cells is a useful biomarker in gastric cancer patients with peritoneal metastasis. Ann Surg Oncol. 2015;22(7):2336–42.
38. Yu JL, Lv P, Han J, Zhu X, Hong LL, Zhu WY, Wang XB, Wu YC, Li P, Ling ZQ. Methylated TIMP-3 DNA in body fluids is an independent prognostic factor for gastric cancer. Arch Pathol Lab Med. 2014;138(11):1466–73.
39. Roviello F, Marrelli D, Neri A, Cerretani D, de Manzoni G, Pedrazzani C, Cioppa T, Nastri G, Giorgi G, Pinto E. Treatment of peritoneal carcinomatosis by cytoreductive surgery and intraperitoneal hyperthermic chemoperfusion (IHCP): postoperative outcome and risk factors for morbidity. World J Surg. 2006;30(11):2033–40. discussion 41–2.
40. Fujimoto S, Takahashi M, Mutou T, Kobayashi K, Toyosawa T. Successful intraperitoneal hyperthermic chemoperfusion for the prevention of postoperative peritoneal recurrence in patients with advanced gastric carcinoma. Cancer. 1999;85(3):529–34.
41. Montori G, Coccolini F, Ceresoli M, Catena F, Colaianni N, Poletti E, Ansaloni L. The treatment of peritoneal carcinomatosis in advanced gastric cancer: state of the art. Int J Surg Oncol. 2014;2014:912418.
42. Di Vita M, Cappellani A, Piccolo G, Zanghi A, Cavallaro A, Bertola G, Bolognese A, Facchini G, D'Aniello C, Di Francia R, Cardi F, Berretta M. The role of HIPEC in the treatment of peritoneal

carcinomatosis from gastric cancer: between lights and shadows. Anticancer Drugs. 2015;26(2):123–38.
43. Desai AD, Hawksworth GM. Cryopreservation of rat hepatocytes with high attachment efficiency and mixed function oxidase activity post thawing. Biochem Soc Trans. 1990;18(6):1214.
44. Brucher BL, Piso P, Verwaal V, Esquivel J, Derraco M, Yonemura Y, Gonzalez-Moreno S, Pelz J, Konigsrainer A, Strohlein M, Levine EA, Morris D, Bartlett D, Glehen O, Garofalo A, Nissan A. Peritoneal carcinomatosis: cytoreductive surgery and HIPEC—overview and basics. Cancer Invest. 2012;30(3):209–24.
45. Hildebrandt B, Wust P, Ahlers O, Dieing A, Sreenivasa G, Kerner T, Felix R, Riess H. The cellular and molecular basis of hyperthermia. Crit Rev Oncol Hematol. 2002;43(1):33–56.
46. Eppink B, Krawczyk PM, Stap J, Kanaar R. Hyperthermia-induced DNA repair deficiency suggests novel therapeutic anti-cancer strategies. Int J Hyperthermia. 2012;28(6):509–17.
47. Spratt JS, Adcock RA, Sherrill W, Travathen S. Hyperthermic peritoneal perfusion system in canines. Cancer Res. 1980;40(2):253–5.
48. Sugarbaker PH, Stuart OA, Yoo D. Strategies for management of the peritoneal surface component of cancer: cytoreductive surgery plus perioperative intraperitoneal chemotherapy. J Oncol Pharm Pract. 2005;11(3):111–9.
49. Graziosi L, Marino E, Donini A. Role of CRS plus HIPEC in gastric cancer peritoneal carcinomatosis. J Surg Oncol. 2015;111(2):248.
50. Glehen O, Gilly FN, Arvieux C, Cotte E, Boutitie F, Mansvelt B, Bereder JM, Lorimier G, Quenet F, Elias D. Peritoneal carcinomatosis from gastric cancer: a multi-institutional study of 159 patients treated by cytoreductive surgery combined with perioperative intraperitoneal chemotherapy. Ann Surg Oncol. 2010;17(9):2370–7.
51. Fujimoto S, Takahashi M, Kobayashi K, Kure M, Mutou T, Masaoka H, Ohkubo H. Relation between clinical and histologic outcome of intraperitoneal hyperthermic perfusion for patients with gastric cancer and peritoneal metastasis. Oncology. 1993;50(5):338–43.
52. Sha H, Zou Z, Xin K, Bian X, Cai X, Lu W, Chen J, Chen G, Huang L, Blair AM, Cao P, Liu B. Tumor-penetrating peptide fused EGFR single-domain antibody enhances cancer drug penetration into 3D multicellular spheroids and facilitates effective gastric cancer therapy. J Control Release. 2015;200:188–200.
53. Glockzin G, Piso P. Current status and future directions in gastric cancer with peritoneal dissemination. Surg Oncol Clin N Am. 2012;21(4):625–33.
54. Cabalag CS, Chan ST, Kaneko Y, Duong CP. A systematic review and meta-analysis of gastric cancer treatment in patients with positive peritoneal cytology. Gastric Cancer. 2015;18(1):11–22.
55. Shitara K, Mizota A, Matsuo K, Sato Y, Kondo C, Takahari D, Ura T, Tajika M, Muro K. Fluoropyrimidine plus cisplatin for patients with advanced or recurrent gastric cancer with peritoneal metastasis. Gastric Cancer. 2013;16(1):48–55.
56. Oshima T, Yamada R, Hatori S, Kunisaki C, Imada T. Pharmacokinetics of S-1 in patients with peritoneal dissemination of gastric cancer. Oncol Rep. 2006;16(2):361–6.
57. Peng YF, Imano M, Itoh T, Satoh T, Chiba Y, Imamoto H, Tsubaki M, Nishida S, Yasuda T, Furukawa H. A phase II trial of perioperative chemotherapy involving a single intraperitoneal administration of paclitaxel followed by sequential S-1 plus intravenous paclitaxel for serosa-positive gastric cancer. J Surg Oncol. 2015;111(8):1041–6.
58. Sautner T, Hofbauer F, Depisch D, Schiessel R, Jakesz R. Adjuvant intraperitoneal cisplatin chemotherapy does not improve long-term survival after surgery for advanced gastric cancer. J Clin Oncol. 1994;12(5):970–4.
59. Morgan Jr RJ, Doroshow JH, Synold T, Lim D, Shibata S, Margolin K, Schwarz R, Leong L, Somlo G, Twardowski P, Yen Y, Chow W, Lin P, Paz B, Chu D, Frankel P, Stalter S. Phase I trial of intraperitoneal docetaxel in the treatment of advanced malignancies primarily confined to the peritoneal cavity: dose-limiting toxicity and pharmacokinetics. Clin Cancer Res. 2003;9(16 Pt 1):5896–901.
60. Tsujimoto H, Hagiwara A, Shimotsuma M, Sakakura C, Osaki K, Sasaki S, Ohyama T, Ohgaki M, Imanishi T, Yamazaki J, Takahashi T. Role of milky spots as selective implantation sites for malignant cells in peritoneal dissemination in mice. J Cancer Res Clin Oncol. 1996;122(10):590–5.
61. Kitayama J, Ishigami H, Yamaguchi H, Yamashita H, Emoto S, Kaisaki S. S-1 plus intravenous and intraperitoneal Paclitaxel for gastric cancer with peritoneal metastasis. Gastrointest Cancer Res. 2012;5(3 Suppl 1):S10–3.
62. Fushida S, Kinoshita J, Kaji M, Hirono Y, Goda F, Yagi Y, Oyama K, Sudo Y, Watanabe Y, Fujimura T. Phase I/II study of intraperitoneal docetaxel plus S-1 for the gastric cancer patients with peritoneal carcinomatosis. Cancer Chemother Pharmacol. 2013;71(5):1265–72.
63. Fujiwara Y, Takiguchi S, Nakajima K, Miyata H, Yamasaki M, Kurokawa Y, Mori M, Doki Y. Intraperitoneal docetaxel combined with S-1 for advanced gastric cancer with peritoneal dissemination. J Surg Oncol. 2012;105(1):38–42.
64. Markman M. Intraperitoneal antineoplastic drug delivery: rationale and results. Lancet Oncol. 2003;4(5):277–83.
65. Turcotte S, Sideris L, Younan R, Drolet P, Dube P. Pharmacokinetics of intraperitoneal irinotecan in a pig model. J Surg Oncol. 2010;101(7):637–42.
66. Chambers SK, Chow HH, Janicek MF, Cragun JM, Hatch KD, Cui H, Laughren C, Clouser MC, Cohen JL, Wright HM, Abu Shahin N, Alberts DS. Phase I trial of intraperitoneal pemetrexed, cisplatin, and paclitaxel in optimally debulked ovarian cancer. Clin Cancer Res. 2012;18(9):2668–78.

67. Bijelic L, Stuart OA, Sugarbaker P. Adjuvant bidirectional chemotherapy with intraperitoneal pemetrexed combined with intravenous Cisplatin for diffuse malignant peritoneal mesothelioma. Gastroenterol Res Pract. 2012;2012:890450.
68. Heiss MM, Murawa P, Koralewski P, Kutarska E, Kolesnik OO, Ivanchenko VV, Dudnichenko AS, Aleknaviciene B, Razbadauskas A, Gore M, Ganea-Motan E, Ciuleanu T, Wimberger P, Schmittel A, Schmalfeldt B, Burges A, Bokemeyer C, Lindhofer H, Lahr A, Parsons SL. The trifunctional antibody catumaxomab for the treatment of malignant ascites due to epithelial cancer: Results of a prospective randomized phase II/III trial. Int J Cancer. 2010;127(9):2209–21.
69. Strohlein MA, Lordick F, Ruttinger D, Grutzner KU, Schemanski OC, Jager M, Lindhofer H, Hennig M, Jauch KW, Peschel C, Heiss MM. Immunotherapy of peritoneal carcinomatosis with the antibody catumaxomab in colon, gastric, or pancreatic cancer: an open-label, multicenter, phase I/II trial. Onkologie. 2011;34(3):101–8.

Part III

Immunotherapy

9 Immune Checkpoint Blockade and Gastric Cancer

Shu Su and Baorui Liu

9.1 Introduction

The term "checkpoints" refers to a broad spectrum of either co-receptors or ligands that are widely expressed by immune cells. Importantly, such checkpoints regulate immune cells' activation. The "inhibitory checkpoints" represent those molecules that play an important role in preventing over-activation of the immune system and are important to maintaining self-tolerance. In this way, immune attack by the host immune system can be prevented. Conversely and in the context of the tumor-immune environment, co-inhibitory receptors may pose a threat to the host's health by preventing an immune response against these malignancies. Both co-inhibitory receptors and ligands are highly expressed in a large number of malignancies. This high expression allows for successful evasion of antitumor immune responses. One of the most promising tumor immunotherapy strategies is to interrupt these immune "brakes" by blocking antibodies that prevent interactions between receptors and their cognate ligands. As shown by recent clinical trials targeting either the PD-1/PD-L1 or CTLA-4, pathways has yielded exciting results. However, there remains very limited study and understanding on gastric cancer when compared to other malignancies such as melanoma or lung cancer.

As such, this chapter seeks to first summarize clinical experiences and outcomes that are based on the use of anti-PD-1, anti-PD-L1, and anti-CTLA-4 monoclonal antibodies. We will then discuss how a selection of promising inhibitory checkpoint function, with a particular focus on their expression landscape in gastric cancer. Finally, we will highlight related clinical studies as well as preclinical research, concentrating on strategies that have been used to disturb them in order to enhance their immunotherapeutic efficacy against gastric cancer.

9.2 PD-1/PD-L1 Axis

9.2.1 Introduction to PD-1/PD-L1

PD-1 is also known as CD279 and is an immunoglobulin superfamily surface molecule sharing homology with both CD28 and CTLA-4 [1, 2]. PD-1 is expressed on activated T cells, B cells, NK cells, and myeloid-derived cells [3–5]. Its expression is relatively low on naïve T cells but can be induced by TCR signaling as well as by cytokines such as IL-2, IL-7, IL-15, and IL-21 [6]. PD-L1 is a ligand for PD-1; it is also known as

S. Su (✉) • B. Liu
The Comprehensive Cancer Centre of Drum Tower Hospital, Medical School of Nanjing University and Clinical Cancer Institute of Nanjing University, Nanjing 210008, China

J. Wei, B. Liu (eds.), *Personalized Management of Gastric Cancer*,
DOI 10.1007/978-981-10-3978-2_9

B7H1 or CD274 and shares significant homology with B7-1 (CD80). It also has a broad distribution on both hematopoietic cells such as T cells, B cells, dendritic cells (DCs), myeloid cells, as well as non-hematopoietic cells such as tumor cells [7]. It is constitutively expressed at low levels, and it is robustly induced by Th1 cytokines such as IFN-γ and TNF-α [8, 9]. PD-L2 is another ligand for PD-1, sharing homology with B7-2 (CD86). It is expressed on DCs and competes with PD-L1 to inactivate T cell functioning.

When compared with PD-L1, much less is known about PD-L2, beyond the fact that it is expressed at much lower levels [10]. PD-1 itself has been shown to recruit the tyrosine phosphatases SHP-2 and SHP-1 to the membrane where PD-1 ligation takes place. As a result, signaling through CD3-TCR and CD28 are inactivated, leading to T cell exhaustion and apoptosis [11]. Simultaneously with PD-1 ligation, PD-L1-positive tumors receive an anti-apoptotic signal, preventing them from succumbing to lysis by cytotoxic T lymphocytes (CTLs) [12] (Fig. 9.1). The past 5 years has seen successful use of a PD-1 blocking antibody in clinical trials and has raised the plausibility of immunotherapy in various kinds cancers [13–18]. Clinical data have revealed that up to 40% of patients with advanced-stage melanoma experienced measurable responses upon treatment with pembrolizumab or nivolumab, two PD-1 blocking antibodies approved by the FDA in 2014. In 2015, nivolumab was also approved for the treatment of squamous cell lung cancer, which is resistant to chemotherapy. Nivolumab and pembrolizumab have since been expanded to the treatment of additional cancers, including NSCLC, RCC, bladder, ovarian, and other malignancies [19]. Promising results have also been shown in patients with hematologic malignancies such as Hodgkin lymphoma [18].

9.2.2 PD-1/PD-L1 in Gastric Cancers

When turning the attention to examining the evidence for PD-1 and PD-L1 blockade in gastric cancers, in this chapter, the clinical significance as well as clinical studies of this pathway in the treatment of gastric cancers will be summarized. Besides, some of the future strategies targeting this pathway will be discussed.

9.2.2.1 Preclinical Studies

Preclinical studies investigating PD-1 and PD-L1 blockade therapy for gastric cancer have focused predominantly on mouse models and have yielded limited results. Some engrafted human tumor cells into T cell-deficient, nude mice to explore their efficacy. However, this model has limited the use for immunotherapy, since the effect of antibody blockade depends entirely on the interaction between immune and tumor cells.

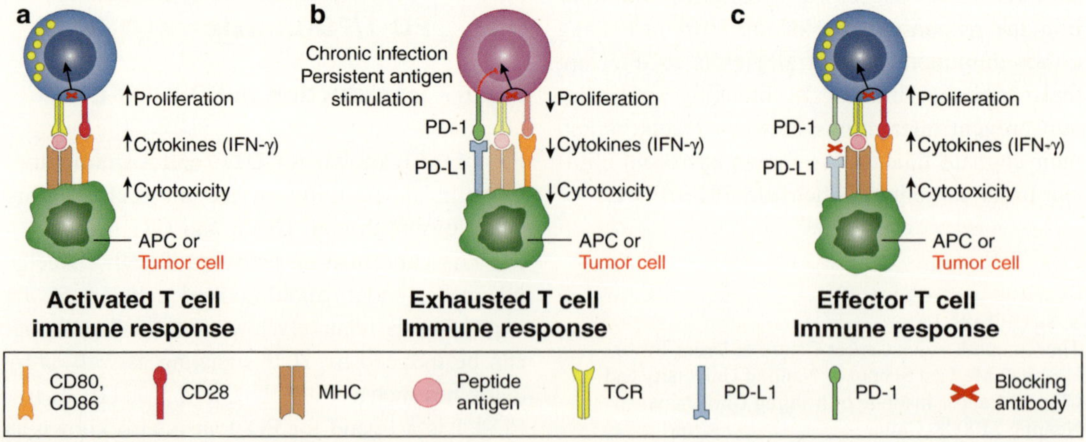

Fig. 9.1 PD-1/PD-L1 in cancer therapy *Cancer Med*, (2013) 2(5): 662–673. (**a**) Activation of T cells by CD28-CD80/86 signal. (**b**) Tolerence of T cells by PD-1-PD-L1 signal. (**c**) Reactivation of T cells by PD-1-PD-L1 blocking (Adapted from PD-1/PD-L1 in cancer therapy Cancer Med, (2013) 2(5): 662–673)

Given this, other studies have focused on immune-competent mice that have been modified to express human immune system components [20, 21]. Other strategies also use human PBMC to reconstitute the immune system of mice in order to validate the efficacy of the immune blocking antibody. Despite this wide array of approaches, models featuring human tumors inoculated onto mice have different signatures from those found in humans. It has also been suggested that most mouse models constitutively express PD-L1 [22]. With these limitations in mind, the following discussion will focus predominantly on human studies.

9.2.2.2 Clinical Significance of PD-1/PD-L1 in Gastric Cancers

Expression, Clinical Associations, and Prognosis

A variety of studies have described the clinical significance of the PD-1/PD-L1 pathway in gastric cancer. In these studies, the expression rates of PD-L1 or PD-1 in gastric cancer tumor tissues or peripheral blood were measured along with their correlated clinical-pathological features. These studies also then described the prognostic value of these biomarkers. Examples of these studies are summarized below and can be found in Tables 9.1 and 9.2.

Wu et al. examined PD-L1 protein expression in 102 cases of gastric cancer using immunohistochemical staining. They found that PD-L1 is detectable in 42.2% of gastric carcinoma tissues and not in healthy tissues. Furthermore, PD-L1 expression is significantly correlated with tumor size, invasion, and lymph node metastasis. Taken together, these results show that PD-L1 could be used as an independent factor to evaluate the possible outcomes of gastric cancer [23].

Hou et al. also used immunohistochemistry to evaluate FOXP3 and PD-L1 expression in tumor sections obtained from 111 gastric cancer patients. Co-expressions of PD-L1 and FOXP3 were found in these tissue samples. Moreover, the expressions of PD-L1 and FOXP3 were found

Table 9.1 Expression of PD-L1 in gastric cancer patients

Time	Author	Country	Journal	Sample size	Positive rate	Associated characteristics	Prognostic factor
2016	Changping Wu	China	Acta histochemica	102	42.2%	Tumor size; invasion; lymph node metastasis	Poor survival
2016	Cristin Boger	Germany	Oncotarget	465	30.1% on tumor cells 88.4% on immune cells	MSI; EBV; PIK3CA mutation Men	Better survival
2016	Elizabeth D Thompson	USA	Gut	34	12% on tumor cells 44% immune stroma	$CD8^+$ T cell density	Poor survival
2015	Kei Muro	Multicenters	ASCO GI symposium	162	40%	–	–
2015	Lin Zhang	China	Int J Clin Exp Pathol	132	50.8%	Tumor size >5 cm	Poor survival
2014	Kim J.W	Korean	Gastric Cancer	243	43.6%	Less advanced stage; intestinal type; well differentiated	Better survival
2014	Jing ying Hou	China	Experimental and Molecular Pathology	111	63% 71%	Lymph node metastase	Poor survival
2014	Zhixue Zheng	China	Chin J Cancer Res	80	Low in 41.2%; high in 58.8% (serum)	Differentiation lymph node metastasis	Better survival

Table 9.2 PD-1 expression on immune cells of gastric cancer patients

Time	Author	Country	Journal	Sample size	Positive rate	Associated characteristics	Prognostic factor
2016	Eto S	Japanese	Gastric Cancer	105	–	PD-L1 expression; Foxp 3 expression	Poor prognosis
2016	Takano S	Japanese	Surg Today	–	–	TIM-3 expression; reduced IFN-ϒ production	–
2016	Cristin Boger	Germany	Oncotarget	465	53.8%	PD-L1 expression	–
2015	Seigo Takaya	Japanese	Yonago Acta medica	33	17.7% on CD4 15.5% on CD8	Post surgery; LAG-3 expression;	–
2013	Hiroaki Saito	Japanese	Journal of Surgical Oncology	40	31~73.4%	Tumor progression; reduced IFN-ϒ production	–

to be correlated with lymph node metastasis and clinical-pathological stages, indicating poor prognosis. This study provided evidence for the idea that depleting Tregs in combination with PD-L1 blockade might improve immunotherapeutic efficacy in gastric cancer [24].

In another study, Kim et al. examined post-tumor resections obtained from 243 gastric cancer patients. PD-L1 was observed in 43.6% of the patients and was related to intestinal type, well-to-moderate differentiation and a less advanced stage. PD-L1 expression was found to be related to better disease-free survival (DFS) (5-year DFS rate: 82.6% vs. 66.9%) and overall survival (OS) (5-year OS rate: 83.0% vs. 69.1%) in gastric cancer. More importantly, patients within higher infiltration of $CD3^+$ cells showed better survival outcomes. In a subsequent multivariate analysis, PD-L1 expression had a better prognostic impact on survival, independent of other clinical variables [25].

Additionally, Zhang et al. reported that PD-L1 expression was observed in 50.8% of 132 surgically resected gastric cancer specimens. There was no relationship between the expression of PD-L1 and any clinical-pathological variables. However, patients with larger tumor size (>5 cm) had a higher positive rate of PD-L1 expression. Also, PD-L1 positively expressing patients had poorer long-term survival rates (5-year survival rates: 83.1% vs. 50.7%) [26].

Elizabeth et al. focused on 34 resections obtained from primary invasive gastroesophageal junction (G/GEJ) adenocarcinomas and performed immunohistochemistry for PD-L1 and CD8 expression. Of these, 12% showed membrane expression of PD-L1 on tumor cells, while 44% showed PD-L1 expression within the immune stroma itself. Increasing $CD8^+$ infiltrations were associated with an increasing percentage of tumor and stromal PD-L1 expression, both within tumors and immune stroma. This finding indicated an adaptive immune resistance pattern. Moreover, they found both tumor, and immune stromal PD-L1 expression was associated with a worsening of disease-free and overall survival rates [27].

Christine et al. also used an immunohistochemical approach to investigate the expression of PD-L1 and PD-1 in samples taken from 465 gastric cancer patients. PD-L1 expression was found in the tumor cells of 140 gastric cancer patients (30.1%) and in 9 (60%) liver metastases from these same patients. PD-L1 expression was also found in the immune cells from 411 (88.4%) of gastric cancer patients and 11 (73.3%) liver metastases from these same patients. PD-L1 expression was significantly more abundant in the following: samples obtained from men, Her2/neu positive, Epstein-Barr virus positive, microsatellite unstable, PIK3CA-mutated, and the proximal, unclassified, papillary gastric cancer. High PD-L1 expression was independently associated with better clinical outcome [28].

In addition to PD-L1 membrane staining, Zheng et al. also examined PD-L1 expression in the circulation of gastric patients using an enzyme-linked immunosorbent assay (ELISA). This approach was tested on 80 advanced gastric cancer patients and 40 health controls. Researchers found that circulating PD-L1 was upregulated in gastric cancer patients and correlated with lymph node metastasis and tumor differentiation. In this study, patients with high PD-L1 expression had a better prognosis than patients with low PD-L1 expression [29].

There are also emerging work examining the relationship between genetic polymorphism of PD-1/PD-L1 and gastric cancer. For instance, Savabkar et al. evaluated the association of PD-1.5 C/T polymorphism in 122 gastric cancer patients and 166 healthy controls. They found that the frequencies of PD-1.5CT genotypes were higher in gastric cancer patients [30]. Other work has also indicated that some PD-L1 genotypes have a strong correlation with the clinical-pathological features of gastric cancer [31].

Despite the relatively stable expression of PD-L1 in the tumor tissue of gastric cancer, there is no definitive conclusion as to whether PD-L1 expression can predict a good or poor disease prognosis. It is likely to be much more complicated in the post-curative resection setting or other specific situations such as infection with the Epstein-Barr-virus status, microsatellite instability, and/or high mutation load gastric cancers. Future work will require expanded cases and additional research to better understand PD-L1's role in the development and prognosis of gastric cancer.

There are fewer studies examining PD-1 expression relative to PD-L1 in gastric cancer patients. For instance, Hiroaki et al. found that PD-1 expressions on both $CD4^+$ T cells and $CD8^+$ T cells were significantly higher in gastric cancer patients than in normal controls. In addition, PD-1 expression on $CD4^+$ T cells and $CD8^+$ T cells in advanced-stage patients was significantly higher than in early-stage patients. Finally, they also found that less IFN-γ was produced by PD-1 positive T cells than by PD-1-negative T cells, indicating that PD-1 upregulation may play a role in the immune evasion capacity of gastric cancer [32].

In another study, Seigo et al. evaluated PD-1 expression on both $CD4^+$ and $CD8^+$ T cells obtained pre- and postoperatively from gastric cancer patients. Total lymphocyte count decreased rapidly postoperation. In contrast, $PD\text{-}1^+CD4^+$ and $PD\text{-}1^+CD8^+$ T cells showed a significant increase postoperation and returned to preoperative levels on day 30. Collectively, these results showed that PD-1 expression was upregulated on T cells after surgery. Moreover, it could be related to the impaired cell-mediated immunity seen in gastric cancer [33].

Christine et al. demonstrated that PD-1 was expressed in tumor-infiltrating lymphocytes in 53.8% of gastric cancer patients and in 73.3% of those with liver metastases. PD-1-positive immune cells were frequently observed in either intra-tumor lymphocyte aggregates or lymph follicles. Moreover, PD-1 expression in TILs was significantly correlated with PD-L1 expression in tumor microenvironments (TME). Higher PD-L1/PD-1 expression was also associated with better clinical outcome. Furthermore, there was a correlation between PD-L1/PD-1 expression and distinct clinical-pathological characteristics such as EBV status, MSI, Her2/neu positivity, and PIK3CA mutation status. These characteristics may instruct the use of immune checkpoint treatment strategies in the treatment of PD-L1-positive gastric cancer [28].

Takano et al. found PD-1 expression on $CD8^+$ T cells obtained from gastric cancer patients was significantly correlated with Tim-3 expression in peripheral blood samples. T cells positive for both PD-1 and Tim-3 had significantly reduced production of IFN-γ than negative cells. This result indicates that PD-1, together with other immune inhibitory checkpoints, mediates the immune tolerance of gastric cancer [34].

Eto et al. evaluated PD-1 expression on tumor tissue obtained from 105, post-curative surgery, gastric cancer patients. PD-1 was found to be correlated with both PD-L1 and Foxp3 expression. Moreover, PD-1-positive patients had poorer survival rates when compared with PD-1-negative patients (3-year DFS: 36.1% vs. 64.7%). In this way, PD-1 expression can be used as an independent prognostic indicator of gastric cancer [35].

Molecular Classification of Gastric Cancer and PD-1/PD-L1 Blockade Strategy

The Cancer Genome Atlas (TCGA) project has classified gastric cancer into four molecular subtypes according to the following characteristics: (1) EBV, tumors positive for Epstein-Barr virus; (2) MSI, microsatellite unstable tumors; (3) GS, genomically stable tumors; and (4) CIN, tumors with chromosomal instability [36]. Christine et al. found that PD-L1 expression in tumor cells was both more intense and extensive in EBV-positive, MSI, papillary-type, and unclassified gastric cancers. In particular, MSI-GCs have peculiar histological MSI features and often showed high PD-L1 expression in tumor cells. Moreover, four different PD-L1 expression patterns were observed: (1) EBV-positive GCs with a heterogeneous, "patchy" expression pattern with a striking accumulation of PD-L1-positive tumor cells around larger blood vessels; (2) MSI-GC were mainly PD-L1 positive at the interface between neoplastic and nonneoplastic tissues; (3) papillary-type GCs often showed PD-L1 positivity within the fibrovascular connective tissue cores and the intra-tumor necrosis; and (4) other cases showed no distinct PD-L1 distribution pattern and were classified as "patternless" [28].

EBV-GCs

Globally, there are approximately 80,000 new cases each year of EBV-associated gastric cancer (EBVaGC), comprising almost 10% of total gastric cancer cases worldwide [37]. Recent evidence has suggested that the immune system may play an important role in the development of EBVaGC, since EBV infection is always accompanied by a high degree of immune cell infiltration [38]. Studies have also revealed that most genetic changes in EBVaGC occur in immune response genes, including significant amplification of PD-L1 and PD-L2 [38]. Immune responses have also been shown to be negatively regulated via PD-1 ligation [39]. Prior investigations have shown PD-L1 overexpression on the cell surface of lymphoma, which inhibited lysis of infected, malignant cells by cytotoxic T cells [40]. Therefore, it is likely that EBV-reactive immune cells may be dysfunctional due to the acquired immune resistance mediated by the PD-1/PD-L1 pathway.

Given this, it was hypothesized that inhibition of the PD-1/PD-L1 pathway might augment anti-tumor immune responses. In a recent study from our lab, the PD-L1 expression on $CD3^+$ T cells that had infiltrated gastric tumor tissues was evaluated. The results indicated that PD-L1 was more prevalent on cells obtained from EBVaGC patients than from patients with EBV nonassociated gastric cancer (EBVnGC) (64% vs. 15%, respectively). Moreover, PD-1 was found to be upregulated on EBV-LMP2A-specific $CD8^+$ T cells. Finally, using CRISPR-Cas9 interference with the PD-1 gene of cytotoxic T cells resulted in a significant enhancement of IFN-γ production and killing ability of T cells.

MSI-GCs

Recently, the literature has discussed the stratification of the tumor microenvironment (TME) and classified it into four types. Of these, it has been reported that type I TME contains PD-1-expressing tumor-specific $CD8^+$ T cells which is in close proximity to PD-L1-expressing cells. These types of tumors with a greater mutation load have been found to be more sensitive to anti-PD-1/PD-L1 therapy [41]. A separate study has also shown that mismatch repair status predicted the clinical benefit of anti-PD-1 therapy [42]. Therefore, accumulating evidence suggests that PD-L1 is expressed at higher levels in the EBV and MSI subgroups, likely due to viral stimulation and elevated mutational load. As such, these represent promising subtypes for the use of PD-1/PD-L1 blockade therapy, as these patients are most likely to benefit from immune inhibitory checkpoint blockade therapy.

9.2.2.3 Clinical Studies of PD-1/PD-L1 Blockade in Gastric Cancer

A growing number of clinical projects aimed at evaluating the use of anti-PD-1 and anti-PD-L1 immune checkpoint inhibitors for advanced gastric cancer are currently recruiting or ongoing.

For instance, the KEYNOTE-012 trial (NCT01848834) enrolled 162 gastric cancer patients for screening. Among them, 65 patients were PD-L1 positive (40%). A total of 39 patients were enrolled in the trial and treated bi-weekly with pembrolizumab (10 mg/kg). The objective response rate (ORR) was 22%, and the clinical response was associated with PD-L1 expression [43, 44]. The most common treatment-associated adverse events (AEs) were hypothyroidism ($n = 5$) and fatigue ($n = 5$). Grade ≥ 3 AEs were observed in three patients, who were treated for hypoxia, peripheral neuropathy, and pneumonitis, respectively. This trial provided the first evidence for the feasibility of clinical application of the PD-1 blocking antibody for use in treating gastric cancer. However, the application of immune checkpoint inhibitors for gastric cancer is still in its infancy, and a growing number of clinical trials targeting PD-1 and PD-L1 are ongoing. It should be noted that there have also been studies of PD-L/PD-L1 blockade in combination with traditional therapy or other immune checkpoint inhibition for the treatment of gastric cancer (Table 9.3). It is unknown whether those patients who responded well belonged to the EBV-positive or MSI-positive subgroups. As such, further investigation into the molecular pattern of patients who could benefit most from the PD-1/PD-L1 blockade will be needed.

Table 9.3 Clinical trials for PD-1/PD-L1 inhibition in gastric cancer

Study	Subject	Agent	Stage	Status
NCT02267343	Study in patients with unresectable advanced or recurrent gastric cancer	Nivolumab	Phase III	Recruiting
NCT02335411	Pembrolizumab as monotherapy and in combination with cisplatin + 5-fluorouracil with recurrent or metastatic gastric or gastroesophageal junction adenocarcinoma (KEYNOTE-059)	Pembrolizumab	Phase I/IIA	Recruiting
NCT02268825	Study of MK-3475 with chemotherapy in patients with advanced GI cancers (MK-3475 GI)	Pembrolizumab	Phase I/II	Recruiting
NCT02340975	Study of MEDI4736 with tremelimumab, MEDI4736, or tremelimumab monotherapy in gastric or GEJ adenocarcinoma	MEDI4736 tremelimumab	Phase I/II	Recruiting
NCT02625610	Avelumab in first-line gastric cancer	Avelumab	Phase III	Recruiting
NCT01848834	Study of pembrolizumab in participants with advanced solid tumors (KEYNOTE-012)	Pembrolizumab	Phase I	Ongoing
NCT02625623	Avelumab in third-line gastric cancer (JAVELIN Gastric 300)	Avelumab	Phase III	Recruiting
NCT02268825	Study of MK-3475 with chemotherapy in patients with advanced GI cancers	Pembrolizumab	Phase I/II	Recruiting
NCT02589496	Study of pembrolizumab with advanced gastric or gastroesophageal junction adenocarcinoma progressed after first-line therapy	Pembrolizumab	Phase II	Recruiting
NCT02340975	Study of MEDI4736 with tremelimumab, MEDI4736, or tremelimumab monotherapy in gastric or GEJ adenocarcinoma	MEDI4736 tremelimumab	Phase I/II	Recruiting
NCT02494583	Study of pembrolizumab as first-line monotherapy and combination therapy for advanced gastric or gastroesophageal junction adenocarcinoma (KEYNOTE-062)	Pembrolizumab	Phase III	Recruiting

(continued)

Table 9.3 (continued)

Study	Subject	Agent	Stage	Status
NCT02370498	Study of pembrolizumab versus paclitaxel for participants with advanced gastric/ gastroesophageal junction adenocarcinoma progressed after first-line therapy (KEYNOTE-061)	Pembrolizumab	Phase III	Recruiting
NCT02689284	Combination margetuximab and pembrolizumab for advanced, metastatic Her2(+) gastric or gastroesophageal junction cancer	Margetuximab Pembrolizumab	Phase I/II	Recruiting
NCT02572687	Study of ramucirumab plus MEDI4736 in advanced gastrointestinal or thoracic malignancies	Ramucirumab MEDI4736	Phase I	Recruiting
NCT02443324	Study of ramucirumab plus pembrolizumab in participants with gastric or GEJ adenocarcinoma, NSCLC or transitional cell carcinoma	Ramucirumab Pembrolizumab	Phase I	Recruiting

9.3 CTLA-4

9.3.1 Introduction to CTLA-4

CTLA-4 is also known as CD152 and was identified as a member of the immunoglobulin superfamily closely related to the CD28 homolog [45]. It is present on the plasma membrane upon antigen recognition at immune synapses between T cells and antigen-presenting cells (APCs) [46, 47]. The CTLA-4 suppressive mechanisms behind T cell dysfunction have been attributed to the following steps: First, CTLA-4 has a 10- to 100-fold higher affinity for CD80 (B7-1) and CD86 (B7-2) than CD28, thus outcompeting CD28 for co-stimulation. Second, CTLA-4 transduces co-inhibitory signals through protein phosphatases. Third, CTLA-4 binds to CD80 and CD86, which leads to their internalization into T cells and results in decreased contact of antigen-presenting dendritic cells from co-stimulatory ligands. Fourth, CTLA-4 shortens the duration of immune synapse responses as a result of signal attenuation and integrin deactivation [48–53]. However, there is a difference in how CTLA-4 affects different T cell subsets [54]. As shown in Treg cells, CTLA-4 activated its function, thereby mediating immune tolerance [55] (Fig. 9.2).

The CTLA-4 blocking antibody Ipilimumab was approved by the FDA in 2011 for treating metastatic melanoma. It was the first immune checkpoint inhibitor approved for cancer treatment. Subsequent to this approval, it has also shown promising clinical responses in several other tumor types [56–58].

9.3.2 CTLA-4 in Gastric Cancers

There is quite a limited amount of preclinical research into CTLA-4 blockade strategy and gastric cancer. To this end, we sought to explore the clinical significance of CTLA-4 expression in gastric cancer. In the following section, we discuss some of the clinical trials that are targeting this pathway, either alone or in combination with other immunotherapies, in the treatment of gastric cancer.

9.3.2.1 Clinical Significance of CTLA-4 in Gastric Cancers

When compared with immune checkpoints PD-1 and PD-L1, there are far fewer studies that have investigated the expression, clinical associations, and prognosis of CTLA-4 in gastric cancer. Summarized below are those studies that have focused on the clinical significance of CTLA-4 in gastric cancer patients.

Kordi et al. analyzed promoter methylation, polymorphisms, and expression levels of CTLA-4 in 25 patients with gastric cancer. The study showed that the methylation of the CTLA-4 gene is associated with higher risk of gastric cancer, with lower gene expression levels in cancer tissues than in their relative normal margins (7.56 ± 17.35 vs. 15.45 ± 7.96, respectively). This study indicated

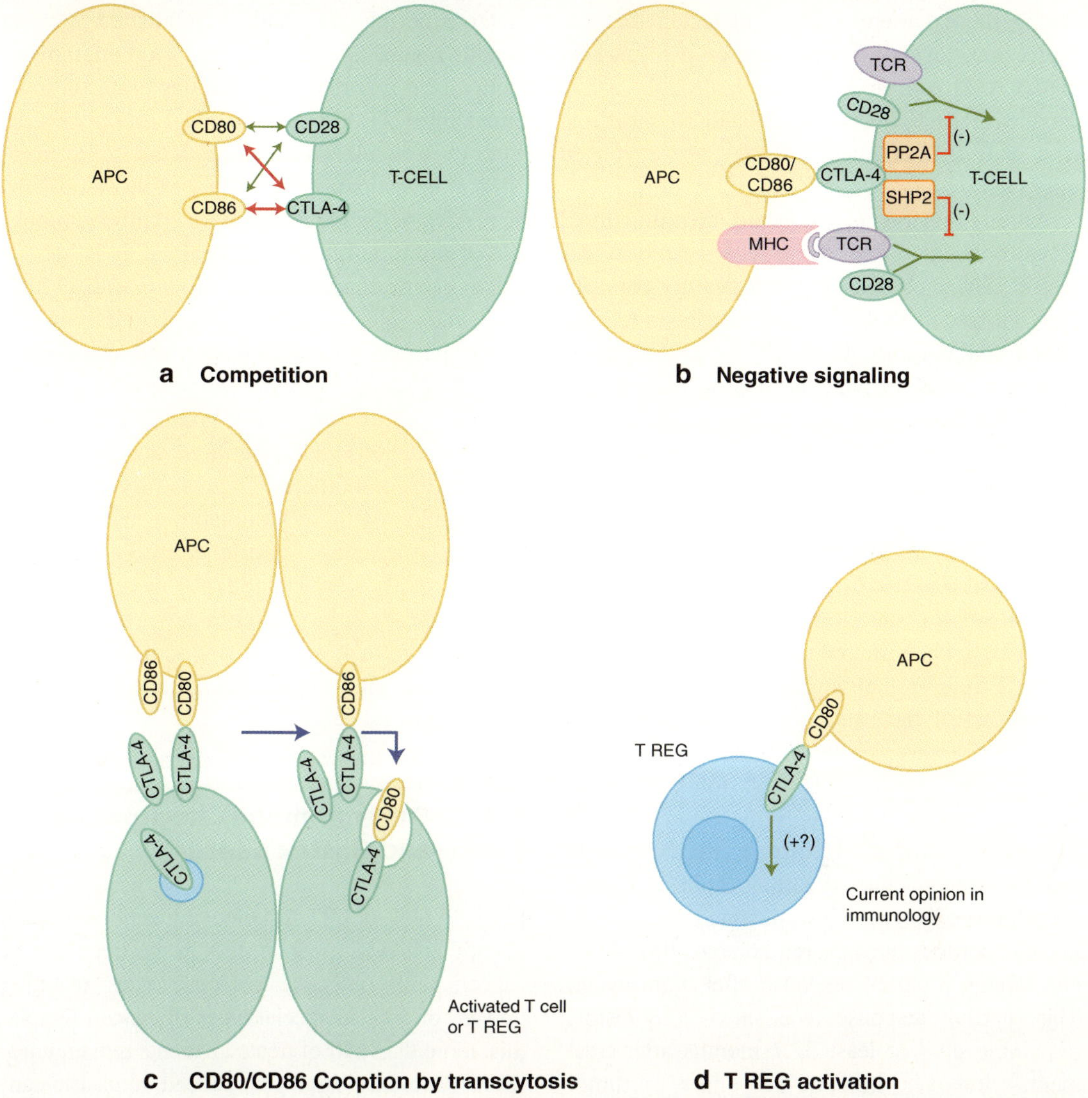

Fig. 9.2 Orchestrating combined immune checkpoint blockade for cancer immunotherapy *Curr Opin Immunol*. (2014) 27: 89–97. (**a**) Competition for CD80/86. (**b**) Transduction of inhibitory signal. (**c**) CD80/86 internazation into T cells. (**d**) Treg activation (Adapted from Orchestrating combined immune checkpoint blockade for cancer immunotherapy Curr Opin Immunol. (2014), Perez-Gracia JL et al. [55])

that gene silencing of CTLA-4 is possibly related to promoter hypermethylation. This could be one of the risk factors for gastric cancer. These results indicated that CTLA-4 is a potential therapeutic target for gastric cancer [59]. However, this study was conducted with a limited number of patients and requires a larger sample size for a more thorough, convincing understanding of the role CTLA-4 plays in the development of gastric cancer.

Suling et al. investigated over 1600 Asian and non-Asian gastric cancer patients and showed that gastric cancers from different genetic backgrounds exhibited distinct genetic signatures. When compared with Asian gastric cancers, non-Asian gastric cancers exhibited enrichment in multiple genes related to T cell biology, including the CD28 and CTLA-4 pathways. These findings indicated that geographical differences could influence patients' clinical outcomes. Moreover, it provided a rationale for future clinical trials targeting CTLA-4 inhibition in non-Asian gastric cancer patients [60].

Jin et al. included 243 gastric cancer patients and reported 65.8% positive CTLA-4 expression among these patients. They suggested that the expression levels of the suppressive markers PD-L1, CTLA-4, and IDO were strongly correlated with each other and related to intestinal type, well-differentiated histology, less advanced stages and reduced vascular invasion [25].

A study by Hou et al. selected three functional polymorphisms within the CTLA-4 gene in 205 gastric cancer patients and 262 healthy controls. They showed that +49A/G polymorphism AG and −1661A/G polymorphism GG were frequently observed in cancer patients than in healthy controls. Based on these results, they suggested that CTLA-4 variation may be an important factor impacting the risk of gastric cancer [61].

9.3.2.2 Clinical Studies of CTLA-4 in Gastric Cancers

Clinical studies centering on CTLA-4 and gastric cancer have been limited until fairly recently. In a Phase II trial, Tremelimumab was investigated in 18 patients of metastatic gastric and esophageal adenocarcinomas as a second-line treatment. The drug-related toxicity was well tolerated in all patients. Among those receiving tremelimumab, four patients had stable disease after treatment, and one patient achieved partial response. Though overall responses were low, the one patient showing a response achieved a remarkable clinical benefit, having a partial response after eight cycles. This partial response was also long-lasting, remaining until at least 32.7 months after treatment. Moreover, immune responses to tumor-associated antigens were also evaluated. To this end, eight patients responded to 5T4 and five patients responded to CEA. Patients with a post-treatment CEA proliferative response had a median survival of 17.1 months, while nonresponders had a median survival of 4.7 months. This difference revealed a correlation between treatment-related immune responses and clinical benefit [62]. Another Phase II trial (NCT01585987) for ipilimumab sought to examine its effects on metastatic gastric cancer and gastroesophageal junction cancer and importantly, to compare the efficacy of ipilimumab with the best supportive care treatment after first-line chemotherapy. This study has been completed, but results have yet to be published.

Considering the limited published clinical benefit regarding anti-CTLA-4 monotherapy as well as the reported high response rate of combined anti-CTLA-4 and anti-PD-1 therapy evaluated in a small group of patients [63], more clinical investigations and longer follow-ups will be needed to decide whether the combined blockade of immune inhibitory checkpoints is beneficial to gastric cancer patients. To this end, a Phase I/IIb study (NCT02340975) is ongoing in gastric cancer patients to evaluate the combined effects of the PD-L1 antibody durvalumab with tremelimumab. Moreover, a Phase I/II study (NCT01928394) is ongoing to investigate nivolumab monotherapy versus nivolumab in combination with ipilimumab for use in solid tumors (including gastric cancer). Finally, another study (NCT02488759) is ongoing to investigate the safety and efficacy of nivolumab plus ipilimumab in virus-associated tumors (CheckMate358)—including Epstein-Barr-virus-positive gastric cancer.

9.4 Other Immune Checkpoints and Gastric Cancer

PD-1, PD-L1, or CTLA-4 blocking antibodies have already achieved great success in the treatment of cancer, with objective response rates reaching upward of 50% in special types of cancer. Despite this, more than half of treated patients remain unresponsive to these strategies. Indeed, in gastric cancer, patients who could benefit from these therapies were much lower until recently. With this in mind, other inhibitory receptors should be investigated as potential treatment options to increase the frequency of objective responses in gastric cancer. In the following sections, the studies of two other immune inhibitory checkpoints, both of which may have potential use in the treatment and/or prognosis of gastric cancer, will be outlined.

9.4.1 Tim-3

9.4.1.1 Introduction to Tim-3

Tim-3 was first discovered in 2002 and was identified on T cells, most of which were either $CD4^+$

T helper type 1 (Th1) or CD8$^+$ T cytotoxic type 1 (Tc1) cells. The endogenous Tim-3 ligand is the S-type lectin galectin-9 (Gal-9), itself a soluble molecule that is widely expressed [64]. The interaction between Tim-3 and Gal-9 induces cell death. Tim-3 is considered to be a negative regulatory molecule for immune responses driven by Th1 and Tc1 [65]. There are eight members of Tim family (Tim-1–8) that have been discovered in mice. Comparatively, humans only express Tim-1, Tim-3, and Tim-4.

9.4.1.2 Preclinical Studies of Tim-3

A considerable amount of literature has been published on the immune inhibitory function of Tim-3 in preclinical cancer models, including gastrointestinal cancers. In murine models of colon carcinoma, Tim-3 blockade performs almost as effectively as PD-1 blockade [66]. Moreover, work has also shown that when combined with PD-1 blockade, the blocking of Tim-3 is more effective in some type of tumors. These include melanoma, sarcoma, and acute myelogenous leukemia [67]. These preclinical data support the potential for Tim-3 pathway blockade as an effective treatment for various types of cancer [68]. Collectively, these results suggest that a combined approach featuring Tim-3 and PD-1 may achieve optimal clinical efficacy.

9.4.1.3 Tim-3 and Gastric Cancer

At present, several attempts have been made to investigate the role of either Tim-3 or Gal-9 in gastric cancer patients as well as to explore their clinical significances.

A growing body of literature suggests that the Tim-3 and Gal-9 may play an important role in gastric carcinogenesis. For example, Jiang et al. used an immunohistochemical approach to investigate Gal-9 and Tim-3 expression in 305 samples of gastric cancer tissue. The percentage of positive expression of Gal-9 and Tim-3 was 86.2% and 60.0%, respectively. This suggests that higher expression of Gal-9 is related to better survival. Conversely, negative expression of Tim-3 was significantly correlated with better patient outcomes. The combination of Gal-9 and Tim-3 expression was an independent prognostic marker for gastric cancer [69]. In another study, Yang et al. assessed Gal-9 mRNA expression in 44 frozen primary gastric cancer tissues and healthy, adjacent tissue. These results showed a significant reduction of both Gal-9 and Tim-3 (> two-fold decrease) in 77% and 59% of the samples of gastric cancer, respectively. Moreover, Gal-9 expression was correlated with TNM stage, tumor differentiation, lymph node metastasis, and survival [70].

Cheng et al. found that Tim-3 expression was significantly upregulated on tumor-infiltrated T cells. Interestingly, on CD4$^+$ T cells, the expression level of Tim-3 was significantly associated with the size of tumor, the depth of tumor invasion, lymph node metastasis, and TNM stage. While on CD8$^+$ T cells, it was only relevant to TNM stage and tumor invasion. In accordance with the above findings, it was also shown that patients with higher Tim-3 levels on T cells had significantly poorer survival rates [71].

Apart from tissue analysis, Tim-3 expression in peripheral blood samples was also analyzed. It was found that PD-1 and Tim-3 were significantly higher on CD8$^+$ T cells of gastric cancer patients than those of healthy controls. In addition, PD-1 and Tim-3 expression on CD8$^+$ T cells was significantly correlated with each other in gastric cancer patients. Furthermore, statistically greater numbers of CD8$^+$ T cells positive for PD-1 and Tim-3 were seen in gastric cancer tissues than in PBMCs. Impaired immune responses were also detected in PD-1$^+$Tim-3$^+$CD8$^+$ T cells [34].

In addition to T cells, Wang et al. also found that Tim-3 levels in NK cells obtained from patients with gastric cancer were significantly higher than those in healthy controls. Tim-3 levels in NK cells were also associated with advanced tumor stage. In a tumor-bearing mouse model, Tim-3 levels in NK cells increased with tumor growth, indicating that tumor progression could induce Tim-3 expression on NK cells. Moreover, they reported that T-bet was a key factor involved in the regulation of Tim-3 [72]. Similarly, Rui et al. also found that the expression of Tim-3 on MDSCs in peripheral blood was higher in patients with gastric cancer [73].

Cao et al. performed a polymorphic screening for Tim-3 gene in gastric cancer in the Chinese population. This analysis revealed that three types of polymorphisms, −574G/T, −882C/T, and −1516G/T, were all located in the promoter region of Tim-3. These results indicate that the Tim-3 haplotypes may also be associated with increased gastric cancer susceptibility [74].

Up until now, there have been no clinical trials specifically investigated the use of anti-Tim-3 antibody for treatment of gastric cancer. A Phase I study (NCT02817633) evaluating the anti-Tim-3 antibody TSR-022 for use as a monotherapy as well as in combination with an anti-PD-1 antibody is currently recruiting patients with advanced solid tumors.

9.4.2 IDO

9.4.2.1 Introduction to IDO

Indoleamine 2,3-dioxygenase (IDO) is a group of negative immune regulators which has attracted much attention in recent years. It plays an important role in the catabolism of tryptophan, which is an essential amino acid in the process of T cell proliferation. Tryptophan degradation via the kynurenine pathway is enzymatically controlled at its first step. Among the IDO groups, IDO1 is most frequently expressed in many tumors and considered as the main contributor of tumor resistance against immune rejection. IDO1 inhibits T cell responses by two mechanisms: (1) local depletion of tryptophan, which is required for T cell proliferation, and (2) induction of apoptosis or growth arrest by tryptophan metabolites. A few years ago, IDO2 was also identified as an IDO1 homolog, but its function is not clearly known [75–78].

9.4.2.2 IDO and Gastric Cancer

Overexpression of IDO1 has been observed in gastric, breast, lung, pancreatic, and colorectal cancers [76, 79–81]. Zhang et al. sought to explore the expression of IDO in different subsets of tumor-infiltrating T cells in gastric cancer. Their results demonstrated that IDO overexpression and memory T cells (Tm) in the tumor microenvironment were correlated with both tumor stage and histological type. More importantly, they showed that patients with a lower percentage of $CD4^+$ Tm and $CD8^+$ Tm cells usually had higher IDO expression. It has been suggested that Tm plays a critical role in the antitumor immunity. The proliferation and the long existence of T cell memory may determine gastric carcinogenesis and carcinogenic progression. Therefore, a strategy targeting the IDO checkpoint might be associated with interfering in T cell memory function [82].

Similarly, Li et al. showed high IDO expression was present in gastric tumor tissue relative to normal tissue. High IDO expression was also related to low percentages of $CD4^+$ Tm/$CD8^+$ Tm and high percentages of $CD8^+$ T effector memory cells (Tem). Clinical characteristics such as larger tumor size, deeper tumor invasion, and lymph node metastasis were also correlated with high IDO expression [83].

Another study conducted by Kim et al. was concerned with the multiple immune suppressive checkpoints of gastric cancer and showed that, together with PD-L1 and CTLA-4, IDO was upregulated in gastric cancer tumor tissue. High IDO expression was also related to less advanced stages and well-to-moderate differentiation. Among these 243 patients, the positive rate of PD-L1, CTLA-4, and IDO expression was 43.6, 65.8, and 47.7%, respectively [25].

Taking into account the limited research on IDO expression and its role in gastric cancer, no clinical trials have been launched to date to target this pathway for the treatment of gastric cancer.

9.5 Conclusion and Future Perspectives

During the past few years, the strategy of checkpoint blockade therapy has achieved great success in a variety of tumor types. This is especially true for the application of PD-1/PD-L1 blocking antibodies. Although our knowledge about immune checkpoint and gastric cancer is largely based on preclinical studies and a limited set of clinical investigations, it is clear that more emphasis should be placed on this approach. A growing body of evidence has supported the hypothesis that aberrant expression of the immune checkpoint molecules in the tumor microenvironment of gastric cancer is correlated with clinical characteristics and prognosis. However, the different clinical settings used in these studies mean that the exact relationship between such aberrant expression and their association with worse or better clinical outcomes is still unclear.

More importantly, we can now comprehensively use molecular classification on certain types of gastric cancer to define some as immune "checkpoint-sensitive" tumors. In the future, using such fine-grained classifications will allow for the personalized application of checkpoint blockade. Ultimately, this will lead to the best therapeutic efficacies. In addition, accumulating preclinical as well as clinical studies has shown that the efficacy of checkpoint inhibition could be amplified through dual blockade or in combination with other immunotherapies such as cancer vaccines or adoptive cell therapy. As such, it is worth combining various immune regents to achieve a maximal effect. Moreover, it is possible that further applications of this approach with traditional chemotherapy or radiation therapy could achieve better clinical responses in patients with gastric cancer. However, this will require further investigation at both the basic and clinical research levels.

In conclusion, PD-1 and PD-L1 blockade as well as other immune checkpoint inhibition strategies are expected to be available in the future, thereby offering more opportunities for the treatment of gastric cancers.

References

1. Ishida Y, Agata Y, Shibahara K, Honjo T. Induced expression of PD-1, a novel member of the immunoglobulin gene superfamily, upon programmed cell death. EMBO J. 1992;11(11):3887–95.
2. Wong RM, Scotland RR, Lau RL, Wang C, Korman AJ, Kast WM, et al. Programmed death-1 blockade enhances expansion and functional capacity of human melanoma antigen-specific CTLs. Int Immunol. 2007;19(10):1223–34.
3. Good-Jacobson KL, Szumilas CG, Chen L, Sharpe AH, Tomayko MM, Shlomchik MJ. PD-1 regulates germinal center B cell survival and the formation and affinity of long-lived plasma cells. Nat Immunol. 2010;11(6):535–42.
4. Terme M, Ullrich E, Aymeric L, Meinhardt K, Desbois M, Delahaye N, et al. IL-18 induces PD-1-dependent immunosuppression in cancer. Cancer Res. 2011;71(16):5393–9.
5. Keir ME, Butte MJ, Freeman GJ, Sharpe AH. PD-1 and its ligands in tolerance and immunity. Annu Rev Immunol. 2008;26:677–704.
6. Kinter AL, Godbout EJ, McNally JP, Sereti I, Roby GA, O'Shea MA, et al. The common gamma-chain cytokines IL-2, IL-7, IL-15, and IL-21 induce the expression of programmed death-1 and its ligands. J Immunol. 2008;181(10):6738–46.
7. Chen DS, Irving BA, Hodi FS. Molecular pathways: next-generation immunotherapy inhibiting programmed death-ligand 1 and programmed death-1. Clin Cancer Res. 2012;18(24):6580–7.
8. Lee SJ, Jang BC, Lee SW, Yang YI, Suh SI, Park YM, et al. Interferon regulatory factor-1 is prerequisite to the constitutive expression and IFN-gamma induced upregulation of B7-H1 (CD274). FEBS Lett. 2006;580(3):755–62.
9. Muhlbauer M, Fleck M, Schutz C, Weiss T, Froh M, Blank C, et al. PD-L1 is induced in hepatocytes by viral infection and by interferon-alpha and -gamma and mediates T cell apoptosis. J Hepatol. 2006;45(4):520–8.
10. Youngnak P, Kozono Y, Kozono H, Iwai H, Otsuki N, Jin H, et al. Differential binding properties of B7-H1 and B7-DC to programmed death-1. Biochem Biophys Res Commun. 2003;307(3):672–7.
11. Yokosuka T, Takamatsu M, Kobayashi-Imanishi W, Hashimoto-Tane A, Azuma M, Saito T. Programmed cell death 1 forms negative costimulatory microclusters that directly inhibit T cell receptor signaling by recruiting phosphatase SHP2. J Exp Med. 2012;209(6):1201–17.
12. Azuma T, Yao S, Zhu G, Flies AS, Flies SJ, Chen L. B7-H1 is a ubiquitous antiapoptotic receptor on cancer cells. Blood. 2008;111(7):3635–43.
13. Weber JS, D'Angelo SP, Minor D, Hodi FS, Gutzmer R, Neyns B, et al. Nivolumab versus chemotherapy in patients with advanced melanoma who progressed after anti-CTLA-4 treatment (CheckMate 037): a randomised, controlled, open-label, phase 3 trial. Lancet Oncol. 2015;16(4):375–84.
14. Le DT, Uram JN, Wang H, Bartlett BR, Kemberling H, Eyring AD, et al. PD-1 Blockade in Tumors with Mismatch-Repair Deficiency. N Engl J Med. 2015;372(26):2509–20.
15. Larkin J, Chiarion-Sileni V, Gonzalez R, Grob JJ, Cowey CL, Lao CD, et al. Combined Nivolumab and Ipilimumab or Monotherapy in Untreated Melanoma. N Engl J Med. 2015;373(1):23–34.
16. Garon EB, Rizvi NA, Hui R, Leighl N, Balmanoukian AS, Eder JP, et al. Pembrolizumab for the treatment of non-small-cell lung cancer. N Engl J Med. 2015;372(21):2018–28.

17. Brahmer J, Reckamp KL, Baas P, Crino L, Eberhardt WE, Poddubskaya E, et al. Nivolumab versus Docetaxel in Advanced Squamous-Cell Non-Small-Cell Lung Cancer. N Engl J Med. 2015;373(2):123–35.
18. Ansell SM, Lesokhin AM, Borrello I, Halwani A, Scott EC, Gutierrez M, et al. PD-1 blockade with nivolumab in relapsed or refractory Hodgkin's lymphoma. N Engl J Med. 2015;372(4):311–9.
19. Khalil DN, Smith EL, Brentjens RJ, Wolchok JD. The future of cancer treatment: immunomodulation, CARs and combination immunotherapy. Nat Rev Clin Oncol. 2016;13(5):273–90.
20. Bartucci M, Ferrari AC, Kim IY, Ploss A, Yarmush M, Sabaawy HE. Personalized medicine approaches in prostate cancer employing patient derived 3D organoids and humanized mice. Front Cell Dev Biol. 2016;4:64.
21. Liu J, Blake SJ, Smyth MJ, Teng MW. Improved mouse models to assess tumour immunity and irAEs after combination cancer immunotherapies. Clin Transl Immunol. 2014;3(8):e22.
22. Lote H, Cafferkey C, Chau I. PD-1 and PD-L1 blockade in gastrointestinal malignancies. Cancer Treat Rev. 2015;41(10):893–903.
23. Wu C, Zhu Y, Jiang J, Zhao J, Zhang XG, Xu N. Immunohistochemical localization of programmed death-1 ligand-1 (PD-L1) in gastric carcinoma and its clinical significance. Acta Histochem. 2006;108(1): 19–24.
24. Hou J, Yu Z, Xiang R, Li C, Wang L, Chen S, et al. Correlation between infiltration of FOXP3+ regulatory T cells and expression of B7-H1 in the tumor tissues of gastric cancer. Exp Mol Pathol. 2014;96(3):284–91.
25. Kim JW, Nam KH, Ahn SH, Park do J, Kim HH, Kim SH, et al. Prognostic implications of immunosuppressive protein expression in tumors as well as immune cell infiltration within the tumor microenvironment in gastric cancer. Gastric Cancer. 2016;19(1):42–52.
26. Zhang L, Qiu M, Jin Y, Ji J, Li B, Wang X, et al. Programmed cell death ligand 1 (PD-L1) expression on gastric cancer and its relationship with clinic pathologic factors. Int J Clin Exp Pathol. 2015;8(9):11084–91.
27. Thompson ED, Zahurak M, Murphy A, Cornish T, Cuka N, Abdelfatah E, et al. Patterns of PD-L1 expression and CD8 T cell infiltration in gastric adenocarcinomas and associated immune stroma. Gut. 2016; doi:10.1136/gutjnl-2015-310839.
28. Böger C, Behrens HM, Mathiak M, Krüger S, Kalthoff H, Röcken C. PD-L1 is an independent prognostic predictor in gastric cancer of Western patients. Oncotarget. 2016;7(17):24269–83.
29. Zheng Z, Bu Z, Liu X, Zhang L, Li Z, Wu A, et al. Level of circulating PD-L1 expression in patients with advanced gastric cancer and its clinical implications. Chung-kuo yen cheng yen chiu (Chin J Cancer Res). 2014;26(1):104–11.
30. Savabkar S, Azimzadeh P, Chaleshi V, Nazemalhosseini Mojarad E, Aghdaei HA. Programmed death-1 gene polymorphism (PD-1.5 C/T) is associated with gastric cancer. Gastroenterol Hepatol Bed Bench. 2013;6(4):178–82.
31. Wang W, Li F, Mao Y, Zhou H, Sun J, Li R, et al. A miR-570 binding site polymorphism in the B7-H1 gene is associated with the risk of gastric adenocarcinoma. Hum Genet. 2013;132(6):641–8.
32. Saito H, Kuroda H, Matsunaga T, Osaki T, Ikeguchi M. Increased PD-1 expression on $CD4^+$ and $CD8^+$ T cells is involved in immune evasion in gastric cancer. J Surg Oncol. 2013;107(5):517–22.
33. Takaya S, Saito H, Ikeguchi M. Upregulation of Immune Checkpoint Molecules, PD-1 and LAG-3, on $CD4^+$ and $CD8^+$ T Cells after Gastric Cancer Surgery. Yonago Acta Med. 2015;58(1):39–44.
34. Takano S, Saito H, Ikeguchi M. An increased number of PD-1+ and Tim-3+ CD8+ T cells is involved in immune evasion in gastric cancer. Surg Today. 2016;46(11):1341–7.
35. Eto S, Yoshikawa K, Nishi M, Higashijima J, Tokunaga T, Nakao T, et al. Programmed cell death protein 1 expression is an independent prognostic factor in gastric cancer after curative resection. Gastric Cancer. 2016;19(2):466–71.
36. Cancer Genome Atlas Research Network. Comprehensive molecular characterization of gastric adenocarcinoma. Nature. 2014;513(7517):202–9.
37. Iizasa H, Nanbo A, Nishikawa J, Jinushi M, Yoshiyama H. Epstein-Barr virus (EBV)-associated gastric carcinoma. Viruses. 2012;4(12):3420–39.
38. Kim SY, Park C, Kim HJ, Park J, Hwang J, Kim JI, et al. Deregulation of immune response genes in patients with Epstein-Barr virus-associated gastric cancer and outcomes. Gastroenterology. 2015;148(1):137–47.
39. Shinozaki-Ushiku A, Kunita A, Fukayama M. Update on Epstein-Barr virus and gastric cancer (review). Int J Oncol. 2015;46(4):1421–34.
40. Gulley ML. Genomic assays for Epstein-Barr virus-positive gastric adenocarcinoma. Exp Mol Med. 2015;47:e134.
41. Smyth MJ, Ngiow SF, Ribas A, Teng MW. Combination cancer immunotherapies tailored to the tumour microenvironment. Nat Rev Clin Oncol. 2016;13(3):143–58.
42. Xiao Y, Freeman GJ. The microsatellite instable subset of colorectal cancer is a particularly good candidate for checkpoint blockade immunotherapy. Cancer Discov. 2015;5(1):16–8.
43. Muro K, Bang Y, Shankaran V, Geva R, Catenacci D, Gupta S, et al. LBA15A phase1B study of pembrolizumab (Pembro; MK-3475) in patients (Pts) with advanced gastric cancer. Ann Oncol. 2014;25(Suppl 4):v1–4.
44. Muro K, Bang YJ, Shankaran V, Geva R, Catenacci DVT, Gupta S, et al. Relationship between PD-L1 expression and clinical outcomes in patients (Pts) with advanced gastric cancer treated with the anti-PD-1 monoclonal antibody pembrolizumab (Pembro; MK-3475) in KEYNOTE-012. Presented at the ASCO 2015 gastrointestinal cancers symposium. 2015.
45. Brunet JF, Denizot F, Luciani MF, Roux-Dosseto M, Suzan M, Mattei MG, et al. A new member of the

immunoglobulin superfamily-CTLA-4. Nature. 1987;328(6127):267–70.
46. Insley PS, Bradshaw J, Greene J, Peach R, Bennett KL, Mittler RS. Intracellular trafficking of CTLA-4 and focal localization towards sites of TCR engagement. Immunity. 1996;4(6):535–43.
47. Pentcheva-Hoang T, Egen JG, Wojnoonski K, Allison JP. B7-1 and B7-2 selectively recruit CTLA-4 and CD28 to the immunological synapse. Immunity. 2004;21(3):401–13.
48. van der Merwe PA, Bodian DL, Daenke S, Linsley P, Davis SJ. CD80 (B7-1) binds both CD28 and CTLA-4 with a low affinity and very fast kinetics. J Exp Med. 1997;185(3):393–403.
49. Mandelbrot DA, Oosterwegel MA, Shimizu K, Yamada A, Freeman GJ, Mitchell RN, et al. B7-dependent T-cell costimulation in mice lacking CD28 and CTLA4. J Clin Invest. 2001;107(7):881–7.
50. Marengere LE, Waterhouse P, Duncan GS, Mittrucker HW, Feng GS, Mak TW. Regulation of T cell receptor signaling by tyrosine phosphatase SYP association with CTLA-4. Science. 1996;272(5265):1170–3.
51. Lee KM, Chuang E, Griffin M, Khattri R, Hong DK, Zhang W, et al. Molecular basis of T cell inactivation by CTLA-4. Science. 1998;282(5397):2263–6.
52. Qureshi OS, Zheng Y, Nakamura K, Attridge K, Manzotti C, Schmidt EM, et al. Trans-endocytosis of CD80 and CD86: a molecular basis for the cell-extrinsic function of CTLA-4. Science. 2011;332(6029):600–3.
53. Schneider H, Downey J, Smith A, Zinselmeyer BH, Rush C, Brewer JM, et al. Reversal of the TCR stop signal by CTLA-4. Science. 2006;313(5795):1972–5.
54. Raufi AG, Klempner SJ. Immunotherapy for advanced gastric and esophageal cancer: preclinical rationale and ongoing clinical investigations. J Gastrointest Oncol. 2015;6(5):561–9.
55. Perez-Gracia JL, Labiano S, Rodriguez-Ruiz ME, Sanmamed MF, Melero I. Orchestrating immune check-point blockade for cancer immunotherapy in combinations. Curr Opin Immunol. 2014;27:89–97.
56. Hodi FS, O'Day SJ, McDermott DF, Weber RW, Sosman JA, Haanen JB, et al. Improved survival with ipilimumab in patients with metastatic melanoma. N Engl J Med. 2010;363(8):711–23.
57. Kyi C, Postow MA. Checkpoint blocking antibodies in cancer immunotherapy. FEBS Lett. 2014;588(2):368–76.
58. Abdel-Rahman O. Immune checkpoints aberrations and gastric cancer; assessment of prognostic value and evaluation of therapeutic potentials. Crit Rev Oncol Hematol. 2016;97:65–71.
59. Kordi-Tamandani DM, Davani SK, Baranzehi T, Hemati S. Analysis of promoter methylation, polymorphism and expression profile of cytotoxic T-lymphocyte-associated antigen-4 in patients with gastric cancer. J Gastrointestin Liver Dis. 2014;23(3):249–53.
60. Lin SJ, Gagnon-Bartsch JA, Tan IB, Earle S, Ruff L, Pettinger K, et al. Signatures of tumour immunity distinguish Asian and non-Asian gastric adenocarcinomas. Gut. 2015;64(11):1721–31.
61. Hou R, Cao B, Chen Z, Li Y, Ning T, Li C, et al. Association of Cytotoxic T Lymphocyte-associated antigen-4 gene haplotype with the susceptibility to gastric cancer. Mol Biol Rep. 2010;37(1):515–20.
62. Ralph C, Elkord E, Burt DJ, O'Dwyer JF, Austin EB, Stern PL, et al. Modulation of lymphocyte regulation for cancer therapy: a phase II trial of tremelimumab in advanced gastric and esophageal adenocarcinoma. Clin Cancer Res. 2010;16(5):1662–72.
63. Wolchok JD, Kluger H, Callahan MK, Postow MA, Rizvi NA, Lesokhin AM, et al. Nivolumab plus ipilimumab in advanced melanoma. N Engl J Med. 2013;369(2):122–33.
64. Monney L, Sabatos CA, Gaglia JL, Ryu A, Waldner H, Chernova T, et al. Th1-specific cell surface protein Tim-3 regulates macrophage activation and severity of an autoimmune disease. Nature. 2002;415(6871):536–41.
65. Sakuishi K, Jayaraman P, Behar SM, Anderson AC, Kuchroo VK. Emerging Tim-3 functions in antimicrobial and tumor immunity. Trends Immunol. 2011;32(8):345–9.
66. Ngiow SF, von Scheidt B, Akiba H, Yagita H, Teng MW, Smyth MJ. Anti-TIM3 antibody promotes T cell IFN-gamma-mediated antitumor immunity and suppresses established tumors. Cancer Res. 2011;71(10):3540–51.
67. Zhou Q, Munger ME, Veenstra RG, Weigel BJ, Hirashima M, Munn DH, et al. Co-expression of Tim-3 and PD-1 identifies a $CD8^+$ T-cell exhaustion phenotype in mice with disseminated acute myelogenous leukemia. Blood. 2011;117(17):4501–10.
68. Anderson AC. Tim-3: an emerging target in the cancer immunotherapy landscape. Cancer Immunol Res. 2014;2(5):393–8.
69. Jiang J, Jin MS, Kong F, Cao D, Ma HX, Jia Z, et al. Decreased galectin-9 and increased Tim-3 expression are related to poor prognosis in gastric cancer. PLoS One. 2013;8(12):e81799.
70. Yang J, Zhu L, Cai Y, Suo J, Jin J. Role of downregulation of galectin-9 in the tumorigenesis of gastric cancer. Int J Oncol. 2014;45(3):1313–20.
71. Cheng G, Li M, Wu J, Ji M, Fang C, Shi H, et al. Expression of Tim-3 in gastric cancer tissue and its relationship with prognosis. Int J Clin Exp Pathol. 2015;8(8):9452–7.
72. Wang Z, Zhu J, Gu H, Yuan Y, Zhang B, Zhu D, et al. The clinical significance of abnormal Tim-3 expression on NK cells from patients with gastric cancer. Immunol Invest. 2015;44(6):578–89.
73. Xia R, Wang F, Gao T, Wen W, Lu B, Zhu Y, et al. The number of myeloid derived suppressor cells in the peripheral blood and tumor tissues in patients with gastric cancer and its clinical significance. Xi Bao Yu Fen Zi Mian Yi Xue Za Zhi. 2014;30(7):740–3.
74. Cao B, Zhu L, Zhu S, Li D, Zhang C, Xu C, et al. Genetic variations and haplotypes in TIM-3 gene and the risk of gastric cancer. Cancer Immunol Immunother. 2010;59(12):1851–7.

75. van Baren N, Van den Eynde BJ. Tumoral immune resistance mediated by enzymes that degrade tryptophan. Cancer Immunol Res. 2015;3(9):978–85.
76. Li R, Wei F, Yu J, Li H, Ren X, Hao X. IDO inhibits T-cell function through suppressing Vav1 expression and activation. Cancer Biol Ther. 2009;8(14):1402–8.
77. Fallarino F, Grohmann U, You S, McGrath BC, Cavener DR, Vacca C, et al. The combined effects of tryptophan starvation and tryptophan catabolites down-regulate T cell receptor zeta-chain and induce a regulatory phenotype in naive T cells. J Immunother. 2006;176(11):6752–61.
78. Munn DH, Shafizadeh E, Attwood JT, Bondarev I, Pashine A, Mellor AL. Inhibition of T cell proliferation by macrophage tryptophan catabolism. J Exp Med. 1999;189(9):1363–72.
79. Yu J, Sun J, Wang SE, Li H, Cao S, Cong Y, et al. Upregulated expression of indoleamine 2, 3-dioxygenase in primary breast cancer correlates with increase of infiltrated regulatory T cells in situ and lymph node metastasis. Clin Dev Immunol. 2011;2011:469135.
80. Creelan BC, Antonia S, Bepler G, Garrett TJ, Simon GR, Soliman HH. Indoleamine 2,3-dioxygenase activity and clinical outcome following induction chemotherapy and concurrent chemoradiation in stage III non-small cell lung cancer. Oncoimmunology. 2013;2(3):e23428.
81. Brandacher G, Perathoner A, Ladurner R, Schneeberger S, Obrist P, Winkler C, et al. Prognostic value of indoleamine 2,3-dioxygenase expression in colorectal cancer: effect on tumor-infiltrating T cells. Clin Cancer Res. 2006;12(4):1144–51.
82. Zhang R, Liu H, Li F, Li H, Yu J, Ren X. The correlation between the subsets of tumor infiltrating memory T cells and the expression of indoleamine 2,3-dioxygenase in gastric cancer. Dig Dis Sci. 2013;58(12):3494–502.
83. Li F, Huang J, Li S, Li H, Yu J, Ren X, et al. The subsets of dendritic cells and memory T cells correspond to indoleamine 2,3-dioxygenase in stomach tumor microenvironment. Tumour Biol. 2014;35(9):8691–8.

10 Therapeutic Vaccine of Gastric Cancer

Fangjun Chen and Fanyan Meng

10.1 Introduction

Gastric cancer is a challenging global health issue with poor outcomes for patients in advanced stages of the disease and, consequently, high mortality rates. Palliative treatment options have remained focused on chemotherapy, even though it only achieves modest survival benefits [1]. Although there have been recent advances in both genetic characterization and development of novel targeting agents, the overall prognosis for advanced cases of the disease remains disappointing. To this end, the median overall survival (OS) has been less than 12 months in the majority of trials [2]. When compared with other cancer types, there has been an increasing interest in the use of immunotherapy to improve gastric cancer outcomes.

Cancer immunotherapy is a treatment that uses activation and/or improvement of a person's immune system as a cancer-fighting entity. Over the past decades, various immunotherapeutic strategies have been developed for cancer treatment, such as immune checkpoint modulators, immune cell therapy, therapeutic antibodies, cancer treatment vaccines, and nonspecific immunotherapies. Briefly, tumor immunity can be divided into active and passive immunization (Fig. 10.1) [3]. Within this binary, cancer vaccines belong to the former immunization mode. Therapeutic cancer vaccines include those based on DNA/RNA, protein, peptide, viral vectors, tumor cells, and peptide-pulsed dendritic cells.

To target and destroy cancer, the immune system must be able to recognize a given cancer antigen and label it as a "foreign invader" [1]. Tumor antigens (TAs) can be roughly divided into two different classes according to the specificity of antigen: tumor-associated antigens (TAAs) and tumor-specific antigens (TSAs). TAAs are expressed in some normal tissues at low levels but overexpressed in tumor cells. In comparison, TSAs are expressed exclusively on tumor cells, including (1) cancer-testis antigens (CTAs), which is shared across multiple tumor types, but is typically restricted to non-MHC-bearing germ cells such as those found in adult testis tissue; (2) viral antigen, which is encoded by viral oncogenes and restrictively expressed in virus-associated tumors; and (3) neoantigen, the immunogenic product of genetic mutation in tumor cells, which can be processed, be presented to T cells, and activate antitumor immune responses.

With this in mind, the following section is focused on the topic of tumor vaccines and its application to gastric cancer immunology. It

F. Chen • F. Meng (✉)
The Comprehensive Cancer Centre of Drum Tower Hospital, Medical School of Nanjing University & Clinical Cancer Institute of Nanjing University, Nanjing 210008, China
e-mail: fanyanmeng@hotmail.com

J. Wei, B. Liu (eds.), *Personalized Management of Gastric Cancer*,
DOI 10.1007/978-981-10-3978-2_10

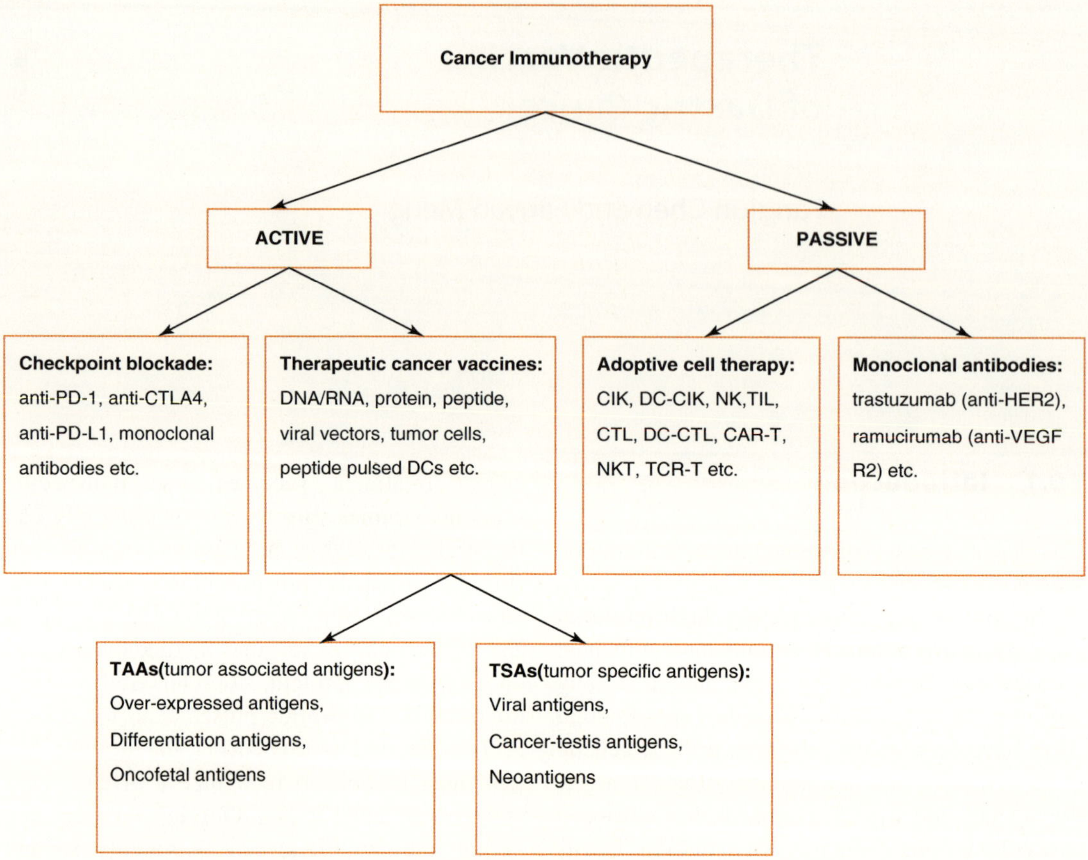

Fig. 10.1 A general classification of tumor immunotherapeutic approaches

seeks to outline the theoretical basis, historical trajectory, present-day status, and potential future applications for vaccine-based immunotherapy.

10.2 Scientific Basis of Immunotherapeutic Tumor Vaccines

10.2.1 MHC Molecules and T-Cell Epitopes

A MHC class I molecule consists of a polymorphic heavy chain, a β2-microglobulin subunit, and a peptide anchored to the binding groove that is located in the heavy chain. Classical MHC class I molecules include HLA-A, HLA-B, and HLA-C, which are encoded by genes at the HLA-A, HLA-B, and HLA-C loci, respectively. There are also some nonclassical MHC molecules with immunomodulatory functions, such as HLA-E, HLA-F, and HLA-G. Several hundred human heavy chain alleles have been discovered (http://www.allelefrequencies.net/). The peptide ligands binding to MHC class I molecules are generally composed of 9–10 amino acids. MHC class I peptides are predominantly derived from endogenous degraded proteins. This process begins with cleavage of the endogenous proteins by canonical proteasome and immunoproteasome with different cleavage preferences. Cleaved peptides in the cytosol are translocated into the endoplasmic reticulum and assembled into MHC class I molecules. Finally, the assembled MHC class I molecules are translocated to the cell membrane and recognized by T-cell receptors on T lymphocytes. Exogenous antigens can also generate MHC class I peptides through cross-presentation pathways. In this case, exogenous proteins are endocytosed into professional antigen-presenting cells (APCs) and then processed and loaded onto MHC class I molecules. MHC class II molecules are comprised of ligands with 12–26 amino acids. MHC class II peptides are mainly produced by professional APCs, such as DCs, macrophages, and B cells. Exogenous proteins are internalized, proteolyzed, and assembled into MHC class II molecules in the endosomes and lysosomes of the professional APCs. MHC class II molecules can also bind peptides originating from endogenous proteins by other processing pathways.

10.2.2 Identification of Tumor Antigens and Their Epitopes

10.2.2.1 Identification of Tumor Antigens

Different methods are developed to identify tumor antigens. Tumor-reactive T cells from cancer patients and tumor cell lines were used in the classical strategy for identifying T-cell antigens and their epitopes. Briefly, the tumor cDNA library is transfected into target cells expressing the appropriate HLA molecules. T cells deriving from tumor-infiltrating lymphocytes (TILs) or the peripheral blood mononuclear cells (PBMCs) are then adopted to identify T-cell antigens. The CTL epitope is subsequently defined through cDNA truncation and peptide recognition. Many T-cell antigens and their epitopes—including MAGE families, MART-1, tyrosinase, and gp100—are defined using this strategy. This direct immunological strategy is still the major strategy for identifying tumor-specific T-cell antigens and epitopes.

Gene-expression profiling is an approach used to identify overexpressed antigens found in tumors. This is because some of the genes overexpressed in tumor cells are involved in tumor growth and metastasis. The corresponding proteins of these overexpressed genes have been postulated to be useful tumor antigens. For example, the telomerase catalytic subunit is overexpressed in tumor cells and can be recognized by cytotoxic T lymphocytes [4].

Another method is serological screening of recombinant cDNA expression libraries (SEREX) and used to analyze B-cell responses in cancer patients in order to identify T-cell targets. NY-ESO-1, tyrosinase, and MAGE are examples of tumor antigens that have been identified via the SEREX strategy.

10.2.2.2 Identifying T-Cell Epitopes

Two strategies are currently being used to define T-cell epitopes and are based on different starting points. One is used in the case of knowing a T-cell reaction against tumor cells, without information regarding its specificity. Another begins with known tumor antigens, with allele-specific peptides being predicted and validated via a reverse immunological approach.

1. Identification of CTL epitopes via T-cell recognition

The classical approach for T-cell epitope identification is to investigate the specificity of a tumor-specific CTL clone in order to define its epitope. Tumor-specific CTL clones from the patients are adopted to screen a tumor cDNA library. The minimal epitope sequences are then revealed by truncation experiments. An alternative approach is to use MHC molecules presenting the relevant peptides. These molecules are then purified using biochemical methods. The mixture of MHC ligands is eluted from the MHC molecules and fractionated using high-performance liquid chromatography (HPLC). Finally, the fractions recognized by T cells are then analyzed using tandem mass spectrometry (MS/MS)-mediated sequencing.

2. Identification of CTL epitopes starting with tumor antigens

In comparison, this approach begins with known tumor antigens rather than preexisting T cells. Epitope prediction is the first and most important step to identifying CTL epitopes. Many software and online programs (e.g.,

BIMAS24, SYFPEITHI, and NetMHC) have been developed to predict peptides that have the possibility to bind with HLA molecules. In addition, other prediction methods can be adopted in order to more accurately predict the epitope. These strategies include proteasomal cleavage site and TAP translocation prediction methods. Once possible epitopes have been selected, they should be validated in order to demonstrate the presentation and immunogenicity of the predicted epitope. Peptide-specific T cells induced from human PBMC or HLA class I transgenic mice are often used as tools to test the natural presentation and immunogenicity of the epitope.

10.3 TAA-Based Tumor Vaccines

10.3.1 Peptides Derived from TAs and Their Properties

Tumor antigens (TAs) are the molecules specifically expressed or overexpressed by tumor cells. There are two types of tumor antigens, defined according to their tumor specificity [5]. Antigens with high tumor specificity include viral antigens, neoantigens, and cancer-testis antigens. Differentiated and/or overexpressed antigens belong to the class of antigens with low tumor specificity.

Some tumors are accompanied by viral infection. For instance, Epstein-Barr virus (EBV) was the first human virus to be directly associated with a wide range of cancers, including Burkitt's lymphoma, Hodgkin's disease, nasopharyngeal carcinoma, and gastric cancer [6]. Moreover, almost all cervical cancer cases (95%) are caused by the human papilloma virus (HPV) [7]. Finally, about 80% of hepatocellular carcinoma (HCC) is due to hepatitis B virus (HBV) or hepatitis C virus (HCV) infections [8]. Importantly, the connection between viral infection and cancer signifies that the virus antigens expressed by infected cells provides a source of distinctive tumor antigens.

Neoantigens are tumor antigens encoded by the mutated genes of tumor cells. They are promising immunogens and immunotherapeutic targets due to their tumor specificity as well as the lack of central tolerance [9]. Along with the development of whole-genome sequencing and the strategies used to systematically identify tumor neoepitopes, personalized tumor vaccines derived from neoantigens have been designed and utilized in both basic and clinical studies.

Cancer test antigens are proteins normally expressed in germline and trophoblastic cells, but are abnormally expressed in various human tumors (e.g., families of MAGE, BAGE, NY-ESO1, and SSX). They are immunogenic and highly tumor specific, so vaccines derived from them have been studied as safe and therapeutically beneficial.

Differentiated antigens are derived from proteins that are expressed in malignant and normal cells with the same lineage. Most of the discovered, differentiated antigens are expressed in melanoma cells. Moreover, melanoma differentiated antigens (MDAs) can be detected in melanoma cells as well as normal melanocytes. Antigen-specific T cells that have a high affinity to MHC complexes and that are loaded with MDA-derived peptides have been identified from the blood and tumors of the melanoma patients. This suggests that there is incomplete central tolerance to these antigens. MART-1, gp100, tyrosinase, and tyrosinase-related protein (TRP) 12 are the common MDAs. Vaccines derived from these proteins have been tested in clinical studies.

Overexpressed antigens are also potential sources of tumor immunotherapeutic vaccines. In comparison to normal cells, some genes are upregulated in tumor cells, ultimately resulting in overexpressed proteins. Peptides derived from these overexpressed proteins (e.g., Her2, MUC1, PRAME, survivin, and telomerase) can be recognized by specific T lymphocytes. This suggests that there is the potential for the development of promising cancer vaccines from them that can be used in the clinic. More specifically, ERBB2, Wilms tumor 1 (WT1), and mucin1 (MUC1) are all examples of these overexpressed antigens.

10.3.2 Single and Polyepitope Vaccines

The simple generations of peptide vaccines only involved single HLA-class I-restricted peptides. Polyepitope vaccines have been developed to enhance the clinical efficiency of vaccines. This is because tumors express multiple tumor antigen epitopes recognized by T cells and a single peptide vaccine targeting only one of them is often inefficient. Simple polyepitope vaccines contain several HLA-class I-restricted peptides from the same HLA type, such as HLA-A24-restricted LY6K-177 and VEGFR1-1084 peptides [10]. Personalized peptide vaccination (PPV) approach with a maximum of four HLA-matched vaccine peptides adopted was developed according to the finding that peptide-specific cellular responses could be detected from the peripheral blood of patients with tumors [11, 12]. A series of Phase I and II PPV clinical trials were performed and showed improved antigen-specific CTL and antibody responses and better clinical outcomes in patients with advanced tumors, such as melanoma, gastric, lung, and prostate cancers [13–16].

It is well-known that Th1 cells promote CTL cell survival and memory response, ultimately resulting in effective CTL-mediated antitumor responses [17]. Simultaneously, tumor-specific T-helper cells can induce tumor senescence and possess direct either antitumor and/or antiangiogenic effects [18, 19]. To this end, a series of studies were performed to study whether peptide vaccines could induce $CD4^+$ T-cell responses. For example, 6 HLA-DR-restricted melanoma helper peptides (6MHP) were used in patients with metastatic melanoma. Results showed that median survival was significantly longer for vaccinated patients. Moreover, that appearance of a specific Th1-dominant $CD4^+$ T-cell response was related with enhanced survival in vaccinated patients [20].

Vaccination using long peptides with both $CD8^+$ and $CD4^+$ epitopes is another proposed strategy for inducing an antitumor response in patients with tumors. Some clinical trials using long peptide cancer vaccines for malignancies have been conducted. For instance, GV1001 is a peptide vaccine with a 16-aa human telomerase reverse transcriptase (hTERT) sequence that can be loaded into multiple HLA class II molecules and may bind the putative HLA class I molecules [21, 22]. A GV1001 Phase II trial in non-small cell lung cancer (NSCLC) patients who had been vaccinated after receiving chemoradiotherapy showed a good toleration to the vaccine. Importantly, it immunized the majority (80%) of NSCLC patients and established a durable T-cell memory [23]. GV1001 vaccination in patients with advanced stage IV melanoma revealed a peptide-specific immune response in 78% (18 out of 23) of the evaluated patients [24].

However, some clinical trials have failed to show effective results in patients with certain types of cancers. For example, a study was performed to explore the safety and immunogenicity in non-resectable pancreatic carcinoma patients using GV1001 vaccination with chemotherapy. Although the combined therapy was safe, the immune responses weren't strong and lasting enough [25]. In a separate study, six cutaneous T-cell lymphoma (CTCL) patients were vaccinated with the GV-peptide. Unfortunately, none demonstrated objective clinical responses to the vaccination [26]. Taken together, it is clear that further studies need to be conducted to definitively state the effectiveness of a GV1001vaccination in cancer. It should also be noted that other studies using both short- and long-peptide vaccinations aimed at inducing both $CD4^+$ and $CD8^+$ responses have been performed [27, 28].

10.3.3 Clinical Application of Vaccination with TAA Peptides in Gastric Cancer

10.3.3.1 Lymphocyte Antigen 6 Complex Locus K (LY6K)

LY6K has been revealed as a tumor-associated antigen in various tumor types, including those found in bladder, breast, and lung cancers. To this end, it has been reported that vaccine therapy with peptide LY6K-177 stimulated an antigen-specific CD8$^+$ CTL response in patients with esophageal carcinoma [29]. This expression was also immunohistochemically identified in about 85% of gastric cancer samples [30]. Given this past work, a Phase I clinical trial featuring vaccination with HLA-A*2402-restricted LY6K-derived peptide LY6K-177 was conducted at Kinki University in patients with advanced or recurrent gastric cancer [30]. Methodologically, LY6K-177 peptide was mixed with incomplete Freund's adjuvant ISA 51 and administered intracutaneously to either the inguinal region or axilla of patients. There was no evidence of systemic toxicology during the observation period, suggesting that the peptide vaccine was safe. Three out of six patents achieved a stable disease (SD) clinical response. Moreover, the presence of more specific spots in an ELISPOT assay was correlated with increased survival rates [30].

10.3.3.2 MAGE-A3

There is positive expression of melanoma antigen-A3 genes (MAGE-A3) in over 50% of gastric cancer tumor tissue [31, 32]. Given this, vaccination of dendritic cells (DCs) loaded with both HLA-A2-restricted peptide MAGE-A3-271 and HLA-A24-restricted peptide MAGE-A3-195 derived from MAGE-A3 was tested in the patients with gastrointestinal carcinomas. Postvaccination, peptide-specific CTL responses were detectable in 50% (4/8) of patients. Moreover, tumor markers declined in seven patients. These results suggest that the treatment is a safe and promising immunotherapeutic method for gastrointestinal carcinomas [33].

10.3.3.3 HER-2

HER-2is a transmembrane tyrosine-specific kinase. It is overexpressed at a median rate of 18% (range, 4–53%) of gastric cancers [34]. A Phase I vaccination trial in patients with gastric cancer via DCs pulsed with HLA-A2-restricted HER-2-derived peptide HER2-369 showed that no serious adverse effects were observed in the patients who had received the vaccination. Furthermore, HER2-369 peptide-specific CTL was shown in six of nine patients after immunization. Of these, one patient underwent a partial clinical response and another showed stabilized disease status [35].

10.3.3.4 VEGFR1 and VEGFR2

Vascular endothelial growth factors (VEGFs) are highly specific mitogens for vascular endothelial cells and important in tumor angiogenesis and vasculogenesis. VEGF receptors (VEGFRs) bind different VEGFs and result in different biological responses, which can include angiogenesis, lymphangiogenesis, and inflammatory cell recruitment [36]. As such, both VEGFR1 and VEGFR2 are important antiangiogenic targets. A Phase I/II study of HLA-A24-restricted peptide vaccines used VEGFR1-1084 and VEGFR2-169 in combination with therapeutic agents S-1 and cisplatin in advanced or recurrent gastric cancer patients. Results indicated that this combined approach was both safe and highly effective to patients with either advanced or recurrent gastric cancer. More specifically, VEGFR1-1084- and VEGFR2-169-specific CTL responses were each induced in 82% (18/22) of patients. Of those tested, twelve patients demonstrated a partial response, while ten showed a stable disease status after two cycles of the combination treatment. Collectively, these results suggest that this combined strategy gives promise for the therapy of advanced cancers.

10.3.3.5 LY6K and VEGFR1

A Phase I trial of a peptide vaccination with HLA-A24-restricted LY6K-177 and VEGFR1-1084 peptides in patients with chemotherapy-resistant, advanced, and unresectable gastric cancer showed that such vaccination was safe for advanced gastric cancer. Four out of 12 patients had a stable disease state after a single treatment course in this study [10].

10.3.3.6 WT1 and MUC1

HLA-A2402-restricted Wilms' tumor gene WT1-modified peptide (CYTWNQMNL) has an amino-acid mutation (M to Y at position 2) to increase the binding affinity to HLA-A*2402 molecules. With this substitution, WT1-specific CTL was more effectively elicited than if the wild-type peptide from PBMC of HLA-A*2402-positive healthy volunteers was used [37]. To this end, vaccination of DC pulsed with MUC1 long peptide (TRPAPGSTAPPAHGVTSAPDTRPAP-GSTAP) was safely used in patients with recurrent ovarian cancer [38]. Furthermore, vaccination of DC pulsed with WT1 peptide and MUC1 long peptide was used in a patient with locally recurrent gastric cancer. The patient had been in remission for 30 months, suggesting the therapeutic benefit of intratumoral injections of DCs into the patients who could not undergo endoscopic submucosal dissection or surgery [39].

10.3.3.7 Personalized TAA Peptide Vaccination

Vaccinations can be made by screening personalized peptides according to preexisting T-cell responses to the given peptide. Patients with advanced gastric cancer were screened using a 16-peptide library for HLA-A2 allele and a 14-peptide library for HLA-A24 allele. Enhanced T-cell and antibody responses to the screened peptides were detected. Crucially, patients with the immune responses to the vaccinated peptides showed prolonged survival [14]. Another study featuring personalized peptide vaccinations with TS-1was done for advanced gastric and/or colorectal carcinoma patients. This study also showed that the combination treatment was well tolerated. Moreover, postvaccination peptide-specific IgG and interferon-gamma production by CTL were both increased in 9/11 and 7/11, respectively [40].

10.4 Neoantigen-Based Tumor Vaccines

10.4.1 Introduction

Over the course of its evolution, the immune system has developed to recognize and destroy foreign invaders. Given this basis, the foundation of a successful immunotherapy is inherently an issue of "self" versus "non-self" discrimination [41]. Until recently, the majority of researches in tumor immunotherapy were placed on tumor-associated antigens and shared antigens expressed in both tumors and normal tissues [42, 43]. However, the low affinity to TCRs resulting from incomplete central tolerance and on-target but off-tumor toxicity limits the application of these antigens. To this end, work in transgenic mice with non-mutated, tumor antigen-specific TCR expressed in all T cells showed they were unable to reject tumors that express the P1A antigen [43]. Highly specific tumor antigens that are displayed exclusively by tumor cells without normal cell expression have the potential to elicit a robust tumor-specific, immune response. This specificity is theorized to result in minimal risk for adverse effects, thus making it a promising target for cancer immunotherapies such as therapeutic vaccines and engineered T cells [44, 45]. On theoretical grounds, cancer rejection epitopes may be derived from one of two antigen classes. A first class of potential cancer rejection antigens is formed by non-mutated proteins to which T-cell tolerance is incomplete—for instance, because of their restricted tissue expression pattern, as seen in cancer-testis antigens (CTAs). A second class of potential cancer rejection antigens is derived from gene segments which are completely absent in normal human genome and include both viral and neoantigens [44]. Among these classes of cancer-specific antigens, neoantigens have received the most attention since they are taken to be strictly tumor specific. With this in mind, scientists have sought to harness this specificity to draw the cancer out of its cloak of immune tolerance. In this manner, it would be visible, allow for a provocation of a T-cell response, and putatively lead to cancer control or eradication.

When compared with non-mutated self-antigens, it has been proposed that neoantigens are more intimately correlated with tumor control [46]. Possible reasons for this are as follows: (1) some somatic mutations may serve as core steps in the process of oncogenesis and could influence or decide biological tumor behaviors [47]; (2) neoantigens are expressed exclusively in tumor tissue and therefore minimize the risk of on-target, off-tumor killing of healthy tissue; (3) finally, given that neoantigens are derived from mutations acquired during in tumorigenesis, the TCR repertoire of T-cell progenitors has not encountered neoantigens during thymic development. In theory, this would lead to a lack of central tolerance toward neoantigens. Neoantigen-specific T cells should not be deleted by negative selection and may be present in circulation [48].

It is known that gastric cancers display a high somatic mutational burden, with only melanoma, lung, and bladder cancers displaying a more mutated profile [47]. There are genetic and etiological features specific to gastric cancers, which may have relevance when considering their suitability for immune-targeting approaches.

In the past two decades, a cDNA library was frequently utilized in screening for unique neoantigens [49]. The classical cDNA library screening approach, which led to the discovery of multiple neoantigens, is a labor-intensive method that inherently low throughput. Collectively, this can lead to failures in identifying some mutated antigens. A large fraction of the mutations found in human tumors is patient specific, meaning that they are not shared between patients. Therefore, technologies that are designed to analyze T-cell reactivity against putative mutation-derived neoantigens should be based on the genome of an individual tumor [44]. Recently, the development of whole-exome sequencing technologies has made the identification of non-synonymous tumor mutations easier and more efficient. To this end, mutated peptide immunogenicity was analyzed using a prediction algorithm. The potential neoantigens that resulted from this analysis underwent further experiments to investigate their inherent T-cell reactivity [50, 51].

The application of modern sequencing technology to the development of personalized neoantigen-based vaccines represents an exciting fusion of genomics and immunotherapy, with potentially important clinical implications for gastric cancer treatment.

10.4.2 Evidence That Neoantigens Are Dominant Tumor Regression Antigens

Long-term follow-up studies have shown that a substantial subset of patients receiving tumor-infiltrating lymphocytes (TILs) for metastatic melanoma experienced complete, lasting, and even curative tumor regression [52]. This field was pioneered by Steven Rosenberg of National Cancer Institute (NCI), whose team developed methods for the isolation and culture of tumor-infiltrating lymphocytes (TILs). After lymhodepleting chemotherapy, TILs were reinfused together with exogenous IL2 to heavily pretreat patients with metastatic melanoma. This approach resulted in objective clinical responses in 52/93 patients (56%) and complete responses in 20/93 patients (22%) [53]. Other medical centers, such as the MD Anderson Cancer Center in Houston, TX, USA, had overall responses in 13/31 patients (42%) [54].

Recent studies have more specifically investigated the tumor antigens recognized by TILs and the probable specificities of the T cells mediating tumor rejection. Early studies identified TILs and other T cells in melanoma with reactivity against the shared tumor/self-melanocyte differentiation antigens (MDAs) (e.g., gp100, MART1, tyrosinase) [52]. However, both melanomas and normal melanocytes in skin and retina express MDAs. Given this, autoimmune toxicities against these normal tissues were rarely observed—even in patients who experienced profound tumor regression. The frequency of MDA-specific T cells in bulk TIL populations was also generally low [55, 56]. Conversely, TCR T-cell therapies that specifically target MDAs with high affinity have been shown to consistently induce autoimmune toxicities and rarely mediate tumor regression [57]. Therefore, the primary approach for TIL antitumor effects should not be ascribed to MDA-specific T cells. In reality, increasing evidence has suggested that neoantigens derived from genetic mutations are the main targets of tumor-reactive TILs and the primary cancer rejection antigens in melanoma. These mutations result in neoepitopes which can be recognized by TILs. Moreover, it is possible that T cells with specificity for these neoepitopes constitute the dominant tumor-reactive populations in TILs [58, 59].

Unlike self-antigens such as MDAs, T-cell affinity for mutated epitopes is not limited by thymic negative selection. TIL clones against mutated gene products routinely display high target antigen avidity and robust recognition of autologous tumor lines [58, 59]. It seems likely, therefore, that melanoma immunogenicity is linked to the high frequency of mutational events in this cancer. Moreover, that T cells specific for mutated gene products are responsible for tumor regression in patients receiving TIL therapy.

Checkpoint inhibitor therapy, such as anti-CTLA-4 and/or anti-PD-1 monoclonal antibody, blocks the inhibitory signals toward T cells. It is a revolutionary cancer treatment and has achieved significant clinical benefits including robust and long-lasting responses in several different malignancies [60–63]. Mechanistically, such checkpoint agents activate the immune system in order to attack tumor cells. To this end, Gubin and colleagues used genomics and bioinformatics approaches to identify neoantigens derived from tumor-specific mutant proteins as a major class of T-cell rejection antigens. This was done following anti-PD-1 and/or anti-CTLA-4 therapy in a sarcoma mouse model. Furthermore, they showed that therapeutic synthetic peptide vaccines incorporating these mutant epitopes induced tumor rejection to levels comparable to those of checkpoint blockade immunotherapy.

It has been recently proposed that the mutation load and neoantigen landscape might serve as biomarkers to predict clinical responsiveness to checkpoint blockade therapy, given that a mutational gene signature was inferred to correlate with the long-term clinical benefits seen in anti-CTLA-4 therapy [64]. Recently, Rizvi and colleagues used whole-exome sequencing of non-small cell lung cancers treated with anti-PD-1 (pembrolizumab). Their results confirmed that they had a higher, non-synonymous mutation burden in tumors associated with improved objective response, robust clinical benefit, and progression-free survival [65]. Subsequently, a separate study enrolling more than 100 patients with metastatic melanoma confirmed that those with the highest neoantigen load were most likely to respond to ipilimumab [66, 67]. Following this study, Diaz, Jr. et al. [68] found that colorectal cancers that had a large number of somatic mutations caused by mismatch-repair defects were susceptible to immune checkpoint blockade. For mismatch repair–deficient colorectal cancers, the immune-related objective response and immune-related progression-free survival rates were 40% and 78%, respectively. For mismatch repair–proficient colorectal cancers, the rates were 0% and 11%, respectively. Whole-exome sequencing revealed a mean of 1782 somatic mutations per tumor in mismatch repair–deficient colorectal cancers, compared with 73 in mismatch repair–proficient tumors. High somatic mutational loads were associated with prolonged progression-free survival.

Taken together, these studies revealed that neoantigens are not only important targets for checkpoint blockade therapy but that they can also be used to develop personalized, cancer-specific vaccines. Mechanistically, they can also be used to probe the underpinnings of different checkpoint blockade treatments. Indeed, neoantigen-specific T cells have been shown to underlie the clinical responses to many current standard treatments and immunotherapeutic interventions.

10.4.3 Neoantigen Identification

Tumor-specific mutations are ideal targets for cancer immunotherapy, as they lack expression in healthy tissues and can potentially be recognized as neoantigens by the mature T-cell repertoire. The predominant obstacle for the clinical use of neoantigen-based vaccine approaches is the fact that every patient's tumor possesses a unique set of mutations ("the mutanome"). In order for such a therapeutic approach to be effective, each mutanome must first be identified. Over the past two decades, classical cDNA library screening has been utilized to screen neoantigens. In this approach, cDNA library and MHC molecules were overexpressed in cell lines and then cocultured with T cells. This was done to identify antigens that could successfully induce T-cell activation, which was monitored by up-regulation of cytokine secretion and active markers [49]. The development of exome sequencing and bioinformatics has allowed for significant technical advances in the rapid identification for personalized cancer neoantigens. As such, they have intrigued immunologists into targeting these mutations for cancer immune therapy.

To this end, the Rosenberg research group at the National Cancer Institute has developed a screening approach involving mining whole-exome sequence data and MHCI/peptide bind prediction algorithm to identify neoantigens expressed in patients with melanoma [59]. Using this approach, they have successfully identified mutated antigens expressed on autologous tumor cells that were recognized by three bulk TIL lines from three individuals with melanoma that were associated with objective tumor regressions following adoptive cell transfer. However, this approach is limited by the accuracy of the predictive algorithms that are used. At times, these algorithms can be adequate, sometimes even resulting in excessively large candidate numbers. Yadav and colleagues developed a screening approach that combines whole-exome and transcriptome sequencing analysis with mass spectrometry to identify neoepitopes in two widely used murine tumor models [69]. Their predictions lead to the generation of peptide-MHC I dextramers, enabling the monitoring of the kinetics and distribution of antitumor T-cell responses both before and after vaccination. Moreover, Kalaora and colleagues [70] also reported on a combined whole-exome sequencing and mass spectrometry method to analyze the mutated HLA-I peptidome of human melanoma cells.

Another method is the use of tandem minigenes (TMGs) that encode polypeptides containing a mutated amino acid residue flanked on their N- and C-termini by 12–13 amino acids. The previous work synthesized tandem minigene constructs, which were then used to transfect autologous APCs or cell lines co-expressing autologous HLA molecules. Using this method, Rosenberg and colleagues reported a patient with widely metastatic cholangiocarcinoma whose lung metastases were resected and adopted as a source for WES. This revealed 26 non-synonymous mutations [71]. Finally, they constructed three TMGs that covered all 26 non-synonymous mutations and demonstrated that TILs from this metastatic cholangiocarcinoma patient contained $CD4^+$ T cells that recognized a mutation in erbb2 interacting protein (ERBB2IP) expressed by the cancer. Using NGS combined with a high-throughput, immunological screening approach constructed of tandem minigenes, they demonstrated that TILs from 9/10 patients with metastatic gastrointestinal cancers contained $CD4^+$ and/or $CD8^+$ T cells that recognized one to three neoepitopes derived from patient-specific somatic mutations [72].

10.4.4 MHC II-Restricted Neoantigens and $CD4^+$ T Cells in Antitumor Immunity

Given that $CD8^+$ CTLs can directly kill tumor cells and destroy tumor masses in vivo, much attention has been paid to the role of $CD8^+$ T cells in tumor immunotherapy. To this end, a series of MHC-class I-restricted TAs have been selected and identified. Although antigen-specific $CD8^+$ T cells are widely considered to be superior, there are many advantages to $CD4^+$ T-cell-mediated responses to tumor antigens over $CD8^+$ T cells [73]. These advantages are as follows: (1) as opposed to the restricted HLA type of $CD8^+$ T-cell-mediated immunity, $CD4^+$ T-cell-mediated immunity is much more HLA promiscuous; (2) independent activation of $CD4^+$ T cells relative to antigen presentation by tumor cells, meaning there is no dampening due to their impaired presentation machinery; (3) $CD4^+$ T cells can play a supporting role like T helper cells; (4) $CD4^+$ T cells are able to directly mediate cytotoxicity, in an IFN-γ and MHC-class II-restricted way that is independent of either $CD8^+$ T or NK cells in host; (5) tumor cells can process and present MHC class II epitopes by autophagy; (6) IFN-γ can induce up-regulation of MHC class II in tumor cells, thus rendering them susceptible to $CD4^+$ T-cell-mediated cytotoxicity [18]; (7) $CD4^+$ Th cells secrete multiple cytokines once antigens are encountered, thereby inducing an inflammatory microenvironment that can provide a co-stimulatory signal for innate and adaptive immune cells; finally, (8) $CD4^+$ T cells help $CD8^+$ T cells to proliferate, maintain their function, and infiltrate tumors.

As mentioned above, MHC class II-restricted neoantigens and neoantigen-reactive CD4+ T cells have the potential to not only realize a broader range of immune responses but also a stronger and longer-lasting immune response when compared with single MHC class I-restricted neoantigens. Tools for identifying MHC class I molecule restricted neoantigens are relatively efficient. However, the algorithms to predict epitopes that bind to MHC class II molecules and engage receptors on CD4+ T cells are far less accurate [67]. More recently, Sahin et al. conducted an experiment that found 80–90% of immunogenic neoepitopes were recognized by CD4+ T rather than CD8+ T cells. This demonstrated that personalized tumor mutant neoantigens are perhaps more likely to bind to MHC II molecules [74]. They then established a process by which mutations screened out by exome sequencing could be identified as vaccine targets simply through bioinformatic prioritization combining expression level and major histocompatibility complex (MHC) class II-binding capacity of neoantigens. Thus, this would enable the production of poly-neoepitope messenger RNA vaccines much more conveniently and rapidly.

The neoantigens identified in the study elicited antitumor immunity in three different mouse models. Based on these results, they showed that the combination of abundant expression and high MHC class II binding could effectively restrict the screening scope of neoantigens. Thus, this approach could offer a simplified screening method for MHC class II-restricted neoantigens.

10.4.5 Potential Clinical Applications of Neoantigen-Based Cancer Vaccines in Gastric Cancer

It is well known that gastric cancer displays a high somatic mutational burden, with only melanoma, lung, and bladder cancers displaying a more mutated profile [47]. Up until now, very few tumor neoantigens have been identified in somatic tumors (Tables 10.1 and 10.2). However, stomach cancers have sufficient mutational loads to generate neoantigens. In 2014, TCGA described a new molecular classification for gastric cancer (GC), dividing it into four subtypes: EBV-positive tumors (EBVaGC), microsatellite-instability (MSI) tumors, tumors with chromosomal instability, and genomically stable tumors [75]. PD-L1 may have higher expression levels within the EBV and MSI subgroups—in the first case, from viral stimulation and, in the second, encouraged by an elevated mutational rate. It is important to further analyze these subtypes prospectively and determine whether they truly enable selection for checkpoint blockade and/or neoantigen-based immunotherapy.

Table 10.1 Already-identified MHC class I-restricted neoantigens in solid tumors

Gene/protein	HLA	Peptide [76]	Position
CTNNB1	A24	SYLDSGIHF [77]	S37F
CDK4	A2	ACDPHSGHFV [78]	R24C
CDK12	A11	CILGKLFTK [59]	E928K
CLPP	A2	ILDKVLVHL [79]	P248L
GAS7	A2	SLADEAEVYL [59]	H149Y
HSP70-2	A2	SLFEGIDIYT [80]	F293I
MART2	A1	FLEGNEVGKTY [81]	G448E
ME1	A2	FLDEFMEGV [82]	A231G
TP53	A2	VVPCEPPEV [83]	Y220C
K-RAS	*B35*	VVVGAVGVG [84]	G12V
	A2	KLVVVGADGV [85]	G12D
	A2	KLVVVGAVGV [85]	G12V
	A3302	VVGACGVGK [86]	G12C
N-RAS	A1	ILDTAGREEY [87]	Q61R

Table 10.2 Already-identified MHC class II-restricted neoantigens in solid tumor

Gene/protein	HLA	Peptide	Position
B-RAF	DR4	EDLTVKIGDFGLATEKSRWSGSHQFEQLS [88]	V600E
KRAS	DRB1*0101	EYKLVVVGAVGVGKS [89]	G12V
	DQA1*0301	CLLDILDTAGLEEYSAMRD [90]	Q61L
	DRB1*0302		Q61L
	DQ8		Q61L
	DQ4		Q61L
	DQ	KLVVVGAVGVGKS [91]	G12V
	DQ7/DP3/DR2	MTEYKLVVVGARGVGKSALTIQLIQ [91]	G12R
	DR	LVVVGARGVGKSAL [92]	G12R
	DR	LVVVGAKGVGKSAL [92]	G12K
	DQ	LVVVGAAGVGKSAL [92]	G12A
	DQ	LVVVGAGVVGKSAL [92]	G13V
PTPRK	DR10	PYYFAAELPPRNLPEP [93]	G677R
IDH1	DRB1*0101	GWVKPIIIGHHAYGDQYRAT [94]	R132H

Muro and colleagues showed that pembrolizumab was active in 40% of pretreated GC patients with PD-L1-expressing tumors, with a response rate of 22%, a 6-month progression free survival rate of 24%, a 6-month OS rate of 69%, and manageable side effects [95]. This was in line with the aforementioned studies, which indicated that checkpoint blockade therapy targets tumor-specific mutant antigens [64]. Collectively, this research indirectly confirms that there are abundant neoantigens in gastric cancer.

The Rosenberg research group used NGS combined with high-throughput immunological screening to show that virtually all patients with metastatic gastrointestinal cancers (9/10) harbor tumor mutation-specific T cells. This finding provides further evidence for the value in developing personalized vaccine and/or adoptive cell therapies targeting immunogenic tumor mutations [72].

10.5 Tumor Vaccine-Based Combined Treatment Strategies

As checkpoint blockade boosts T-cell recognition of tumor antigens, the two approaches should theoretically potentiate each other. Thus, this combined approach might even increase the percentage of people who benefit from checkpoint inhibitor therapy [67]. The immune modulating effect of checkpoint inhibitors may help vaccine-activated T cells overcome the notoriously tumor immunosuppressive microenvironment. Although checkpoint inhibitors may solve the microenvironment problem, it is not clear whether checkpoint inhibitors are able to modify and/or modulate the T cell's ability for tumor infiltration.

There is a significant improvement in the therapeutic response if (1) the antigen is overexpressed or (2) if the adoptive therapy is combined with irradiation, where complete rejection without recurrence has been observed in a high proportion of mice with large tumor burdens [96]. This similarity suggests that immune evasion is an obstacle faced not only by therapy based on unmutated tumor antigens but also for neoantigens. To this end, Leisegang and colleagues have demonstrated that such evasion can be largely avoided by combining it with irradiation therapy [97]. Sublethal and lethal doses of radiation have been shown to induce immunogenic tumor cell death, thus leading to a more robust immune tumor response [98, 99]. In addition to killing tumor cells directly, radiotherapy has been shown to induce expression of MHC class I and ICAM-1, which are proteins important to antigen presentation. In this way, tumor cells become more susceptible to the recognition of immune system and CD8^{+} T-cell-mediated cytotoxicity. Past work has also shown that radiotherapy can induce CXCL16 expression by tumor cells, thus promoting the recruitment of activated CD4 and CD8 effector T cells to sites of inflammation [100].

Other factors besides the tumor microenvironment will undoubtedly also affect neoantigen vaccines' efficacy. Going forward, it is likely that researchers will find many therapeutic cancer vaccines that were previously deemed ineffective will return to the therapeutic forefront if applied in combination with contemporary, immune modulating approaches. It is reasonable to expect that, in the near future, immunotherapy will achieve considerable effects in combination with conventional cancer therapies—potentially in ways that have not yet been conceived [100]. To this end, there has already been work to suggest that immunotherapy is even more effective when used with radiotherapy, cytotoxic chemotherapy, checkpoint inhibitors, inhibitory small molecules, and tumor antigen-targeting mAbs.

10.6 Conclusions and Future Prospects for Cancer Vaccines

Tumor cells commonly express tumor-associated antigens (TAAs) or mutation-derived antigens (neoantigens). These can be regarded as foreign antigens and can elicit antitumor immune responses in cancer patients. In order to elicit tumor-specific immune responses, many TAAs and neoantigens have been identified and utilized as targets for cancer vaccines. There have been several forms of cancer vaccines that are dependent on certain effector cells (e.g., CTLs or CD4^{+} T-helper cells) that can be targeted and activated. A series of tumor vaccine clinical trials based on immunotherapeutic approaches have inconsistently shown survival advantages with few side adverse effects when compared with conventional approaches. However, vaccine-based monotherapy is considered to be insufficient to elicit robust cancer regression [101]. By combining cancer vaccines with immune-checkpoint blockade therapy, radiation therapy, cytotoxic chemotherapy, and/or tumor antigen-targeting mAbs designed to concurrently inactivate immunosuppressive factors in tumor microenvironment, it may be possible to overcome the current tumor vaccine ineffectiveness, thus leading to the induction of stronger antitumor responses.

References

1. Davidson M, Chau I. Immunotherapy for oesophagogastric cancer. Expert Opin Biol Ther. 2016;16(10):1197–207.
2. Wagner AD, Unverzagt S, Grothe W, Kleber G, Grothey A, Haerting J, et al. Chemotherapy for advanced gastric cancer. Cochrane Database Syst Rev. 2010;3:CD004064.
3. Chen DS, Mellman I. Oncology meets immunology: the cancer-immunity cycle. Immunity. 2013;39(1):1–10.
4. Vonderheide RH, Hahn WC, Schultze JL, Nadler LM. The telomerase catalytic subunit is a widely expressed tumor-associated antigen recognized by cytotoxic T lymphocytes. Immunity. 1999;10(6):673–9.
5. Vigneron N. Human tumor antigens and cancer immunotherapy. Biomed Res Int. 2015;2015:948501.
6. Thompson MP, Kurzrock R. Epstein-Barr virus and cancer. Clin Cancer Res. 2004;10(3):803–21.
7. Kreiter S, Vormehr M, van de Roemer N, Diken M, Lower M, Diekmann J, et al. Mutant MHC class II epitopes drive therapeutic immune responses to cancer. 2015 [updated Apr 22]. Available from http://www.ncbi.nlm.nih.gov/pubmed/25901682.
8. Arzumanyan A, Reis HM, Feitelson MA. Pathogenic mechanisms in HBV- and HCV-associated hepatocellular carcinoma. Nat Rev Cancer. 2013;13(2):123–35.
9. Rajasagi M, Shukla SA, Fritsch EF, Keskin DB, DeLuca D, Carmona E, et al. Systematic identification of personal tumor-specific neoantigens in chronic lymphocytic leukemia. Blood. 2014;124(3):453–62.
10. Higashihara Y, Kato J, Nagahara A, Izumi K, Konishi M, Kodani T, et al. Phase I clinical trial of peptide vaccination with URLC10 and VEGFR1 epitope peptides in patients with advanced gastric cancer. Int J Oncol. 2014;44(3):662–8.
11. Maeda Y, Hida N, Niiya F, Katagiri K, Harada M, Yamana H, et al. Detection of peptide-specific CTL-precursors in peripheral blood lymphocytes of cancer patients. Br J Cancer. 2002;87(7):796–804.
12. Mine T, Sato Y, Noguchi M, Sasatomi T, Gouhara R, Tsuda N, et al. Humoral responses to peptides correlate with overall survival in advanced cancer patients vaccinated with peptides based on preexisting, peptide-specific cellular responses. Clin Cancer Res. 2004;10(3):929–37.

13. Tanaka S, Harada M, Mine T, Noguchi M, Gohara R, Azuma K, et al. Peptide vaccination for patients with melanoma and other types of cancer based on pre-existing peptide-specific ctotoxic T-lymphocyte precursors in the periphery. J Immunother. 2003;26(4):357–66.
14. Sato Y, Shomura H, Maeda Y, Mine T, Une Y, Akasaka Y, et al. Immunological evaluation of peptide vaccination for patients with gastric cancer based on pre-existing cellular response to peptide. Cancer Sci. 2003;94(9):802–8.
15. Takayama K, Sugawara S, Saijo Y, Maemondo M, Sato A, Takamori S, et al. Randomized phase II study of docetaxel plus personalized peptide vaccination versus docetaxel plus placebo for patients with previously treated advanced wild type EGFR non-small-cell lung cancer. J Immunol Res. 2016;2016:1745108.
16. Yoshimura K, Minami T, Nozawa M, Kimura T, Egawa S, Fujimoto H, et al. A phase 2 randomized controlled trial of personalized peptide vaccine immunotherapy with low-dose dexamethasone versus dexamethasone alone in chemotherapy-naive castration-resistant prostate cancer. Eur Urol. 2016;70(1):35–41.
17. Huang H, Hao S, Li F, Ye Z, Yang J, Xiang J. CD4+ Th1 cells promote CD8+ Tc1 cell survival, memory response, tumor localization and therapy by targeted delivery of interleukin 2 via acquired pMHC I complexes. Immunology. 2007;120(2):148–59.
18. Quezada SA, Simpson TR, Peggs KS, Merghoub T, Vider J, Fan X, et al. Tumor-reactive CD4(+) T cells develop cytotoxic activity and eradicate large established melanoma after transfer into lymphopenic hosts. J Exp Med. 2010;207(3):637–50.
19. Teramoto K, Kontani K, Fujita T, Ozaki Y, Sawai S, Tezuka N, et al. Successful tumor eradication was achieved by collaboration of augmented cytotoxic activity and anti-angiogenic effects following therapeutic vaccines containing helper-activating analog-loaded dendritic cells and tumor antigen DNA. Cancer Immunol Immunother. 2007;56(3):331–42.
20. Hu Y, Kim H, Blackwell CM, Slingluff Jr CL. Long-term outcomes of helper peptide vaccination for metastatic melanoma. Ann Surg. 2015;262(3):456–64. discussion 62-4
21. Inderberg-Suso EM, Trachsel S, Lislerud K, Rasmussen AM, Gaudernack G. Widespread CD4+ T-cell reactivity to novel hTERT epitopes following vaccination of cancer patients with a single hTERT peptide GV1001. Oncoimmunology. 2012;1(5):670–86.
22. Kyte JA. Cancer vaccination with telomerase peptide GV1001. Expert Opin Investig Drugs. 2009;18(5):687–94.
23. Brunsvig PF, Kyte JA, Kersten C, Sundstrom S, Moller M, Nyakas M, et al. Telomerase peptide vaccination in NSCLC: a phase II trial in stage III patients vaccinated after chemoradiotherapy and an 8-year update on a phase I/II trial. Clin Cancer Res. 2011;17(21):6847–57.
24. Kyte JA, Gaudernack G, Dueland S, Trachsel S, Julsrud L, Aamdal S. Telomerase peptide vaccination combined with temozolomide: a clinical trial in stage IV melanoma patients. Clin Cancer Res. 2011;17(13):4568–80.
25. Staff C, Mozaffari F, Frodin JE, Mellstedt H, Liljefors M. Telomerase (GV1001) vaccination together with gemcitabine in advanced pancreatic cancer patients. Int J Oncol. 2014;45(3):1293–303.
26. Schlapbach C, Yerly D, Daubner B, Yawalkar N, Hunger RE. Telomerase-specific GV1001 peptide vaccination fails to induce objective tumor response in patients with cutaneous T cell lymphoma. J Dermatol Sci. 2011;62(2):75–83.
27. Sayem MA, Tomita Y, Yuno A, Hirayama M, Irie A, Tsukamoto H, et al. Identification of glypican-3-derived long peptides activating both CD8+ and CD4+ T cells; prolonged overall survival in cancer patients with Th cell response. Oncoimmunology. 2016;5(1):e1062209.
28. Gross S, Lennerz V, Gallerani E, Mach N, Bohm S, Hess D, et al. Short peptide vaccine induces CD4+ T helper cells in patients with different solid cancers. Cancer Immunol Res. 2016;4(1):18–25.
29. Iwahashi M, Katsuda M, Nakamori M, Nakamura M, Naka T, Ojima T, et al. Vaccination with peptides derived from cancer-testis antigens in combination with CpG-7909 elicits strong specific CD8+ T cell response in patients with metastatic esophageal squamous cell carcinoma. Cancer Sci. 2010;101(12):2510–7.
30. Ishikawa H, Imano M, Shiraishi O, Yasuda A, Peng YF, Shinkai M, et al. Phase I clinical trial of vaccination with LY6K-derived peptide in patients with advanced gastric cancer. Gastric Cancer. 2014;17(1):173–80.
31. Chen XH, Liu BY, Zhang DQ, Zhang Y, Zhang Y, Li JF, et al. [Expression of MAGE-1 and MAGE-3 genes in gastric cancer and gastric biopsy tissues and its clinical significance]. Xi bao yu fen zi mian yi xue za zhi (Chinese Journal of Cellular and Molecular Immunology). 2004;20(3):310–3.
32. Ofuji S, Ikeda M, Tsujitani S, Ikeguchi M, Kaibara N, Yuasa I, et al. Expression of MAGE-1, MAGE-2 and MAGE-3 genes in human gastric carcinomas; lack of evidence for cytotoxic effects in cases with simultaneous expression of MAGE-3 and HLA-A2. Anticancer Res. 1998;18(5B):3639–44.
33. Sadanaga N, Nagashima H, Mashino K, Tahara K, Yamaguchi H, Ohta M, et al. Dendritic cell vaccination with MAGE peptide is a novel therapeutic approach for gastrointestinal carcinomas. Clin Cancer Res. 2001;7(8):2277–84.
34. Chua TC, Merrett ND. Clinicopathologic factors associated with HER2-positive gastric cancer and its impact on survival outcomes—a systematic review. Int J Cancer. 2012;130(12):2845–56.

35. Kono K, Takahashi A, Sugai H, Fujii H, Choudhury AR, Kiessling R, et al. Dendritic cells pulsed with HER-2/neu-derived peptides can induce specific T-cell responses in patients with gastric cancer. Clin Cancer Res. 2002;8(11):3394–400.
36. Rapisarda A, Melillo G. Role of the VEGF/VEGFR axis in cancer biology and therapy. Adv Cancer Res. 2012;114:237–67.
37. Tsuboi A, Oka Y, Udaka K, Murakami M, Masuda T, Nakano A, et al. Enhanced induction of human WT1-specific cytotoxic T lymphocytes with a 9-mer WT1 peptide modified at HLA-A*2402-binding residues. Cancer Immunol Immunother. 2002;51(11-12):614–20.
38. Kobayashi M, Chiba A, Izawa H, Yanagida E, Okamoto M, Shimodaira S, et al. The feasibility and clinical effects of dendritic cell-based immunotherapy targeting synthesized peptides for recurrent ovarian cancer. J Ovarian Res. 2014;7:48.
39. Kobayashi M, Sakabe T, Chiba A, Nakajima A, Okamoto M, Shimodaira S, et al. Therapeutic effect of intratumoral injections of dendritic cells for locally recurrent gastric cancer: a case report. World J Surg Oncol. 2014;12:390.
40. Sato Y, Fujiwara T, Mine T, Shomura H, Homma S, Maeda Y, et al. Immunological evaluation of personalized peptide vaccination in combination with a 5-fluorouracil derivative (TS-1) for advanced gastric or colorectal carcinoma patients. Cancer Sci. 2007;98(7):1113–9.
41. Burnet FM. The clonal selection theory of acquired immunity. Nashville: Vanderbilt University Press; 1959. p. xiii, 209.
42. Boon T, Cerottini JC, Van den Eynde B, van der Bruggen P, Van Pel A. Tumor antigens recognized by T lymphocytes. Annu Rev Immunol. 1994;12:337–65.
43. Brichard V, Van Pel A, Wolfel T, Wolfel C, De Plaen E, Lethe B, et al. The tyrosinase gene codes for an antigen recognized by autologous cytolytic T lymphocytes on HLA-A2 melanomas. J Exp Med. 1993;178(2):489–95.
44. Schumacher TN, Schreiber RD. Neoantigens in cancer immunotherapy. Science (New York, NY). 2015;348(6230):69–74. Epub 2015/04/04.
45. Coulie PG, Van den Eynde BJ, van der Bruggen P, Boon T. Tumour antigens recognized by T lymphocytes: at the core of cancer immunotherapy. Nat Rev Cancer. 2014;14(2):135–46.
46. Gilboa E. The makings of a tumor rejection antigen. Immunity. 1999;11(3):263–70.
47. Alexandrov LB, Nik-Zainal S, Wedge DC, Aparicio SA, Behjati S, Biankin AV, et al. Signatures of mutational processes in human cancer. Nature. 2013;500(7463):415–21.
48. Klebanoff CA, Rosenberg SA, Restifo NP. Prospects for gene-engineered T cell immunotherapy for solid cancers. Nat Med. 2016;22(1):26–36. Epub 2016/01/07.
49. Takenoyama M, Baurain JF, Yasuda M, So T, Sugaya M, Hanagiri T, et al. A point mutation in the NFYC gene generates an antigenic peptide recognized by autologous cytolytic T lymphocytes on a human squamous cell lung carcinoma. Int J Cancer. 2006;118(8):1992–7.
50. Matsushita H, Vesely MD, Koboldt DC, Rickert CG, Uppaluri R, Magrini VJ, et al. Cancer exome analysis reveals a T-cell-dependent mechanism of cancer immunoediting. Nature. 2012;482(7385):400–4.
51. Castle JC, Kreiter S, Diekmann J, Lower M, van de Roemer N, de Graaf J, et al. Exploiting the mutanome for tumor vaccination. Cancer Res. 2012;72(5):1081–91.
52. Hinrichs CS, Rosenberg SA. Exploiting the curative potential of adoptive T-cell therapy for cancer. Immunol Rev. 2014;257(1):56–71.
53. Rosenberg SA, Yang JC, Sherry RM, Kammula US, Hughes MS, Phan GQ, et al. Durable complete responses in heavily pretreated patients with metastatic melanoma using T-cell transfer immunotherapy. Clin Cancer Res. 2011;17(13):4550–7.
54. Mahony DE, Li A. Comparative study of ten bacteriocins of Clostridium perfringens. Antimicrob Agents Chemother. 1978;14(6):886–92.
55. Dudley ME, Yang JC, Sherry R, Hughes MS, Royal R, Kammula U, et al. Adoptive cell therapy for patients with metastatic melanoma: evaluation of intensive myeloablative chemoradiation preparative regimens. J Clin Oncol Off J Am Soc Clin Oncol. 2008;26(32):5233–9.
56. Kvistborg P, Shu CJ, Heemskerk B, Fankhauser M, Thrue CA, Toebes M, et al. TIL therapy broadens the tumor-reactive CD8(+) T cell compartment in melanoma patients. Oncoimmunology. 2012;1(4):409–18.
57. Johnson LA, Morgan RA, Dudley ME, Cassard L, Yang JC, Hughes MS, et al. Gene therapy with human and mouse T-cell receptors mediates cancer regression and targets normal tissues expressing cognate antigen. Blood. 2009;114(3):535–46.
58. Lu YC, Yao X, Li YF, El-Gamil M, Dudley ME, Yang JC, et al. Mutated PPP1R3B is recognized by T cells used to treat a melanoma patient who experienced a durable complete tumor regression. J Immunol. 2013;190(12):6034–42.
59. Robbins PF, Lu YC, El-Gamil M, Li YF, Gross C, Gartner J, et al. Mining exomic sequencing data to identify mutated antigens recognized by adoptively transferred tumor-reactive T cells. Nat Med. 2013;19(6):747–52.
60. Wolchok JD, Kluger H, Callahan MK, Postow MA, Rizvi NA, Lesokhin AM, et al. Nivolumab plus ipilimumab in advanced melanoma. N Engl J Med. 2013;369(2):122–33.
61. Hamid O, Robert C, Daud A, Hodi FS, Hwu WJ, Kefford R, et al. Safety and tumor responses with lambrolizumab (anti-PD-1) in melanoma. N Engl J Med. 2013;369(2):134–44.

62. Topalian SL, Hodi FS, Brahmer JR, Gettinger SN, Smith DC, McDermott DF, et al. Safety, activity, and immune correlates of anti-PD-1 antibody in cancer. N Engl J Med. 2012;366(26):2443–54.
63. Hodi FS, O'Day SJ, McDermott DF, Weber RW, Sosman JA, Haanen JB, et al. Improved survival with ipilimumab in patients with metastatic melanoma. N Engl J Med. 2010;363(8):711–23.
64. Gubin MM, Zhang X, Schuster H, Caron E, Ward JP, Noguchi T, et al. Checkpoint blockade cancer immunotherapy targets tumour-specific mutant antigens. Nature. 2014;515(7528):577–81.
65. Rizvi NA, Hellmann MD, Snyder A, Kvistborg P, Makarov V, Havel JJ, et al. Cancer immunology. Mutational landscape determines sensitivity to PD-1 blockade in non-small cell lung cancer. Science. 2015;348(6230):124–8.
66. Van Allen EM, Miao D, Schilling B, Shukla SA, Blank C, Zimmer L, et al. Genomic correlates of response to CTLA-4 blockade in metastatic melanoma. Science. 2015;350(6257):207–11.
67. Katsnelson A. Mutations as munitions: Neoantigen vaccines get a closer look as cancer treatment. Nat Med. 2016;22(2):122–4.
68. Le DT, Uram JN, Wang H, Bartlett BR, Kemberling H, Eyring AD, et al. PD-1 Blockade in Tumors with Mismatch-Repair Deficiency. N Engl J Med. 2015;372(26):2509–20.
69. Yadav M, Jhunjhunwala S, Phung QT, Lupardus P, Tanguay J, Bumbaca S, et al. Predicting immunogenic tumour mutations by combining mass spectrometry and exome sequencing. Nature. 2014;515(7528):572–6.
70. Kalaora S, Barnea E, Merhavi-Shoham E, Qutob N, Teer JK, Shimony N, et al. Use of HLA peptidomics and whole exome sequencing to identify human immunogenic neo-antigens. Oncotarget. 2016;7(5):5110–7.
71. Tran E, Turcotte S, Gros A, Robbins PF, Lu YC, Dudley ME, et al. Cancer immunotherapy based on mutation-specific CD4+ T cells in a patient with epithelial cancer. Science. 2014;344(6184):641–5.
72. Tran E, Ahmadzadeh M, Lu YC, Gros A, Turcotte S, Robbins PF, et al. Immunogenicity of somatic mutations in human gastrointestinal cancers. Science. 2015;350(6266):1387–90.
73. Schumacher T, Bunse L, Wick W, Platten M. Mutant IDH1: An immunotherapeutic target in tumors. Oncoimmunology. 2014;3(12):e974392.
74. Kreiter S, Vormehr M, van de Roemer N, Diken M, Lower M, Diekmann J, et al. Mutant MHC class II epitopes drive therapeutic immune responses to cancer. Nature. 2015;520(7549):692–6.
75. Cancer Genome Atlas Research Network. Comprehensive molecular characterization of gastric adenocarcinoma. Nature. 2014;513(7517):202–9.
76. Vigneron N, Stroobant V, Van den Eynde BJ, van der Bruggen P. Database of T cell-defined human tumor antigens: the 2013 update. Cancer Immun. 2013;13:15.
77. Robbins PF, El-Gamil M, Li YF, Kawakami Y, Loftus D, Appella E, et al. A mutated beta-catenin gene encodes a melanoma-specific antigen recognized by tumor infiltrating lymphocytes. J Exp Med. 1996;183(3):1185–92.
78. Wolfel T, Hauer M, Schneider J, Serrano M, Wolfel C, Klehmann-Hieb E, et al. A p16INK4a-insensitive CDK4 mutant targeted by cytolytic T lymphocytes in a human melanoma. Science. 1995;269(5228):1281–4.
79. Kaiser E, Loch EG. Newer aspects of hormonal therapy in gynecology. Z Allgemeinmed. 1975;51(13):600–5.
80. Gaudin C, Kremer F, Angevin E, Scott V, Triebel F. A hsp70-2 mutation recognized by CTL on a human renal cell carcinoma. J Immunol. 1999;162(3):1730–8.
81. Kawakami Y, Wang X, Shofuda T, Sumimoto H, Tupesis J, Fitzgerald E, et al. Isolation of a new melanoma antigen, MART-2, containing a mutated epitope recognized by autologous tumor-infiltrating T lymphocytes. J Immunol. 2001;166(4):2871–7.
82. Karanikas V, Colau D, Baurain JF, Chiari R, Thonnard J, Gutierrez-Roelens I, et al. High frequency of cytolytic T lymphocytes directed against a tumor-specific mutated antigen detectable with HLA tetramers in the blood of a lung carcinoma patient with long survival. Cancer Res. 2001;61(9):3718–24.
83. Ito D, Visus C, Hoffmann TK, Balz V, Bier H, Appella E, et al. Immunological characterization of missense mutations occurring within cytotoxic T cell-defined p53 epitopes in HLA-A*0201+ squamous cell carcinomas of the head and neck. Int J Cancer. 2007;120(12):2618–24.
84. Gjertsen MK, Bjorheim J, Saeterdal I, Myklebust J, Gaudernack G. Cytotoxic CD4+ and CD8+ T lymphocytes, generated by mutant p21-ras (12Val) peptide vaccination of a patient, recognize 12Val-dependent nested epitopes present within the vaccine peptide and kill autologous tumour cells carrying this mutation. Int J Cancer. 1997;72(5):784–90.
85. Abrams SI, Khleif SN, Bergmann-Leitner ES, Kantor JA, Chung Y, Hamilton JM, et al. Generation of stable CD4+ and CD8+ T cell lines from patients immunized with ras oncogene-derived peptides reflecting codon 12 mutations. Cell Immunol. 1997;182(2):137–51.
86. Gjertsen MK, Saeterdal I, Saeboe-Larssen S, Gaudernack G. HLA-A3 restricted mutant ras specific cytotoxic T-lymphocytes induced by vaccination with T-helper epitopes. J Mol Med. 2003;81(1):43–50.
87. Linard B, Bezieau S, Benlalam H, Labarriere N, Guilloux Y, Diez E, et al. A ras-mutated peptide targeted by CTL infiltrating a human melanoma lesion. J Immunol. 2002;168(9):4802–8.
88. Sharkey MS, Lizee G, Gonzales MI, Patel S, Topalian SL. CD4(+) T-cell recognition of mutated

B-RAF in melanoma patients harboring the V599E mutation. Cancer Res. 2004;64(5):1595–9.
89. Nishimura Y, Chen YZ, Uemura Y, Tanaka Y, Tsukamoto H, Kanai T, et al. Degenerate recognition and response of human CD4+ Th cell clones: implications for basic and applied immunology. Mol Immunol. 2004;40(14-15):1089–94.
90. Gedde-Dahl 3rd T, Spurkland A, Eriksen JA, Thorsby E, Gaudernack G. Memory T cells of a patient with follicular thyroid carcinoma recognize peptides derived from mutated p21 ras (Gln→Leu61). Int Immunol. 1992;4(11):1331–7.
91. Gedde-Dahl 3rd T, Spurkland A, Fossum B, Wittinghofer A, Thorsby E, Gaudernack G. T cell epitopes encompassing the mutational hot spot position 61 of p21 ras. Promiscuity in ras peptide binding to HLA. Eur J Immunol. 1994;24(2):410–4.
92. Gedde-Dahl 3rd T, Eriksen JA, Thorsby E, Gaudernack G. T-cell responses against products of oncogenes: generation and characterization of human T-cell clones specific for p21 ras-derived synthetic peptides. Hum Immunol. 1992;33(4):266–74.
93. Novellino L, Renkvist N, Rini F, Mazzocchi A, Rivoltini L, Greco A, et al. Identification of a mutated receptor-like protein tyrosine phosphatase kappa as a novel, class II HLA-restricted melanoma antigen. J Immunol. 2003;170(12):6363–70.
94. Schumacher T, Bunse L, Pusch S, Sahm F, Wiestler B, Quandt J, et al. A vaccine targeting mutant IDH1 induces antitumour immunity. Nature. 2014;512(7514):324–7.
95. Moehler M, Delic M, Goepfert K, Aust D, Grabsch HI, Halama N, et al. Immunotherapy in gastrointestinal cancer: recent results, current studies and future perspectives. Eur J Cancer. 2016;59:160–70.
96. Liu Y. Neoantigen: a long march toward cancer immunotherapy. Clin Cancer Res. 2016;22(11):2602–4.
97. Leisegang M, Engels B, Schreiber K, Yew PY, Kiyotani K, Idel C, et al. Eradication of large solid tumors by gene therapy with a T-cell receptor targeting a single cancer-specific point mutation. Clin Cancer Res. 2016;22(11):2734–43.
98. Apetoh L, Ghiringhelli F, Tesniere A, Obeid M, Ortiz C, Criollo A, et al. Toll-like receptor 4-dependent contribution of the immune system to anticancer chemotherapy and radiotherapy. Nat Med. 2007;13(9):1050–9.
99. Panaretakis T, Kepp O, Brockmeier U, Tesniere A, Bjorklund AC, Chapman DC, et al. Mechanisms of pre-apoptotic calreticulin exposure in immunogenic cell death. EMBO J. 2009;28(5):578–90.
100. Khalil DN, Budhu S, Gasmi B, Zappasodi R, Hirschhorn-Cymerman D, Plitt T, et al. The new era of cancer immunotherapy: manipulating T-cell activity to overcome malignancy. Adv Cancer Res. 2015;128:1–68.
101. Hirayama M, Nishimura Y. The present status and future prospects of peptide-based cancer vaccines. Int Immunol. 2016;28(7):319–28.

Adoptive Cell Therapy of Gastric Cancer

11

Zhengyun Zou, Lianjun Zhao, Yu Ren, and Shiyao Du

11.1 Introduction

Tremendous progress has been made in the field of immunotherapy through various research studies and clinical trials. This work has led to significant breakthroughs in the treatment of malignant tumors. Immunotherapy treatment is an additional treatment option to other novel approaches, including immune checkpoint inhibitors and signaling pathway inhibitors; those have demonstrated clear efficacy in the treatment of numerous cancer types. Some examples include malignant melanoma, kidney cancer, lung cancer, and urinary bladder cancer. Adoptive cell therapy (ACT) has also shown clear effects in the treatment of different malignant diseases. ACT is a highly personalized cancer therapy that takes advantage of immune cells that infiltrate tumors for direct anticancer activities. ACT utilizes either natural host cells, such as lymphokine-activated killer cells (LAK), cytokine-induced killer cells (CIK), tumor-infiltrating lymphocytes (TIL), and cytotoxic T lymphocytes (CTL), or host cells that have been genetically engineered to possess antitumor T cell receptors (TCRs) or chimeric antigen receptors (CARs). This chapter profiles ACT in cancer immunotherapy based on reliable data, some of which demonstrates the use of this cell therapy for the treatment of gastric cancer.

Z. Zou (✉) • L. Zhao • Y. Ren • S. Du
The Comprehensive Cancer Center of Drum Tower Hospital, Medical School of Nanjing University and Clinical Cancer Institute of Nanjing University, Zhongshan Road 321, Nanjing 210008, Jiangsu, China
e-mail: zouzhengyun@medmail.com.cn

11.2 CIK

CIK cells are $CD3^+CD56^+$ phenotype T cells, first identified by Schmidt-Wolf IG in 1991. CIK cells have been shown to not be restricted by major histocompatibility complex (MHC) and are easily developed in vitro by growing peripheral blood mononuclear cells in the presence of anti-CD3 mAb, interferon γ(IFN-γ), and interleukin 2 (IL-2) [1]. There are three potential mechanisms for the therapeutic anticancer effect seen with CIK cells. First, CIK cells proliferate abundantly in vitro and haven been shown to directly kill tumor cells. Second, CIK cells are able to release high levels of IFN-γ and TNF-α but not IL-2 or IL-4, enabling them to regulate and increase host cell immune function in vivo. Finally, CIK cells have been shown to be able to induce necrosis and apoptosis of tumor cells [2, 3].

In the past two decades, there has been great interest in the use of CIK-based immunotherapy for the treatment of numerous cancers, including hepatocellular carcinoma [4], colon cancer [5], advanced non-small cell lung cancer [6], gastric cancer [3], and others. The Liangrong Shi group

J. Wei, B. Liu (eds.), *Personalized Management of Gastric Cancer*,
DOI 10.1007/978-981-10-3978-2_11

demonstrated that the use of immunotherapy with CIK cells resulted in an improved response rate and an increased survival rate of patients suffering from advanced gastric cancer [7].

Six relevant clinical trials with case-control studies were utilized for a meta-analysis. The studies used included 318 patients who received CIK cell therapy and 369 patients who received conventional therapy. The results from this study suggested that CIK cell therapy significantly increased 5-year OS (27 ± 2.44% vs. 49 ± 7.62%, $p < 0.05$) and 5-year OR (increased to 1.77, $p < 0.05$). The increased 5-year survival rate was found to be highly correlated with increased $CD3^+$ T cell numbers and an increased $CD4^+/CD8^+$ ratio in CIK-treated patients [3].

In conclusion, CIK-cell therapy was found to improve the host's immune function; however, multiple treatment cycles are necessary for a long-term therapeutic efficacy. Therefore, other novel treatment technologies are gradually replacing CIK-based immunotherapy.

11.3 TIL

In 1986, the Rosenberg, S.A. group identified a subpopulation of lymphocytes that are able to infiltrate growing cancers, named tumor-infiltrating lymphocytes (TILs). TILs have been shown to be 50–100 times more potent than LAK cells when used as treatment in mice bearing various types of tumors [8]. TILs are a type of a potential lymphocytes, with some able to recognize tumor-specific antigens, especially mutated antigens of the tumor. A retrospective analysis of patients with melanoma at the Surgery Branch, National Cancer Institute (NCI) showed that viable TILs were able to be grown from 94% of patients following resection. In addition, specific, active TILs screened by IFN-γ production following coculture with an autologous tumor cell line were identified in 67% of patients. Importantly, human TILs were able to be generated on a large scale from the majority of tumor types in experiments using mice.

The first reported use of TILs for the treatment of patients was carried out by the Surgery Branch, NCI in 1988 [9]. A total of 20 patients with metastatic melanoma participated in this study. These patients were treated with non-myeloablative (NMA) chemotherapy before their treatment with TILs and IL-2. A total of 11/20 (55%) of the patients exhibited objective responses, including one case of a complete response (CR). Toxicity was found to be similar to that observed with the administration of IL-2 alone. These toxicity issues included hypotension, nausea, anemia, as well as others. Nearly half of all of the patients treated with TILs experienced objective tumor regressions, making adoptive immunotherapy with TILs one of the most effective treatments for malignant melanoma [10]. Despite these examples of success, previous trials demonstrated limited success of TIL therapy in the treatment of solid tumors, including breast cancer, ovarian cancer (OC), cervical cancer, renal cell carcinoma (RCC), colorectal cancer, pancreatic cancer, hepatocellular carcinoma, cholangiocarcinoma cancer, gastric cancer [11–14], and others. TILs have been used in the immunotherapy treatment of gastric cancer since 1990. Yamaue H. [15] demonstrated that activated TIL by adoptive transfer could result in the near complete regression of malignant ascites in gastric cancer patients. A clinical study examining the use of adoptive immunotherapy with tumor-associated lymphocytes (TALs) in combination with chemotherapy in gastric cancer patients showed a greater survival rate (50%) than seen with chemotherapy alone [16]. A clinical trial has been registered on the Clinical Trials website (ClinicalTrials.gov identifier NCT01174121) where patients with digestive tract, urothelial, breast, or ovarian/endometrial cancers will receive the standard non-myeloablative lymphocyte-depleting preconditioning regimen of cyclophosphamide and fludarabine, followed by young TIL and aldesleukin infusion. We expect that this trial will yield promising results.

TIL has been shown to be able to exhibit antitumor effects in the absence of IL-2, which reduces the side effects of adoptive cell therapy. However, a low dose of IL-2 has been shown to enhance the effects of TIL. Novel approaches including the use of phenotypic markers, such as PD-1 and 4-1BB, to select for tumor-reactive cells in TILs, TILs that are able to target mutated antigens, as well as the local secretion of IL-12 to alter the tumor microenvironment, will be critical areas of research in the near future [10, 17–19].

The adoptive transfer of TILs has been shown to be an effective means of therapy for the treatment of patients with metastatic melanoma. The effort to extend TIL therapy for the treatment of gastric cancer patients is an ongoing effort.

11.4 CTL

The most potent killing machinery of our immune system is the $CD8^+$ lymphocyte, which is referred to as the cytotoxic T lymphocyte (CTL) [20]. CTLs specifically recognize MHC-I-peptide complexes that are presented on the surface of target cells through T cell receptors (TCRs). CTLs then release biological substances such as perforin and granzymes into tumor cells to dissolve them. HLA class-I-restricted and tumor-specific CTL have been both observed in PBMC stimulated with autologous tumor cells or IL-2-activated TIL in patients with several different types of cancer, including melanoma, ovarian cancer, nasopharyngeal carcinoma (NPC), breast cancer, gastric cancer, and others [9, 21].

The search for tumor-specific antigens has been a primary focus of CTL research. There exist two types of tumor antigens, tumor-associated antigen (TAA) and tumor-specific antigen (TSA). However, it has been shown that it is possible to generate tumor antigen-specific CTL to achieve therapeutic efficacy, including MAGE-A1~MAGE-A12, New York esophageal squamous cell carcinoma-1(NY-ESO-1), gp100, EBV, β-catenin, MUC-1, and others.

In 1997, the Tomoaki Hoshino group demonstrated the existence of HLA class-I-restricted and tumor-specific CTL in IL-2-activated TIL of four different gastric cancer patients. However, the level of cytotoxicity of these CTLs over a 6-hour cytotoxicity assay was found to be relatively low. This could be due in part to the fact that only one-third of the T cells in the CTL lines tested were $CD8^+$ T cells or the low affinity of the peptide antigens to the HLA A alleles recognized by these CTL clones [21].

A team from Baylor College of Medicine has shown that adoptive transfer of EBV-specific T cells to patients with NPC can induce a durable antitumor response. This group carried out a clinical study in which eight patients with recurrent NPC received CD45 mAbs followed by an EBV-specific CTL infusion. Following the CTL infusion, increased levels of interleukin-15 (IL-15) was detected in six of the eight patients. All patients exhibited increased numbers of EBV-specific T cells in their peripheral blood. A total of three patients demonstrated clinical benefits from this treatment regimen, including one patient with a complete response (> 24 months) and two patients whose condition stabilized (for 12 and 15 months) [22]. In another research study, Bollard CM et al. [23] administered EBV cytotoxic T lymphocyte (CTL) cell lines to 14 patients being treated for relapsed EBV^+ Hodgkin's disease. Five patients were in complete remission for up to 40 months, two of whom had a clearly measurable tumor at the time of treatment. One additional patient exhibited a partial response, and five had stable disease. Importantly, EBV CTLs were found to be well tolerated in patients and were found to be able to control type B symptoms (fever, night sweats, and weight loss). A meta-analysis supported the idea that EBV infection increases the risk of gastric cancer [24]. Thus, we believe the therapeutic effect of EBV-specific CTLs in gastric cancer is an important area of study.

11.5 Genetically Engineered Lymphocytes

With the rapid progression of gene engineering technology, the ability to introduce receptors which specifically recognize tumor antigens into autologous T cells isolated from the peripheral blood is an achievable goal [25]. These specific receptors would include T cell receptors (TCR) or synthetic recognition structures termed chimeric antigen receptors (CAR) [26]. Numerous clinical trials have obtained exciting results demonstrating success in this area, particularly in the application of TCR-T cells for melanoma and CAR-T cells for hematological malignancies. The adoptive transfer of CAR-T/TCR-T is currently a promising cancer therapy approach, as vectors expressing specific receptors could become "off-the-shelf" products for wide therapeutic applications if the patient has a matched antigen and HLA type.

11.5.1 TCR-T

The genetic transfer of TCR-mediated potential tumor recognition has been shown to enable the creation of antigen-specific lymphocytes from circulating normal T cells. An inserted TCR, which is similar to an endogenous TCR, is able to recognize the processed peptide presented by antigen-presenting cells. It is important to note that the specific recognition of an antigen is MHC restricted [27], whereas targets of engineered TCR are more widely selected in solid tumors. Tumor-associated antigens (TAAs), such as melanoma antigens recognized by T cells 1 (MART-1) and gp-100, were consistently chosen to be used in early clinical trials. However, these targeted tumor antigens that are co-expressed in noncancerous cells resulted in obvious on-target, off-tumor toxicity in this therapeutic approach [28, 29]. A different type of antigen, referred to as cancer testis (CT) antigens, has become the current ideal antigen choice. These CT antigens are not expressed in adult normal tissue, with the exception of immune privileged testis [27]. The fact that CT antigen expression is specific toward tumor cells is advantageous in that it greatly reduces damage to noncancerous cells. The first CT antigen selected to express on T cells is NY-ESO-1. This antigen is expressed in 80% of patients with synovial cell sarcoma and in approximately 25% of patients with melanoma and common epithelial tumors [30]. The fact that this antigen is expressed across a wide range of cancer types, but is restricted to tumors, makes this adoptive immunotherapy beneficial for more cancer patients. A total of eleven out of 20 patients with NY-ESO-1 positive melanomas (55%) and 11 out of 18 patients with NY-ESO-1 positive synovial cell sarcomas (61%) who were infused with autologous T cells transfected with an NY-ESO-1-reactive TCR demonstrated an objective clinical response [31]. The encouraging therapeutic efficacy observed in this trial was also found to occur with NY-ESO-1$^+$ multiple myeloma, with a complete response observed in 14 out of 20 patients (70%) [32]. The successful application of T cells with genetically modified TCR is attributed to the rational antigen selection and the reconstruction and selection for high-avidity TCR. Single and dual amino acid substitution variants in the TCR CDRs are thought to contribute to the enhancement of antigen-specific T cell function by improving the TCR affinity [33]. The TCR targeting NY-ESO-1 used in the clinical trials possesses a single amino acid substitution that increases the avidity of the corresponding original TCR and leads to a further sustained response in patients with antigen-positive tumors [31–33]. It is important to note that not all CT antigens are as safe to use as HLA-A2-restricted NY-ESO-1 [25]. Among nine patients who were treated with ACT using lymphocytes engineered with an HLA-A2-restricted and affinity-enhanced MAGE-A3-specific TCR, two patients went on to develop lethal neurologic toxicities. This was explained by a low-level expression of MAGE-A12 within the brain of these patients, which caused the TCR to cross-react with a HLA-A2-restricted MAGE-12 epitope that has yet to be identified [34]. Another clinical trial which utilized a HLA-A1-restricted and affinity-enhanced MAGE-A3-specific TCR was found to result in lethal cardiac toxicity, with this adverse event found to be due to the recognition of an unrelated peptide originated from the striated muscle-specific protein titin, causing an off-tumor toxicity [35]. With the improvement in a receptor's affinity, the specificity for unrelated antigen recognition should, in theory, decrease. With this knowledge, it must be kept in mind that the benefits versus the risk of infusing high-avidity antigen-specific TCR should first be carefully considered [25].

Low expression levels of some CT antigens in certain cancers have encouraged scientists to search for alternative immunogenic antigens.

Increasing evidence supports the fact that neoantigens are better targets for successful immunotherapy, which more likely mediate a clinical response by T cells to target somatic mutations that are unique to each patient's tumor [36]. Tumor neoantigens are the result of genetic alterations that are accumulated by cancer cells during the process of tumorigenesis. Thus, these antigens are potentially specific and therefore ideal targets, which would minimize the risk of on-target, off-tumor toxicity in healthy tissue [37]. It should be noted that the TCR induced by neoantigens should not be deleted by negative selection, as the somatic mutated neoantigens are not expressed during thymic development [10]. Reinfusing natural neoantigen-reactive T cells or lymphocytes stimulated with neoantigen epitopes are feasible approaches for the treatment of cancer. An alternative method would be to acquire the coding gene of neoantigen-specific TCR through high-throughput TCR sequencing and transfect this gene into autologous circulating T cells. Adoptive T cells which target neoantigens carrying immunogenic mutations will be exploited for the further development of highly personalized immunotherapies in the future [25, 37].

11.5.2 Car-T

The genetic engineering of lymphocytes to express chimeric antigen receptors (CAR) is another approach. A CAR consists of an antigen-binding domain and intracellular activation signaling motifs. The antigen-binding domain is comprised of a single-chain variable fragment (scFv) from a mAb, which will recognize only structures present on the cell surface [38]. Importantly, this recognition is MHC independent, compared with TCR. Utilizing CARs to target the B cell lineage differentiation antigen, CD19, has resulted in remarkable tumor regressions in a range of different hematologic malignancies. In addition, the administration of autologous T cells expressing CD19-specific CAR as a therapeutic approach for patients with hematological malignancies has generated remarkable success in clinical trials [39–41]. The first successful application of this gene therapy was demonstrated in the case of a follicular lymphoma treatment [42]. Currently, CAR-modified therapy has been expanded for use in cancer treatment of other B cell malignant diseases, including chronic lymphocytic leukemia (CLL) [43, 44] and adult and pediatric acute lymphoblastic B cell leukemias (ALLs) [45, 46]. These successes that have made using CAR therapy as a treatment for cancer have stimulated intense research into ACT in recent years.

However, the effect of CARs against solid tumors is not as significant due to both the lack of antigens that are specifically expressed on the surface of solid tumors and the presence of the tumor microenvironment [25]. Numerous studies of CAR-T have been used in several clinical trials for the treatment of different types of malignant tumors, including myeloma, colon cancer, renal cell carcinoma, and neuroblastoma [47–50]. The response rates to this treatment are usually found to be mild, sometimes with serious and deadly toxicities associated. These toxicities could be due to the on-target/off-tumor activity, which is attributed to the fact that the antigens targeted in the majority of these cases are shared by both tumors and noncancerous tissues. Another factor at play in the observed toxicity is cytokine release syndrome (CRS), a syndrome caused by cytokines such as interleukin-6 and interferon-gamma being released excessively [25, 51]. Thus, improvements in the safety of these treatments are in need of greater attention. Antigens that are exclusive to cancer cells, but not normal tissues, could be ideal options that could help minimize undesired toxicities associated with this treatment. Recent studies have identified several potential excellent targets, including mutations such as PI3K, BRAF, human papilloma virus (HPV) E6 and E7, and cancer germ line antigens (CGAs) such as MAGE and NY-ESO-1 [25]. A recent study using animal models has surprisingly identified a neoantigen found to be expressed in a variety of tumors. The neoantigen, Tn-MUC1, is not expressed on the cell surface of normal human tissue and is an abnormal glycoform of cancer-associated membrane mucin MUC1. Engineered CAR-T cells targeting Tn-MUC1 were demonstrated to successfully exhibit therapeutic efficacy, thus indicating aberrantly glycosylated antigens as a novel class of targets for ACT using CARs [52].

Based on the achievements described above, TCR and CAR genetically modified therapies have emerged as promising clinical approaches for gastric cancer treatment in comparison with the poor survival rates witnessed with conventional therapies. According to years of studies, tumor-associated antigens (TAAs) including HER-2, HER-3, MAGE-3, c-MET, VEGF, PIK3/mTOR, and gastrin-17 (G17), which are overexpressed in gastric cancers, are considered to be promising targets [53–56]. For example, HER-2, an antigen that is commonly observed to be overexpressed in multiple gastric cancer tumors (up to 9–38 percent), has been widely studied in gene-modified therapy [57]. Preclinical trials where humanized anti-HER-2 CARs were structured have demonstrated that these CAR-modified T cells are able to resist HER-2-positive tumor cells in in vitro experiments, inhibiting the growth and progress of HER-2-positive tumors in in vivo animal models [58]. However, in 2010, the first case of a colorectal cancer patient that received second-generation CAR directed against HER-2 died of respiratory distress 5 days following the cell transfusion [48]. But in the treatment of HER-2-positive sarcoma patients, 4 of the 17 patients treated exhibited a stabilization of their disease state [59]. This indicates that HER-2/neu is a promising target for gastric cancer therapy. An additional class of antigens that is observed in multiple investigations is mutated antigen. The frequently mutated genes include PIK3CA, KRAS, TP53, and CTNNB1, as well as others [60]. In addition, the negative co-stimulatory molecule, B7-H4, a new member of the B7 family, is thought to be expressed in tumor cells as well as some infiltrating immune cells of gastric cancer tumors, while not expressed in normal tissues. Thus, this molecule is believed to be able to negatively regulate the immune response induced by T cells [61]. This makes B7-H4 a promising target for the treatment of gastric carcinoma.

A summary of engineered T cells used in clinical trials is shown in Table 11.1. Although the promising improvements mentioned above have been achieved, numerous investigations remain to be carried out to determine effective applications of gene-modified therapy for the treatment of gastric cancer.

Table 11.1 Summary of engineered T cells in clinical trials

Engineered T cells	Target antigen	Cancer	Number of patients treated in trial	Results	Reference	Year reported
TCR-T	gp100	Melanoma	Sixteen	One CR and two PR	[29]	2009
	MART-1/ Melan-A	Melanoma	Thirty-one	Four OR	[28, 62]	2006, 2009
			Twenty	Six PR	[29]	2009
	p53	Melanoma	Fourteen	One PR	[63]	2010
	NY-ESO-1	Melanoma and synovial sarcoma	Seventeen	Two CR and seven PR	[30]	2011
		Synovial cell sarcomas	Eighteen	Eleven RR	[31]	2015
		Melanoma	Twenty	Eleven RR	[31]	2015
		Multiple myeloma	Twenty	Sixteen RR	[32]	2015
	CEA	Colorectal	Three	One PR	[64]	2011
	MAGE-A3	Melanoma, esophageal and synovial sarcoma	Nine	One CR and four PR	[65]	2013
		Melanoma and MM	Two	Lethal cardiac toxicity	[35]	2013

Table 11.1 (continued)

Engineered T cells	Target antigen	Cancer	Number of patients treated in trial	Results	Reference	Year reported
CAR-T	CD19	CLL	Three	Two CR and one PR	[44, 66]	2011
		Lymphoma and CLL	Seven	One CR, five PR, and one SD	[42, 67]	2012, 2010
		ALL	Sixteen	Fourteen CR	[45]	2014
		Pediatric and adult ALLs	Thirty	Twenty-seven CR	[39]	2014
		NHL	Six	Two SD to 10 months	[68]	2011
	CD20	NHL and mantle cell lymphoma	Seven	Two CR, one PR, four SD	[69]	2008
		NHL	Three	One PR, two NED maintained	[70]	2012
	CD171	Neuroblastoma	Six	One PR	[71]	2007
	GD2	Neuroblastoma	Nineteen	Three CR	[50]	2011
	ERBB2	HNSCC	Proposed		[72]	2013
		Colorectal cancer	One	Died of respiratory distress	[48]	2010
		Sarcoma	Seventeen	Four SD	[59]	2015
	CEA	Colorectal and breast cancer	Seven	Two minor response	[73]	2002
		Gastrointestinal cancer	Nine	One SD	[74]	2015
	Lewis Y	AML	Four	One cytogenetic remission	[75]	2013
	CAIX	Renal cell carcinoma	Twelve	No clinical response	[49]	2013

Abbreviations: *MART-1* melanoma antigen recognized by T cells 1, *Melan-A* melanocyte antigen, *MAGE-A3* melanoma-associated antigen 3, *CEA* carcinoembryonic antigen, *NY-ESO-1* New York esophageal squamous cell carcinoma-1, *ALL* acute lymphoblastic leukemia, *CLL* chronic lymphocytic leukemia, *MM* multiple myeloma, *ERBB2* erythroblastosis oncogene B2, *GD2* ganglioside, *CAIX* carbonic anhydrase-IX, *NHL* non-Hodgkin's lymphoma, *HNSCC* head and neck squamous cell carcinoma, *CR* complete response, *PR* partial response, *OR* objective response, *SD* stable disease, *RR* response rate, *NED* no evidence of disease

11.6 Conclusions and Future Perspectives

According the remarkable clinical trial results described here, we strongly believe that ACT, including TIL, CTL, TCR-T, and CAR-T transfer therapy, is the most promising "living" treatment for targeting human tumors, in which T cells are the terminator. However, there remains a need to improve the killing ability of transfer cells, while reducing the side effects of ACT, such as on-target/off-tumor toxicities, cytokine release syndrome, and, at the same time, develop an ability to harness the immune microenvironment, in order to make ACT an even more successful treatment option.

In order to prevent the on-target/off-tumor toxicities, target antigens that are only expressed on tumor cells, and not on normal tissue cells, must be selected. The tumor-specific "nonself" immunogenic neoantigens encoded by either viral genes or through somatic mutations possess the potential to induce specific anticancer immunity, including cellular and humoral immune responses. Today, numerous clinical trials demonstrate that although these "nonself" antigens initiate the antigen-specific immunoglobulin G antibodies and $CD4^+/CD8^+$ T cells response, not all of them show a clinical benefit in the response rate, progression-free survival, or overall survival [76–78].

Personalized cell therapy is the key to cure human malignant diseases. There are five steps required to reach this goal. First, cancer mutations must be identified through exome sequencing. Second, tandem minigenes or synthetic peptides of all identified mutations must be created and introduced to autologous APC. Third, mature autologous APCs coculture with T cells form peripheral blood or tumor. Fourth, tumor-reactive T cells must accumulate together through 4-1BB or OX40 positive selection. Fifth, rapid expansion of such cells in vitro must be carried out and used to treat the tumor in vivo, or a PCR of the TCR of such cells must be carried out for TCR-T treatment (Figs. 11.1 and 11.2) [26].

Moreover, there exists accumulating correlative data which suggests that directly sorting PD-1$^+$ lymphocytes in peripheral blood could function as an alternative noninvasive strategy to develop neoantigen-reactive lymphocytes or TCRs to treat melanomas (Fig. 11.3) [79].

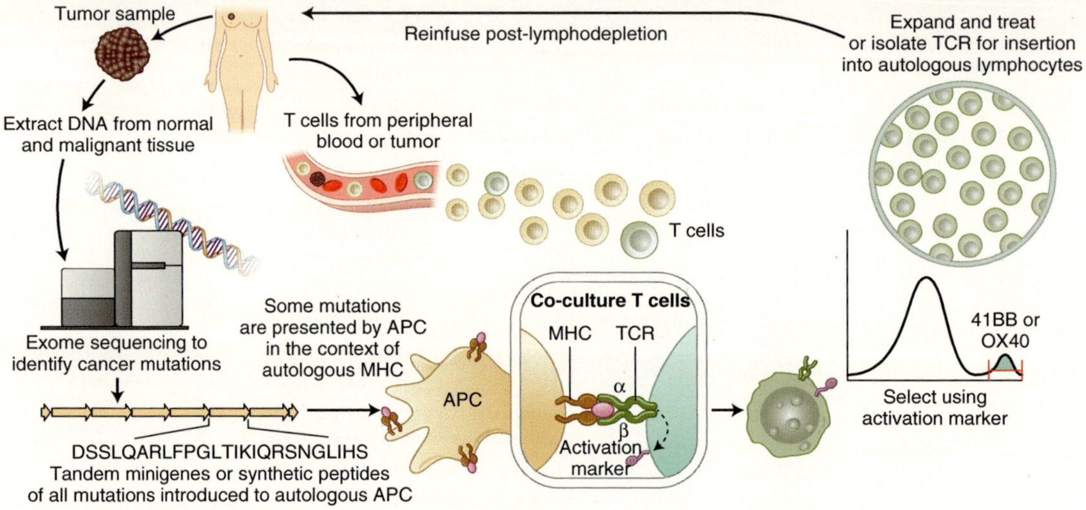

Fig. 11.1 A "blueprint" for T cells treatment targeting tumor-specific mutations (Adapted from Adoptive cell transfer as personalized immunotherapy for human cancer (2015), Rosenberg SA, Restifo NP, [26])

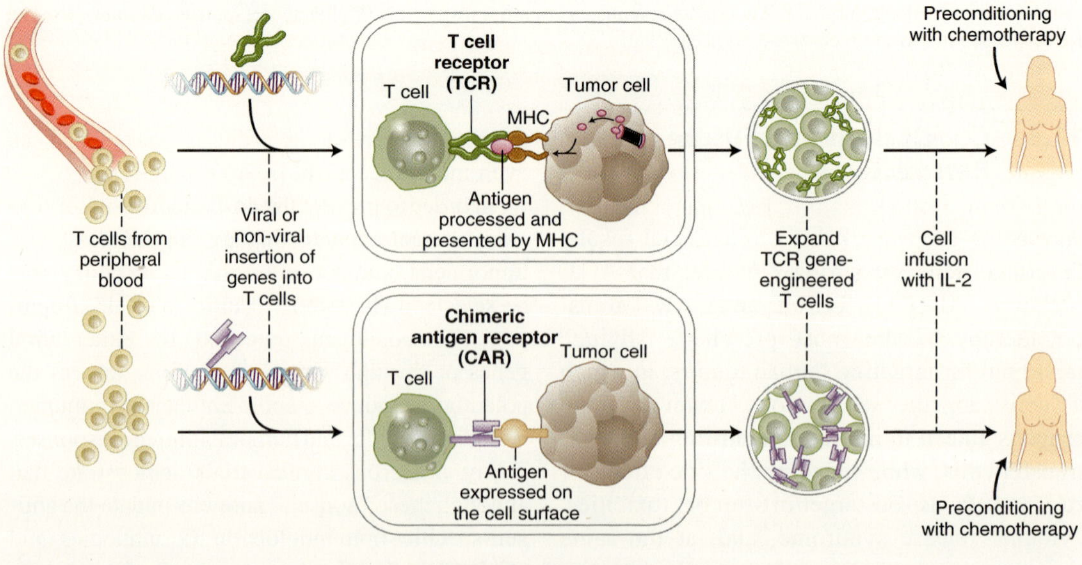

Fig. 11.2 Gene-engineered peripheral blood lymphocytes (Adapted from Adoptive cell transfer as personalized immunotherapy for human cancer (2015), Rosenberg SA, Restifo NP, [26])

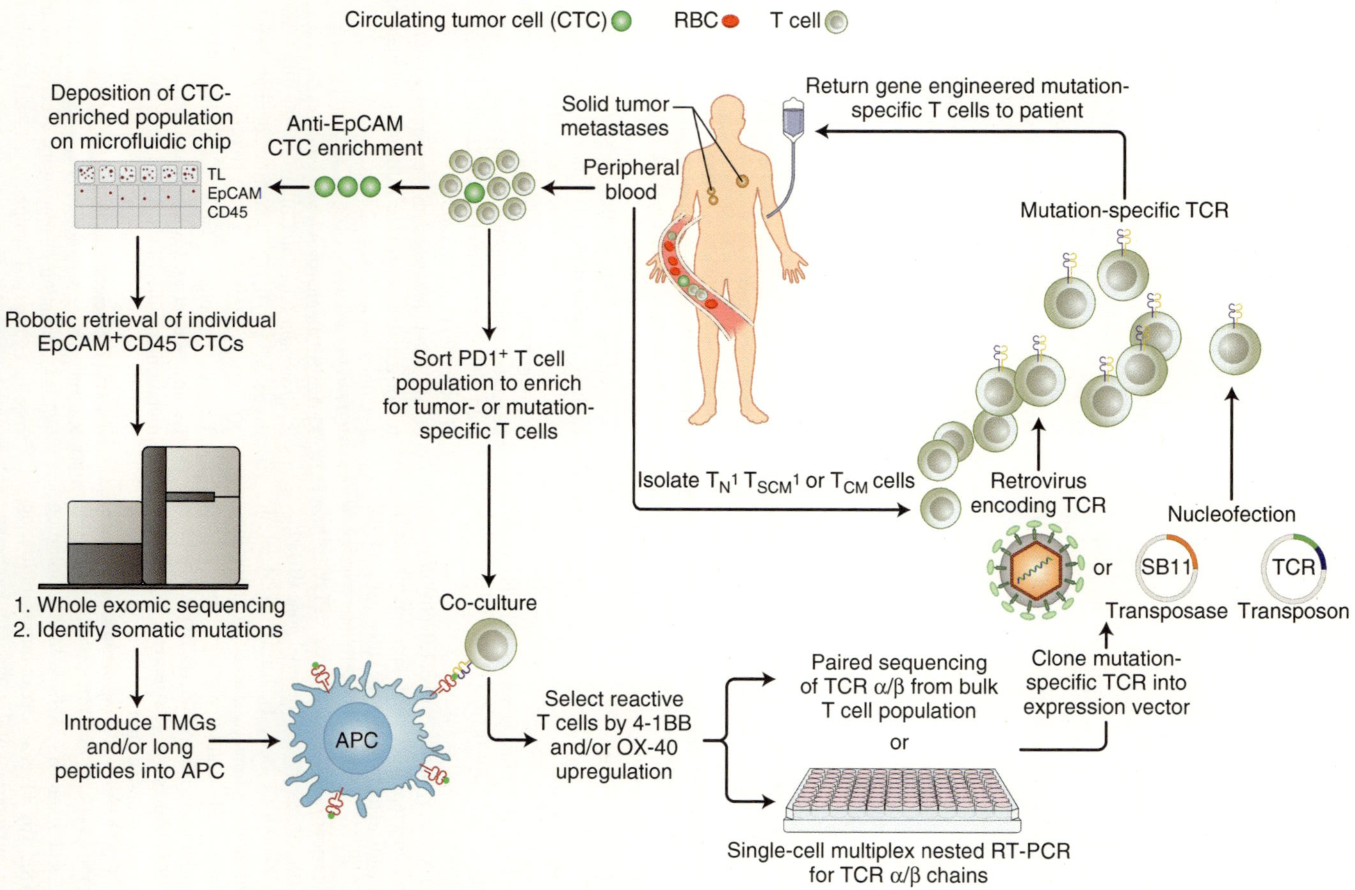

Fig. 11.3 A new strategy for generating autologous TCR gene treatments targeting neoantigens of advanced epithelial cancers (Adapted from Prospective identification of neoantigen-specific lymphocytes in the peripheral blood of melanoma patients (2016), Gros A et al. [79])

Gastric cancer tumors have been shown to exhibit a high prevalence of mutations, with many occurring with EB virus infection. Both mutation antigens and viral antigens are ideal antigen targets for gastric cancer immunotherapy. Thus, we can use the abovementioned strategies to prepare T cells in clinical ACT for gastric cancer.

References

1. Schmidt-Wolf IG, Negrin RS, Kiem HP, Blume KG, Weissman IL. Use of a SCID mouse/human lymphoma model to evaluate cytokine-induced killer cells with potent antitumor cell activity. J Exp Med. 1991;174(1):139–49.
2. Shi L, Zhou Q, Wu J, Ji M, Li G, Jiang J, et al. Efficacy of adjuvant immunotherapy with cytokine-induced killer cells in patients with locally advanced gastric cancer. Cancer Immunol Immunother. 2012;61(12):2251–9. doi:10.1007/s00262-012-1289-2.
3. Liu K, Song G, Hu X, Zhou Y, Li Y, Chen Q, et al. A positive role of cytokine-induced killer cell therapy on gastric cancer therapy in a chinese population: a systematic meta-analysis. Med Sci Monit. 2015;21:3363–70.
4. Li X, Dai D, Song X, Liu J, Zhu L, Xu W. A meta-analysis of cytokine-induced killer cells therapy in combination with minimally invasive treatment for hepatocellular carcinoma. Clin Res Hepatol Gastroenterol. 2014;38(5):583–91. doi:10.1016/j.clinre.2014.04.010.
5. Wang ZX, Cao JX, Liu ZP, Cui YX, Li CY, Li D, et al. Combination of chemotherapy and immunotherapy for colon cancer in China: a meta-analysis. World J Gastroenterol. 2014;20(4):1095–106. doi:10.3748/wjg.v20.i4.1095.
6. Han RX, Liu X, Pan P, Jia YJ, Yu JC. Effectiveness and safety of chemotherapy combined with dendritic cells co-cultured with cytokine-induced killer cells in the treatment of advanced non-small-cell lung cancer: a systematic review and meta-analysis. PLoS One. 2014;9(9):e108958. doi:10.1371/journal.pone.0108958.
7. Jiang J, Xu N, Wu C, Deng H, Lu M, Li M, et al. Treatment of advanced gastric cancer by chemotherapy combined with autologous cytokine-induced killer cells. Anticancer Res. 2006;26(3B):2237–42.
8. Rosenberg SA, Spiess P, Lafreniere R. A new approach to the adoptive immunotherapy of cancer with tumor-infiltrating lymphocytes. Science. 1986;233(4770):1318–21.
9. Rosenberg SA, Packard BS, Aebersold PM, Solomon D, Topalian SL, Toy ST, et al. Use of tumor-infiltrating lymphocytes and interleukin-2 in the immunotherapy of patients with metastatic melanoma. A preliminary report. N Engl J Med. 1988;319(25):1676–80. doi:10.1056/NEJM198812223192527.
10. Feldman SA, Assadipour Y, Kriley I, Goff SL, Rosenberg SA. Adoptive cell therapy—tumor-infiltrating lymphocytes, T-cell receptors, and chimeric antigen receptors. Semin Oncol. 2015;42(4):626–39. doi:10.1053/j.seminoncol.2015.05.005.
11. Andersen R, Donia M, Westergaard MC, Pedersen M, Hansen M, Svane IM. Tumor infiltrating lymphocyte therapy for ovarian cancer and renal cell carcinoma. Hum Vaccin Immunother. 2015;11(12):2790–5. doi:10.1080/21645515.2015.1075106.
12. Turcotte S, Gros A, Hogan K, Tran E, Hinrichs CS, Wunderlich JR, et al. Phenotype and function of T cells infiltrating visceral metastases from gastrointestinal cancers and melanoma: implications for adoptive cell transfer therapy. J Immunol. 2013;191(5):2217–25. doi:10.4049/jimmunol.1300538.
13. Webb JR, Milne K, Watson P, Deleeuw RJ, Nelson BH. Tumor-infiltrating lymphocytes expressing the tissue resident memory marker CD103 are associated with increased survival in high-grade serous ovarian cancer. Clin Cancer Res. 2014;20(2):434–44. doi:10.1158/1078-0432.CCR-13-1877.
14. Yannelli JR, Hyatt C, McConnell S, Hines K, Jacknin L, Parker L, et al. Growth of tumor-infiltrating lymphocytes from human solid cancers: summary of a 5-year experience. Int J Cancer. 1996;65(4):413–21. doi:10.1002/(SICI)1097-0215(19960208)65:4<413::AID-IJC3>3.0.CO;2-#.
15. Yamaue H, Tanimura H, Tsunoda T, Iwahashi M, Tani M, Inoue M, et al. Clinical application of adoptive immunotherapy by cytotoxic T lymphocytes induced from tumor-infiltrating lymphocytes. Nihon Gan Chiryo Gakkai Shi. 1990;25(5):978–89.
16. Kono K, Takahashi A, Ichihara F, Amemiya H, Iizuka H, Fujii H, et al. Prognostic significance of adoptive immunotherapy with tumor-associated lymphocytes in patients with advanced gastric cancer: a randomized trial. Clin Cancer Res. 2002;8(6):1767–71.
17. Gros A, Robbins PF, Yao X, Li YF, Turcotte S, Tran E, et al. PD-1 identifies the patient-specific CD8(+) tumor-reactive repertoire infiltrating human tumors. J Clin Invest. 2014;124(5):2246–59. doi:10.1172/JCI73639.
18. Kerkar SP, Leonardi AJ, van Panhuys N, Zhang L, Yu Z, Crompton JG, et al. Collapse of the tumor stroma is triggered by IL-12 induction of Fas. Mol Ther. 2013;21(7):1369–77. doi:10.1038/mt.2013.58.
19. Tran E, Turcotte S, Gros A, Robbins PF, Lu YC, Dudley ME, et al. Cancer immunotherapy based on mutation-specific CD4+ T cells in a patient with epithelial cancer. Science. 2014;344(6184):641–5. doi:10.1126/science.1251102.
20. Karimi S, Chattopadhyay S, Chakraborty NG. Manipulation of regulatory T cells and antigen-specific cytotoxic T lymphocyte-based tumour immunotherapy. Immunology. 2015;144(2):186–96. doi:10.1111/imm.12387.
21. Hoshino T, Seki N, Kikuchi M, Kuramoto T, Iwamoto O, Kodama I, et al. HLA class-I-restricted and tumor-

specific CTL in tumor-infiltrating lymphocytes of patients with gastric cancer. Int J Cancer. 1997;70(6):631–8.
22. Louis CU, Straathof K, Bollard CM, Gerken C, Huls MH, Gresik MV, et al. Enhancing the in vivo expansion of adoptively transferred EBV-specific CTL with lymphodepleting CD45 monoclonal antibodies in NPC patients. Blood. 2009;113(11):2442–50. doi:10.1182/blood-2008-05-157222.
23. Bollard CM, Aguilar L, Straathof KC, Gahn B, Huls MH, Rousseau A, et al. Cytotoxic T lymphocyte therapy for Epstein-Barr virus+ Hodgkin's disease. J Exp Med. 2004;200(12):1623–33. doi:10.1084/jem.20040890.
24. Bae JM, Kim EH. Epstein-Barr Virus and gastric cancer risk: a meta-analysis with meta-regression of case-control studies. J Prev Med Public Health. 2016;49(2):97–107. doi:10.3961/jpmph.15.068.
25. Klebanoff CA, Rosenberg SA, Restifo NP. Prospects for gene-engineered T cell immunotherapy for solid cancers. Nat Med. 2016;22(1):26–36. doi:10.1038/nm.4015.
26. Rosenberg SA, Restifo NP. Adoptive cell transfer as personalized immunotherapy for human cancer. Science. 2015;348(6230):62–8. doi:10.1126/science.aaa4967.
27. Zhang L, Morgan RA. Genetic engineering with T cell receptors. Adv Drug Deliv Rev. 2012;64(8):756–62. doi:10.1016/j.addr.2011.11.009.
28. Morgan RA, Dudley ME, Wunderlich JR, Hughes MS, Yang JC, Sherry RM, et al. Cancer regression in patients after transfer of genetically engineered lymphocytes. Science. 2006;314(5796):126–9. doi:10.1126/science.1129003.
29. Johnson LA, Morgan RA, Dudley ME, Cassard L, Yang JC, Hughes MS, et al. Gene therapy with human and mouse T-cell receptors mediates cancer regression and targets normal tissues expressing cognate antigen. Blood. 2009;114(3):535–46. doi:10.1182/blood-2009-03-211714.
30. Robbins PF, Morgan RA, Feldman SA, Yang JC, Sherry RM, Dudley ME, et al. Tumor regression in patients with metastatic synovial cell sarcoma and melanoma using genetically engineered lymphocytes reactive with NY-ESO-1. J Clin Oncol. 2011;29(7):917–24. doi:10.1200/JCO.2010.32.2537.
31. Robbins PF, Kassim SH, Tran TL, Crystal JS, Morgan RA, Feldman SA, et al. A pilot trial using lymphocytes genetically engineered with an NY-ESO-1-reactive T-cell receptor: long-term follow-up and correlates with response. Clin Cancer Res. 2015;21(5):1019–27. doi:10.1158/1078-0432.CCR-14-2708.
32. Rapoport AP, Stadtmauer EA, Binder-Scholl GK, Goloubeva O, Vogl DT, Lacey SF, et al. NY-ESO-1-specific TCR-engineered T cells mediate sustained antigen-specific antitumor effects in myeloma. Nat Med. 2015;21(8):914–21. doi:10.1038/nm.3910.
33. Robbins PF, Li YF, El-Gamil M, Zhao Y, Wargo JA, Zheng Z, et al. Single and dual amino acid substitutions in TCR CDRs can enhance antigen-specific T cell functions. J Immunol. 2008;180(9):6116–31.
34. Morgan RA. Risky business: target choice in adoptive cell therapy. Blood. 2013;122(20):3392–4. doi:10.1182/blood-2013-09-527622.
35. Linette GP, Stadtmauer EA, Maus MV, Rapoport AP, Levine BL, Emery L, et al. Cardiovascular toxicity and titin cross-reactivity of affinity-enhanced T cells in myeloma and melanoma. Blood. 2013;122(6):863–71. doi:10.1182/blood-2013-03-490565.
36. Tran E, Ahmadzadeh M, Lu YC, Gros A, Turcotte S, Robbins PF, et al. Immunogenicity of somatic mutations in human gastrointestinal cancers. Science. 2015;350(6266):1387–90. doi:10.1126/science.aad1253.
37. Desrichard A, Snyder A, Chan TA. Cancer neoantigens and applications for immunotherapy. Clin Cancer Res. 2016;22(4):807–12. doi:10.1158/1078-0432.CCR-14-3175.
38. Eshhar Z, Waks T, Gross G, Schindler DG. Specific activation and targeting of cytotoxic lymphocytes through chimeric single chains consisting of antibody-binding domains and the gamma or zeta subunits of the immunoglobulin and T-cell receptors. Proc Natl Acad Sci U S A. 1993;90(2):720–4.
39. Maude SL, Frey N, Shaw PA, Aplenc R, Barrett DM, Bunin NJ, et al. Chimeric antigen receptor T cells for sustained remissions in leukemia. N Engl J Med. 2014;371(16):1507–17. doi:10.1056/NEJMoa1407222.
40. Gill S, Tasian SK, Ruella M, Shestova O, Li Y, Porter DL, et al. Preclinical targeting of human acute myeloid leukemia and myeloablation using chimeric antigen receptor-modified T cells. Blood. 2014;123(15):2343–54. doi:10.1182/blood-2013-09-529537.
41. Brentjens RJ, Davila ML, Riviere I, Park J, Wang X, Cowell LG, et al. CD19-targeted T cells rapidly induce molecular remissions in adults with chemotherapy-refractory acute lymphoblastic leukemia. Sci Transl Med. 2013;5(177):177ra38. doi:10.1126/scitranslmed.3005930.
42. Kochenderfer JN, Wilson WH, Janik JE, Dudley ME, Stetler-Stevenson M, Feldman SA, et al. Eradication of B-lineage cells and regression of lymphoma in a patient treated with autologous T cells genetically engineered to recognize CD19. Blood. 2010;116(20):4099–102. doi:10.1182/blood-2010-04-281931.
43. Porter DL, Hwang WT, Frey NV, Lacey SF, Shaw PA, Loren AW, et al. Chimeric antigen receptor T cells persist and induce sustained remissions in relapsed refractory chronic lymphocytic leukemia. Sci Transl Med. 2015;7(303):303ra139. doi:10.1126/scitranslmed.aac5415.
44. Porter DL, Levine BL, Kalos M, Bagg A, June CH. Chimeric antigen receptor-modified T cells in chronic lymphoid leukemia. N Engl J Med. 2011;365(8):725–33. doi:10.1056/NEJMoa1103849.
45. Davila ML, Riviere I, Wang X, Bartido S, Park J, Curran K, et al. Efficacy and toxicity management of 19-28z CAR T cell therapy in B cell acute lymphoblastic leukemia. Sci Transl Med. 2014;6(224):224ra25. doi:10.1126/scitranslmed.3008226.

46. Lee DW, Kochenderfer JN, Stetler-Stevenson M, Cui YK, Delbrook C, Feldman SA, et al. T cells expressing CD19 chimeric antigen receptors for acute lymphoblastic leukaemia in children and young adults: a phase 1 dose-escalation trial. Lancet. 2015;385(9967):517–28. doi:10.1016/S0140-6736(14)61403-3.
47. Garfall AL, Maus MV, Hwang WT, Lacey SF, Mahnke YD, Melenhorst JJ, et al. Chimeric antigen receptor T Cells against CD19 for multiple myeloma. N Engl J Med. 2015;373(11):1040–7. doi:10.1056/NEJMoa1504542.
48. Morgan RA, Yang JC, Kitano M, Dudley ME, Laurencot CM, Rosenberg SA. Case report of a serious adverse event following the administration of T cells transduced with a chimeric antigen receptor recognizing ERBB2. Mol Ther. 2010;18(4):843–51. doi:10.1038/mt.2010.24.
49. Lamers CH, Sleijfer S, van Steenbergen S, van Elzakker P, van Krimpen B, Groot C, et al. Treatment of metastatic renal cell carcinoma with CAIX CAR-engineered T cells: clinical evaluation and management of on-target toxicity. Mol Ther. 2013;21(4):904–12. doi:10.1038/mt.2013.17.
50. Louis CU, Savoldo B, Dotti G, Pule M, Yvon E, Myers GD, et al. Antitumor activity and long-term fate of chimeric antigen receptor-positive T cells in patients with neuroblastoma. Blood. 2011;118(23):6050–6. doi:10.1182/blood-2011-05-354449.
51. Lee DW, Gardner R, Porter DL, Louis CU, Ahmed N, Jensen M, et al. Current concepts in the diagnosis and management of cytokine release syndrome. Blood. 2014;124(2):188–95. doi:10.1182/blood-2014-05-552729.
52. Posey Jr AD, Schwab RD, Boesteanu AC, Steentoft C, Mandel U, Engels B, et al. Engineered CAR T cells targeting the cancer-associated Tn-glycoform of the membrane mucin MUC1 control adenocarcinoma. Immunity. 2016;44(6):1444–54. doi:10.1016/j.immuni.2016.05.014.
53. Yang J, Li ZH, Zhou JJ, Chen RF, Cheng LZ, Zhou QB, et al. Preparation and antitumor effects of nanovaccines with MAGE-3 peptides in transplanted gastric cancer in mice. Chin J Cancer. 2010;29(4):359–64.
54. Kono K, Takahashi A, Sugai H, Fujii H, Choudhury AR, Kiessling R, et al. Dendritic cells pulsed with HER-2/neu-derived peptides can induce specific T-cell responses in patients with gastric cancer. Clin Cancer Res. 2002;8(11):3394–400.
55. Amemiya H, Pena A, Chiurillo M, Moscoso J, Useche A, Baffi R. Increased expression of the c-Met receptor mRNA in gastric cancer. Invest Clin. 2013;54(3):284–98.
56. Ajani JA, Hecht JR, Ho L, Baker J, Oortgiesen M, Eduljee A, et al. An open-label, multinational, multicenter study of G17DT vaccination combined with cisplatin and 5-fluorouracil in patients with untreated, advanced gastric or gastroesophageal cancer: the GC4 study. Cancer. 2006;106(9):1908–16. doi:10.1002/cncr.21814.
57. Li ZY, Shan F, Zhang LH, Bu ZD, Wu AW, Wu XJ, et al. Preoperative chemotherapy with a trastuzumab-containing regimen for a patient with gastric cancer and hepatic metastases. Genet Mol Res. 2014;13(4):10952–7. doi:10.4238/2014.December.19.17.
58. Sun M, Shi H, Liu C, Liu J, Liu X, Sun Y. Construction and evaluation of a novel humanized HER2-specific chimeric receptor. Breast Cancer Res. 2014;16(3):R61. doi:10.1186/bcr3674.
59. Ahmed N, Brawley VS, Hegde M, Robertson C, Ghazi A, Gerken C, et al. Human epidermal growth factor receptor 2 (HER2)-specific chimeric antigen receptor-modified T cells for the immunotherapy of HER2-positive sarcoma. J Clin Oncol. 2015;33(15):1688–96. doi:10.1200/JCO.2014.58.0225.
60. Lee J, van Hummelen P, Go C, Palescandolo E, Jang J, Park HY, et al. High-throughput mutation profiling identifies frequent somatic mutations in advanced gastric adenocarcinoma. PLoS One. 2012;7(6):e38892. doi:10.1371/journal.pone.0038892.
61. Wang L, Heng X, Lu Y, Cai Z, Yi Q, Che F. Could B7-H4 serve as a target to activate anti-cancer immunity? Int Immunopharmacol. 2016;38:97–103. doi:10.1016/j.intimp.2016.05.020.
62. Burns WR, Zheng Z, Rosenberg SA, Morgan RA. Lack of specific gamma-retroviral vector long terminal repeat promoter silencing in patients receiving genetically engineered lymphocytes and activation upon lymphocyte restimulation. Blood. 2009;114(14):2888–99. doi:10.1182/blood-2009-01-199216.
63. Davis JL, Theoret MR, Zheng Z, Lamers CH, Rosenberg SA, Morgan RA. Development of human anti-murine T-cell receptor antibodies in both responding and nonresponding patients enrolled in TCR gene therapy trials. Clin Cancer Res. 2010;16(23):5852–61. doi:10.1158/1078-0432.CCR-10-1280.
64. Parkhurst MR, Yang JC, Langan RC, Dudley ME, Nathan DA, Feldman SA, et al. T cells targeting carcinoembryonic antigen can mediate regression of metastatic colorectal cancer but induce severe transient colitis. Mol Ther. 2011;19(3):620–6. doi:10.1038/mt.2010.272.
65. Morgan RA, Chinnasamy N, Abate-Daga D, Gros A, Robbins PF, Zheng Z, et al. Cancer regression and neurological toxicity following anti-MAGE-A3 TCR gene therapy. J Immunother. 2013;36(2):133–51. doi:10.1097/CJI.0b013e3182829903.
66. Kalos M, Levine BL, Porter DL, Katz S, Grupp SA, Bagg A, et al. T cells with chimeric antigen receptors have potent antitumor effects and can establish memory in patients with advanced leukemia. Sci Transl Med. 2011;3(95):95ra73. doi:10.1126/scitranslmed.3002842.
67. Kochenderfer JN, Dudley ME, Feldman SA, Wilson WH, Spaner DE, Maric I, et al. B-cell depletion and remissions of malignancy along with cytokine-associated toxicity in a clinical trial of anti-CD19 chimeric-antigen-receptor-transduced T cells. Blood. 2012;119(12):2709–20. doi:10.1182/blood-2011-10-384388.
68. Savoldo B, Ramos CA, Liu E, Mims MP, Keating MJ, Carrum G, et al. CD28 costimulation improves expansion and persistence of chimeric antigen receptor-

modified T cells in lymphoma patients. J Clin Invest. 2011;121(5):1822–6. doi:10.1172/JCI46110.
69. Till BG, Jensen MC, Wang J, Chen EY, Wood BL, Greisman HA, et al. Adoptive immunotherapy for indolent non-Hodgkin lymphoma and mantle cell lymphoma using genetically modified autologous CD20-specific T cells. Blood. 2008;112(6):2261–71. doi:10.1182/blood-2007-12-128843.
70. Till BG, Jensen MC, Wang J, Qian X, Gopal AK, Maloney DG, et al. CD20-specific adoptive immunotherapy for lymphoma using a chimeric antigen receptor with both CD28 and 4-1BB domains: pilot clinical trial results. Blood. 2012;119(17):3940–50. doi:10.1182/blood-2011-10-387969.
71. Park JR, Digiusto DL, Slovak M, Wright C, Naranjo A, Wagner J, et al. Adoptive transfer of chimeric antigen receptor re-directed cytolytic T lymphocyte clones in patients with neuroblastoma. Mol Ther. 2007;15(4):825–33. doi:10.1038/sj.mt.6300104.
72. van Schalkwyk MC, Papa SE, Jeannon JP, Guerrero Urbano T, Spicer JF, Maher J. Design of a phase I clinical trial to evaluate intratumoral delivery of ErbB-targeted chimeric antigen receptor T-cells in locally advanced or recurrent head and neck cancer. Hum Gene Ther Clin Dev. 2013;24(3):134–42. doi:10.1089/humc.2013.144.
73. Ma Q, Gonzalo-Daganzo RM, Junghans RP. Genetically engineered T cells as adoptive immunotherapy of cancer. Cancer Chemother Biol Response Modif. 2002;20:315–41.
74. Katz SC, Burga RA, McCormack E, Wang LJ, Mooring W, Point GR, et al. Phase I hepatic immunotherapy for metastases study of intra-arterial chimeric antigen receptor-modified T-cell therapy for CEA+ liver metastases. Clin Cancer Res. 2015;21(14):3149–59. doi:10.1158/1078-0432.CCR-14-1421.
75. Ritchie DS, Neeson PJ, Khot A, Peinert S, Tai T, Tainton K, et al. Persistence and efficacy of second generation CAR T cell against the LeY antigen in acute myeloid leukemia. Mol Ther. 2013;21(11):2122–9. doi:10.1038/mt.2013.154.
76. Kruit WH, Suciu S, Dreno B, Mortier L, Robert C, Chiarion-Sileni V, et al. Selection of immunostimulant AS15 for active immunization with MAGE-A3 protein: results of a randomized phase II study of the european organisation for research and treatment of cancer melanoma group in metastatic melanoma. J Clin Oncol. 2013;31(19):2413–20. doi:10.1200/JCO.2012.43.7111.
77. Vansteenkiste J, Zielinski M, Linder A, Dahabreh J, Gonzalez EE, Malinowski W, et al. Adjuvant MAGE-A3 immunotherapy in resected non-small-cell lung cancer: phase II randomized study results. J Clin Oncol. 2013;31(19):2396–403. doi:10.1200/JCO.2012.43.7103.
78. Vansteenkiste JF, Cho BC, Vanakesa T, De Pas T, Zielinski M, Kim MS, et al. Efficacy of the MAGE-A3 cancer immunotherapeutic as adjuvant therapy in patients with resected MAGE-A3-positive non-small-cell lung cancer (MAGRIT): a randomised, double-blind, placebo-controlled, phase 3 trial. Lancet Oncol. 2016;17(6):822–35. doi:10.1016/S1470-2045(16)00099-1.
79. Gros A, Parkhurst MR, Tran E, Pasetto A, Robbins PF, Ilyas S, et al. Prospective identification of neoantigen-specific lymphocytes in the peripheral blood of melanoma patients. Nat Med. 2016;22(4):433–8. doi:10.1038/nm.4051.

Combinational Immunotherapy of Gastric Cancer

12

Juan Du and Baorui Liu

12.1 Introduction

Results from recent clinical trials using many novel immunotherapy strategies, including immune checkpoint blockade and adoptive T-cell therapy approaches (CAR T-cell and TCR T-cell therapy), have clearly demonstrated the importance of immunotherapy as a critical treatment strategy for gastric cancer patients. These therapies are additional options to the traditional treatment approaches of surgery, chemotherapy, radiotherapy, and targeted therapy. However, until now, immunotherapy has demonstrated clinical benefits in only a small fraction of patients. To improve the potential benefit of cancer immunotherapy, synergistic combinations of different immunotherapy approaches are currently being explored.

There exist numerous examples in the history of medicine where the combination of different therapeutic strategies results in an improved patient response. Currently, several preclinical and clinical trial studies are underway which aim to explore the therapeutic utility of combinational immunotherapy in gastric cancer patients [1–3]. However, limited data have been reported from these trials so far, preventing firm conclusions from being made.

J. Du (✉) • B. Liu
The Comprehensive Cancer Centre of Drum Tower Hospital, Medical School of Nanjing University and Clinical Cancer Institute of Nanjing University, Nanjing 210008, China
e-mail: dujuanglyy@163.com

Cancer is a disease that evolves to exploit multiple mechanisms in an effort to avoid immune cell recognition, preventing an innate or adaptive immune response. These mechanisms include the downregulation of MHC expression, which renders tumor cells insensitive to T-cell recognition, and the secretion of factors that suppress T-cell responsiveness [4, 5]. Over the last decade, treatment has been developed to specifically target these mechanisms, generating a great deal of enthusiasm for cancer immunotherapy. However, a critical issue remains, which is the best way to combine these different immunotherapy treatments. Here, we will discuss strategies for the development and personalization of combinational cancer immunotherapy strategies.

12.2 Combination of Immunotherapy with Chemotherapy

The clinical efficacy of current tumor immunotherapy and vaccination methods is unsatisfactory. One reason which addresses the lack of clinical efficacy with these treatment options is that immunosuppressive mechanisms predominate in patients with advanced cancer [6]. Because chemotherapy is often associated with potent immunosuppressive effects, the combined use of conventional cancer chemotherapy and cancer immunotherapy has been questioned.

J. Wei, B. Liu (eds.), *Personalized Management of Gastric Cancer*,
DOI 10.1007/978-981-10-3978-2_12

Until recently, it was the generalized belief that chemotherapy and immunotherapy should not be combined due to myelosuppressive effects associated with most cytotoxic agents [7].

However, it has recently been discovered that chemotherapeutics can exhibit several beneficial effects on the immune system [8, 9]. Certain cytotoxic agents, including cyclophosphamide, gemcitabine, and paclitaxel, have been linked to increased primary cell-mediated immunity [10–13]. In addition, both preclinical and clinical findings have suggested that conventional chemotherapy can result in the induction of immune responses against antigens generated by tumor cells undergoing cell death. These antigens include the tumor-cell secreted high-mobility group box 1 (HMGB1) alarmin proteins on Toll-like receptor 4 (TLR4) expressed by dendritic cells [14, 15]. In addition, chemotherapy treatment is thought to induce the release of tumor-specific antigens from tumor cells undergoing cell death, resulting in an improvement in the immunogenicity of the tumor microenvironment. Increased antigen exposure within the tumor microenvironment after chemotherapy is sufficient to generate a productive immune response [8]. In a series of preclinical trials, it was found that treatment with various cytotoxic agents, such as paclitaxel and cisplatin, rendered tumor cells more susceptible to the cytotoxic effect of T lymphocytes and resulted in an induction of apoptosis in a broader range of tumor cells.

Cyclophosphamide has been shown to result in the depletion of suppressive regulatory T cells (Treg), generating enhanced T-cell reactivity [16]. Studies have also shown that a low dosage cyclophosphamide treatment selectively depleted Treg in cancer patients, while a high dosage treatment lost this specificity [17].

Gemcitabine has been shown to selectively deplete Treg cells as well. Gemcitabine treatment alone was shown to increase the number of $CD8^+$ T cells within tumors, which is necessary for the eradication of solid tumors [18]. With the use of gemcitabine in conjunction with cytokine or vaccine treatments, synergistic antitumor activity can result in a reduction in MDSC numbers [19]. Immunotherapeutics aimed at stimulating antigen-presenting cells (APC) have also been shown to benefit from the coadministration of gemcitabine, as observed in studies where gemcitabine treatment was combined with an anti-CD40 agonist antibody [20].

Paclitaxel has been shown to alter the cytokine network at the site of the tumor, while 5-fluorouracil has been shown to exhibit a pronounced effect on the depletion of myeloid-derived suppressor cells (MDSC) [21]. Doxorubicin has been demonstrated to induce immunogenic cell death and activate antitumor T-cell immune responses. Enhanced therapeutic efficacy was discovered when patients were preconditioned with a single low dose of doxorubicin or paclitaxel, followed by adoptive T-cell transfer therapy [22].

Oxaliplatin, a platinum-based drug, was recently demonstrated to induce immunogenic cell death, resulting in increased levels of tumor antigen presented by APC [23]. The use of oxaliplatin in combination with an inducible adenoviral IL-12 (Ad-IL-12) system was demonstrated to result in less of an immunosuppressive microenvironment, as characterized by a reduction of MDSC in intratumoral and an increased ratio of $CD8^+$/Treg cells [24].

Using this strategy, better clinical results have been obtained. Proof-of-concept clinical trials indicated that the efficacy of immunotherapy is likely enhanced by chemotherapy.

In a phase II trial launched in metastatic colon cancer patients, a polychemotherapeutic treatment strategy with gemcitabine and FOLFOX-4 (oxaliplatin, fluorouracil, and folinic acid) combined with GM-CSF and IL-2 demonstrated that a tumor antigen-specific immune response was elicited, with a high objective response and disease control rates [25].

A phase I/II clinical study aimed to test the effectiveness of peptides derived from vascular endothelial growth factor receptor (VEGFR) 1 and 2 in association with cisplatin and S-1 chemotherapy in patients with advanced gastric cancer. This combination therapy was found to be well tolerated and highly effective in advanced or recurrent gastric cancer patient populations [26]. In an additional randomized phase II clinical trial, the effect of metronomic cyclophosphamide (CPA) combined with personalized peptide vaccination (PPV) was investigated. The overall survival of patients with positive immune responses was determined

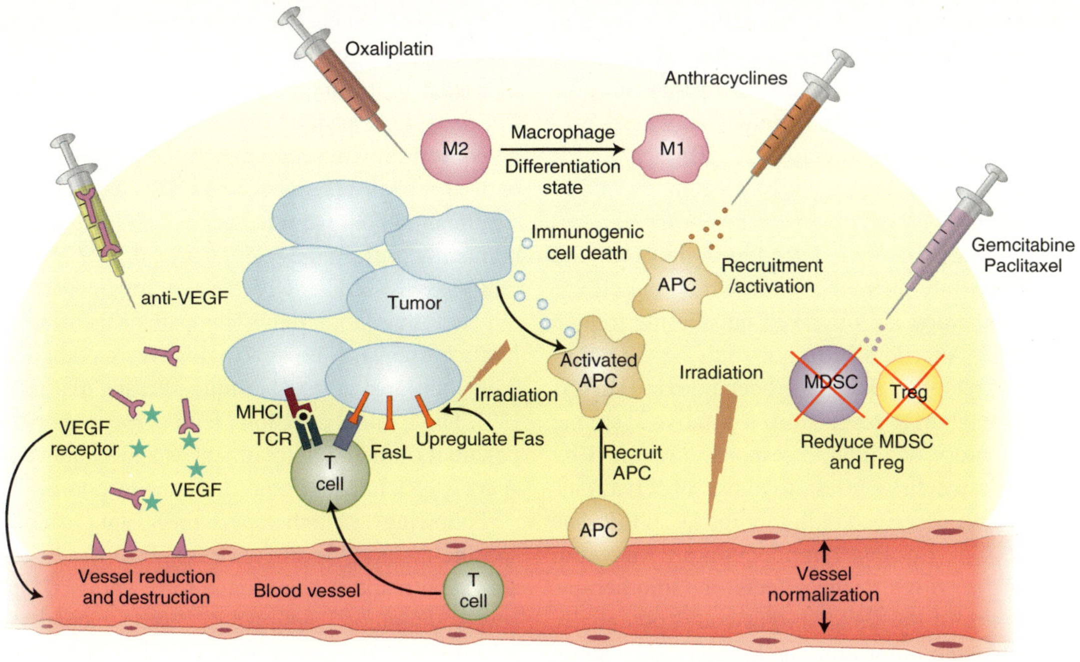

Fig. 12.1 The effects of chemotherapy and radiotherapy on the tumor microenvironment. A range of chemotherapeutic agents can affect the tumor microenvironment in a variety of ways. Oxaliplatin can induce immunogenic cell death in a proportion of tumor cells, which can lead to the release of tumor antigens for uptake and processing by antigen presenting cells (APC). Anthracyclines can recruit APCs and enhance their differentiation to an activated phenotype, better able to present antigen to lymphocytes. Oxaliplatin can also lead to an increased proportion of proinflammatory, M1, macrophages relative to alternatively activated, M2, macrophages. Gemcitabine, oxaliplatin and paclitaxel can reduce the frequency of myeloidderived suppressor cells (MDSC) and/or regulatory T cells (Treg) infiltrating tumors, thereby reducing their immunosuppressive effects. Tumor cells can upregulate expression of immune target molecules such as Fas and MHCI following irradiation, thereby rendering them sensitive to attack by T cells. Irradiation can also normalize dilated and chaotic blood vessels to enable T cells to access tumors. Increases in intratumoral T cells can also be achieved using antibodies against vascular endothelial growth factor (VEGF) (Adapted from Enhancing immunotherapy using chemotherapy and radiation to modify the tumor microenvironment (2013), Kershaw MH et al. [6])

to be longer compared with those having negative immune responses [27].

Another study was carried out to evaluate the efficacy and safety of cellular immunotherapy (CIT) in combination with chemotherapy treatment in patients with GC [28]. The median PFS of the chemo/CIT group was found to be significantly longer compared to that of the control group. This was especially evident in the case of GC patients with advanced stage, poorly differentiated carcinoma or lymph node metastasis. The QOL was found to be improved in patients treated with chemo/CIT compared with those of the control group.

Thus, a better understanding of the effect of these drugs on the immune system and tumor microenvironment will enable the design of more effective combination treatments for gastric cancer patients [6]. This combinational therapy approach combining chemotherapy and immunotherapy may be widely applicable to cancer patients (Fig. 12.1).

12.3 Combination of Immunotherapy with Radiotherapy

Ionizing radiation induces both direct and indirect killing of cancer cells. For a long time, this treatment approach has been considered to be immunosuppressive. However, this concept has evolved over the past few years as it has been demonstrated that irradiation increases tumor immunogenicity, favoring the killing effect of an immune response against tumor cells [29]. Several studies have demonstrated that the efficacy of immunotherapy is enhanced when combined with radiation therapy [10, 30].

The term abscopal, derived from the Latin term *ab* (away from) and the ancient Greek term *skopos* (target), was introduced in 1953 to describe a rare phenomenon in which the effects of radiotherapy are observed outside the treated area [31]. Anecdotally, tumors outside the radiotherapy treatment field have been noted to shrink. This is thought to result from a putative systemic inflammatory or immune response provoked by radiotherapy. In contrast to these observations, others have described radiotherapy as an immune suppressant. Because lymphocytes are known to be very sensitive to the effects of radiotherapy, irradiation of the tumor target could potentially eliminate antitumor immune activity. This, along with the fact that there exists limited local control of radiotherapy and of early immune therapies on systemic disease, has dampened enthusiasm for pursuing this treatment combination [29].

In recent years, two case reports have highlighted the immune adjuvant effect of radiotherapy treatment in melanoma patients. In the first case, the melanoma patient had a presumed abscopal response following radiotherapy alone and a second abscopal response following a combined treatment of both radiotherapy and targeted immunotherapy [32]. In the second case, the patient initially progressed slowly despite treatment with targeted immunotherapy. This patient then exhibited a response following palliative radiotherapy with additional targeted immunotherapy treatment [33]. These initial anecdotal reports focused on the potential of radiation treatment as a mechanism to spark a systemic antitumor immune response.

Following radiotherapy, preexisting tumor-specific antibody levels were found to rise, T-cell activation markers were found to be enriched, and new antitumor antibodies were identified. Augmenting immune activity is also thought to potentiate the local effects of radiotherapy. The possibility of improving the treatment of both local and widespread disease makes this combinational treatment worthy of further investigation (Fig. 12.2).

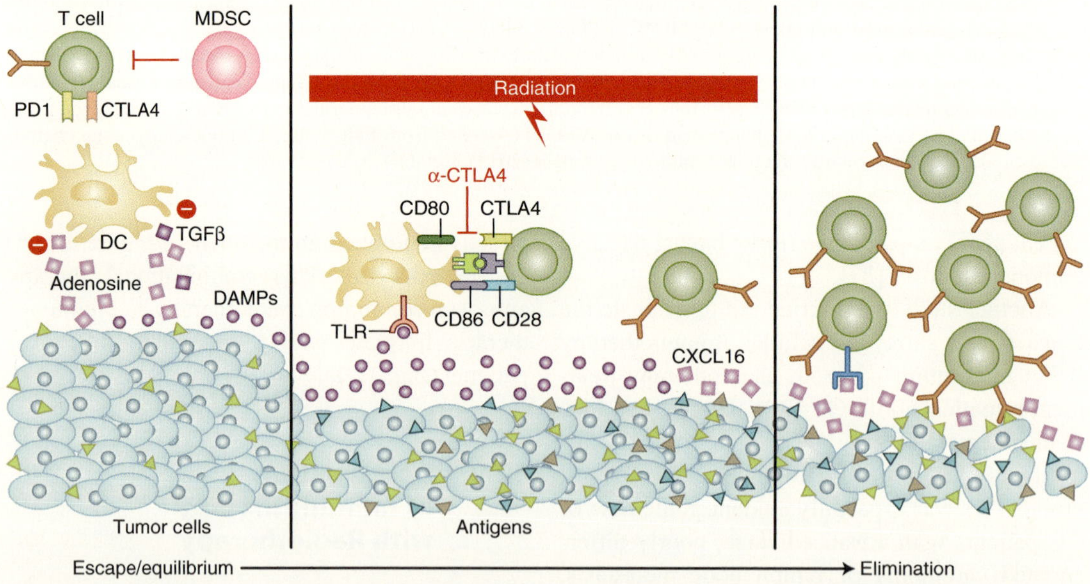

Fig. 12.2 The role of RT in induction of the antitumor immune response. At baseline, both the tumor immune microenvironment and the poor antigenicity of the tumor allow it to escape immune recognition. Targeted RT can induce increased antigenic expression, release pro-inflammatory cytokines (e.g., CXCL16) that recruit immune cells, promote antigen cross-presentation (HMGB-1 via TLR4), and induce tumor expression of death receptors. Anti-CTLA4–targeted immunotherapy can enhance the adaptive immune component by promoting antigen crosspresentation and T cell activation. Used together, RT and immunotherapy may have synergistic effects and may shift the tumor immune system balance toward elimination (Adapted from Radiation and immunotherapy: a synergistic combination (2013), Kalbasi A et al. [29])

The development of a systemic antitumor immune response has been described as concomitant immunity. Evidence suggests that radiotherapy could induce concomitant immunity where it did not exist previously (e.g., RT-induced in situ vaccination). Numerous animal models have demonstrated augmentation of systemic antitumor immunity following local radiotherapy, resulting in the reduction, control, or elimination of distant metastases, especially when used in combination with immunotherapy [32–34]. Thus, the combination of radiotherapy and immunotherapy for the treatment of locally advanced disease is currently being studied in several clinical trials, with the majority of patients being melanoma and prostate cancer patients [29, 35].

In addition to promoting recognition of tumor by preexisting tumor-specific T cells, radiotherapy has also been demonstrated to generate tumor-specific cytotoxic T cells. A recent clinical trial showed that the combination of radiotherapy with intranodal injection of low-dose rituximab resulted in the induction of systemic $CD8^+$ T-cell immunity and regression of disseminated follicular lymphoma in immature dendritic cells and GM-CSF [12]. Irradiated tumors have been shown to upregulate death receptors (e.g., FAS), which could promote the cytotoxic effect of T cells at the tumor site. The immune system, which is devoid of its negative regulatory pathways at the site of the irradiated tumor, can function as a powerful local antitumor agent. These studies suggest a promising role for immune modulatory agents in the generation of improved radiotherapy efficacy.

Moreover, radiotherapy has been shown to cause an inflammatory response in the tumor microenvironment, resulting in the release of cytokines and chemokines and the upregulation of adhesion molecules. Recruitment of cytotoxic T cells to the irradiated tumor site is enhanced due to the release of chemokines, such as CXCL16 [36]. Irradiation was found to cause tumor vasculature remodeling, a result of the upregulation of CXCL9 and CXCL10, which enhances the density and alters the diameter of blood vessels within tumors such that they resemble capillaries. Following irradiation, T cells were found to be able to access and penetrate the tumor, inducing complete tumor regression in some cases. So, irradiation could be followed by the adoptive transfer of activated, tumor-specific lymphocytes, which previously unable to adhere to endothelium and thus access the tumor [37].

12.4 Combination of Cancer Vaccine with Immune Checkpoint Inhibitor

Immune checkpoint inhibitors have contributed great progress to cancer treatment. However, numerous challenges remain, limiting the further development of these immunotherapy drugs. Specifically, only approximately 10–30% of cancer patients with some certain types of solid tumors have exhibited an objective response to treatments using immune checkpoint inhibitors. Such challenges are attributed to properties of the tumor microenvironment (TME) [38].

The TME generates immune-tolerant conditions, posing an obvious challenge for the induction of antitumor immune responses. If the early influx of $CD8^+$ T cells fails to clear the tumor in the TME, tumor cells which express high levels of PD-L1 will induce T-cell anergy, leading to decreased effector T-cell activity. Therapeutically blocking this pathway is thought to enable the reactivation of effector T cells in the tumor.

T cells are often the primary target of therapeutic immune checkpoint inhibitors. Effector T-cell infiltration of solid tumors is considered a signature trait of patients who have responded positively to immune checkpoint inhibitor treatment [39]. Using this marker of T-cell infiltration, it has been determined that only a fraction of solid tumor patients respond to immune checkpoint inhibitors. Thus, the remaining cancer patients would unlikely respond to immune checkpoint inhibitors when used as a single-agent treatment due to the lack of targets [40]. The TME in immune checkpoint inhibitor resistant tumors has been described to resemble that of an engine without gas. Specifically, even if the "brake" set by immune checkpoints is released with immune checkpoint inhibitor immunotherapy, no effective antitumor immune response would be elicited in this case [38].

Cancer vaccines have been demonstrated to enhance the infiltration of effector T cells into tumors in preclinical models. All vaccine-based therapies have been designed such that antigens are delivered to the patients in order to induce tumor-specific effector T cells. A vaccine-based therapy could possibly be the most efficient way to induce T-cell infiltration into tumors.

The formation of immune regulatory structures within the TME is just the first step toward the establishment of an enhanced anticancer immune response. This is attributed to the ability of lymphoid aggregates to express both effector-activating and deactivating immune signatures. Interestingly, PD-L1 expression was found to be induced in all lymphoid aggregates [41]. This observation is consistent with adaptive immune resistance, which occurs with activation of PD-L1 signaling by vaccine-induced adaptive immune response [42]. Thus, vaccine-based therapies may prime advanced tumors for anti-PD-1/PD-L1 treatments [43].

It is thought that vaccines would help stimulate the initiation of the T-cell response, while checkpoint therapies would enhance the activated T-cell response. A blockade of PD-1 or CTLA-4 combined with vaccine treatments was shown to effectively eradicate tumors in multiple preclinical models [44, 45]. Two clinical trials have been initiated which have been designed to test the pancreatic cancer vaccine-based therapy in combination with nivolumab, a treatment for advanced pancreatic cancer (ClinicalTrials.gov identifier: NCT02243371 and NCT02451982). Whether anti-PD-1 therapeutic antibodies can enhance the efficacy of cancer vaccines in the treatment of cancer remains to be studied. The combination treatment using GVAX and the anti-CTLA-4 antibody, ipilimumab, has also been demonstrated to be potentially effective in the treatment of metastatic pancreatic cancer [46]. Preclinical studies showed that the combined treatment of GVAX and ipilimumab resulted in a dramatic increase in the number of effector CD8 T cells in the tumor region, with enhanced tumor-antigen directed lytic function. These effects were found to be maximized when the CTLA-4 blockade was applied following vaccination, but not before. Moreover, the incorporation of a low-dosage cyclophosphamide treatment into this combined treatment regimen was found to provide additional preclinical benefits [47].

In summary, cancer vaccine-based immunotherapy may provide a treatment option to overcome the resistance of certain cancers to immune checkpoint inhibitors, while immune checkpoint inhibitors may further enhance the efficacy of existing cancer-vaccine therapies. Combination immunotherapy merges the strengths of each individual immunotherapy approach, with the cancer vaccine functioning to fuel the engine and the immune checkpoint inhibitors functioning to release the brake [38]. The combination of cancer vaccines and immune checkpoint inhibitors may function synergistically to induce more effective antitumor immune responses (Fig. 12.3).

12.5 Combination of ACT with Immune Checkpoint Inhibitor

Adoptive cell transfer (ACT) is thought to be a promising avenue for cancer treatment. However, despite ongoing improvements in this field, many patients do not experience clinical benefits. The tumor microenvironment is a critical limiting factor in immunotherapy that has not been fully addressed in ACT treatments. Because PD-1 has been shown to attenuate T-cell-mediated antitumor responses, blocking the PD-1 pathway in vivo could function to restore defective effector function of tumor-infiltrating T cells. Thus, an anti-PD-1 antibody could function to enhance the antitumor activity of ACT. The limited preclinical data available supports the use of combination of cellular and immune-modulating mAb therapies in syngeneic cancer models. In these models, the combination of a PD-1 blockade with murine CAR-T cells showed a significantly enhanced antitumor effect compared with either treatment method alone [48]. In addition, treatment with the anti-PD-1 antibody was found to increase expression levels of IFN-γ and IFN-γ inducible chemokine production at the tumor site. This resulted in an increased chemokine-dependent trafficking of immune cells to malignant disease sites [49]. A blockade of PD-1 in combination with ACT demonstrates therapeutic synergy and could provide a potential strategy for the improvement of clinical response rates to ACT.

We predict that, in patients with tumors containing an intermediate neoantigen-presentation

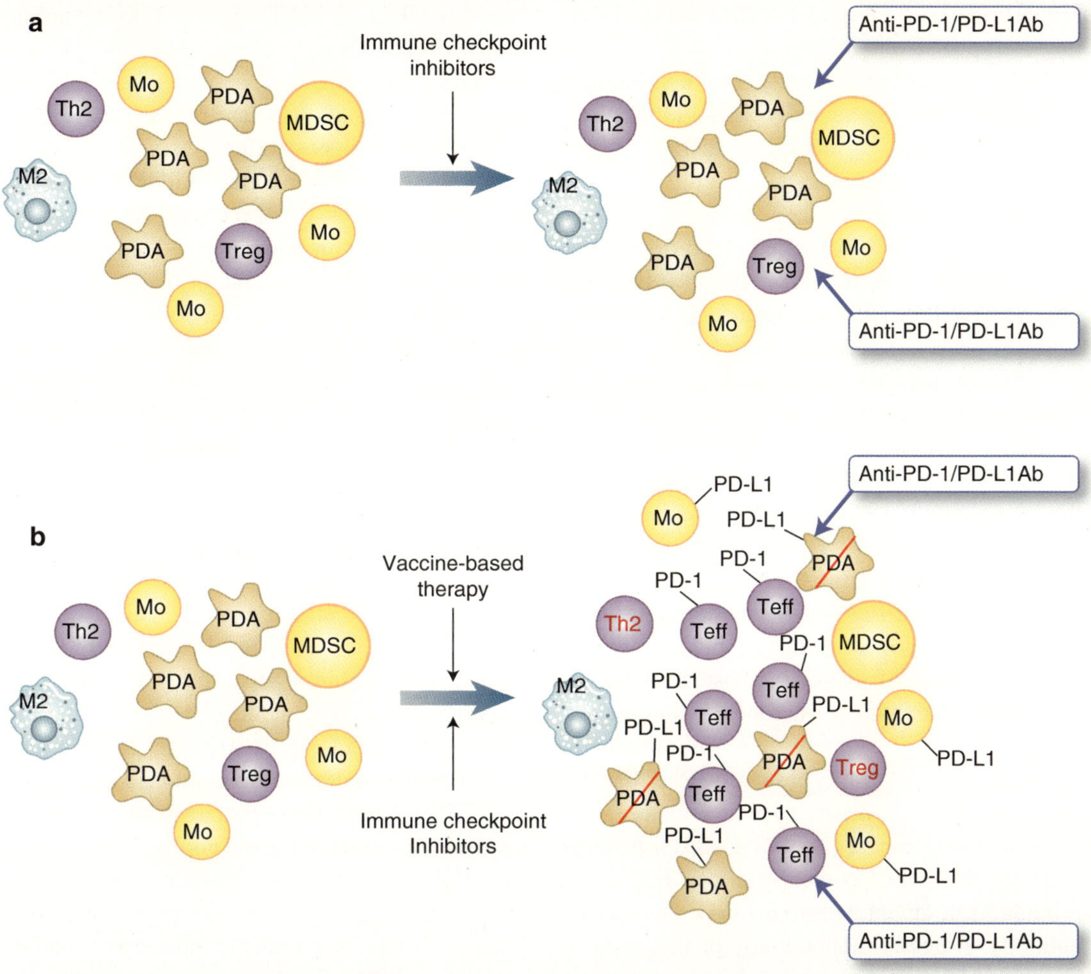

Fig. 12.3 Model for the combination of vaccine-based therapy and immune checkpoint inhibitors. (A) Pancreatic ductal adenocarcinoma (PDA) is infiltrated primarily with M2 macrophages (M2), type 2 T helper cells (Th2), myeloid-derived suppressive cells (MDSC), and regulatory T cells (Treg) but with few effector T cells (Teffs). Lacking PD-1/PD-L1 targets, PDA does not respond to single-agent checkpoint inhibitor treatments, such as anti-PD-1 or PD-L1 therapeutic antibodies (anti-PD-1/PD-L1 Ab). (B) Following vaccine-based therapy, vaccine induced Teffs are infiltrated into PDA; however, PD-L1/PD-L1-mediated immune checkpoint pathways are also induced. By targeting PD-L1/PD-L1 signals on PDA tumor cells and monocytes (Mo) induced by vaccine-based therapy, anti-PD-1/PD-L1 therapeutic antibodies enhance vaccine-induced antitumor immune responses (Adapted from Fueling the engine and releasing the break: combinational therapy of cancer vaccines and immune checkpoint inhibitors (2015), Kleponis J et al. [38])

capacity, the maximal immune-mediated antitumor responses would be achieved best in patients where the microenvironment can be modified and HLA-independent targeted effectors can be added, such as observed with combination immune-modulating mAbs plus ACT therapy or, potentially, CAR-T-cell therapy. However, it is important to note that a risk of toxicities could be exacerbated when these approaches are utilized. We eagerly await the results of ongoing clinical trials aimed to investigate the combination treatment of immune checkpoint inhibitors with ACT.

12.6 Combination of Various Immune Checkpoint Inhibitors

Early results from the use of combination immunotherapy strategies to block multiple immune resistance mechanisms demonstrate that a greater proportion of patients may benefit from combination therapies. Combination of anti-CTLA-4 and anti-PD-1 therapy has already shown significant clinical promise. Specifically, in a global phase III trial, combination therapy of nivolumab and ipilimumab has demonstrated an unprecedented 61% response rate and a 22% complete response rate in patients with advanced stage melanoma. These results compare with a 10–30% response rate observed in patients treated with a single agent. However, it should be noted that combination therapy was associated with a higher incidence of immune-related adverse events [50].

Based on these encouraging results, several phase I/II trials are currently underway to test the combination treatment of an anti-CTLA-4 and an anti-PD-1/PD-L1 antibody, with promising preliminary results. A phase I trial exploring the combination of tremelimumab with durvalumab treatment with GC patients is currently ongoing. An ongoing phase Ib/II trial is aimed at investigating the activity of single-agent nivolumab or nivolumab plus ipilimumab in patients with metastatic gastric cancer, pancreatic cancer, triple-negative breast cancer, and small-cell lung cancer (NCT01975831). Another ongoing phase Ib/II clinical trial of MEDI4736, a human immunoglobulin (Ig) G1κ anti-PD-L1 antibody, either as monotherapy or in combination with the CTLA-4 inhibitor, tremelimumab, monotherapy in gastric or GEJ adenocarcinoma patients (NCT02340975) is also underway.

The combination of agents that enhance effector T-cell function with agents that suppress immune-suppressive elements, such as MDSC, Tregs, and macrophages, in the tumor microenvironment may prove to be complementary, and possibly synergistic. Thus, many of these avenues are being actively investigated for cancer therapy.

12.7 Combination of Immune Checkpoint Inhibitor with Co-stimulation mAbs

The concept of increasing T-cell activity with co-stimulatory mAbs while simultaneously liberating activated T cells to lyse malignant cells by blocking PD-1 or PD-L1 is a promising antitumor approach. Numerous ongoing clinical trials involving patients across various solid tumor and hematological malignancies are being carried out to investigate this possibility.

The generation of optimal "killer" CD8 T-cell responses requires T-cell receptor activation and co-stimulation. This can be provided by the ligation of tumor necrosis factor receptor family members, including OX40 (CD134) and 4-1BB (CD137). OX40 is of particular interest as it has been shown that treatment with an activating (agonist) anti-OX40 mAb results in increased T-cell differentiation and cytolytic function. This leads to an enhanced antitumor immunity against a variety of tumor types. When given as single-agent treatments, these drugs have been shown to induce potent clinical and immunologic responses in patients with metastatic cancer. However, each of these singular agents benefits only a subset of patients. This highlights the importance of research aimed at identifying more effective combinatorial therapeutic strategies [51].

Recent data indicates that combined anti-OX40/anti-CTLA-4 mAb therapy dramatically improved survival rates observed in the poorly immunogenic TRAMP-C1 prostate and the more immunogenic MCA-205 sarcoma models. Specifically, this combination therapy was found to induce robust effector CD4 and CD8 T-cell responses required for the induction of tumor regression [52]. Marabelle et al. recently demonstrated that combined anti-OX40 and anti-CTLA-4 (with adjuvant CpG) therapy successfully induced the regression of local and distant tumors using several aggressive tumor models when the drugs were administered intra-tumorally. The mechanism by which this combination therapy functions is thought to be through the depletion of Treg cells at the tumor site, allowing for a greater inburst of CD8 T cells into the tumor [53].

Moreover, promising results from a study carried out by Guo et al. showed that the PD-1 blockade synergized with the agonistic anti-OX40 mAb to promote the regression of an implantable murine ovarian cancer, which was demonstrated to be nonresponsive to either monotherapy. This study reported that the combination therapy significantly increased the ratio of CD8 T cells present at the tumor site (peritoneal cavity), relative to both myeloid-derived suppressor cells (MDSCs) and Treg cells [54]. Another separate study showed that triple combination therapy, using co-stimulatory anti-OX40 and anti-4-1BB mAbs along with an inhibitory anti-PD-1 mAb, was also effective in a murine hepatocellular carcinoma model, with enhanced tumor infiltration of cytotoxic effector T cells observed [55].

In the near future, more data will be available that will enable the evaluation of the toxicity-benefit ratio of different immunotherapeutic combinations. We anticipate that this knowledge will provide new insights, leading to the design of novel therapies for advanced stage gastric cancer.

12.8 Combination of Molecularly Targeted Agents with Immunotherapy

Molecularly targeted agents provide selectivity and are the cornerstone for "precision medicine." However, while targeted agents are associated with high effective rates, patients are known to often develop resistance to these drugs inevitably. Immunotherapies exploit the endogenous immune system of patients to eradicate tumors, providing a mechanism for sustained treatment resulting in long-term treatment-free survival in some patients. Combination treatment regimens provide the sustained clinical benefit of immunotherapy along with the rapid and high response rates provided by molecularly targeted therapy. This combinatorial approach could potentially offer both short- and long-term benefit to cancer patients. In this vain, numerous efforts have been initiated to combine molecularly targeted agents (MTAs) with immunotherapy.

The use of targeted agents that efficiently kill tumor cells, initiating the concomitant release of tumor antigens, should activate a specific immune response. It is possible that strategies bringing together immune checkpoint agents and MTAs would result in the induction of an immune memory, with all of its benefits. If this is the case, it would lead to a more sustained inhibition of tumor growth than would be achieved with either treatment modality alone. A great interest has developed in gaining an understanding of how immune checkpoint inhibitors can be used in conjunction with molecularly targeted agents to improve clinical outcomes for patients with advanced stage cancer. The advent of novel immunotherapeutic and molecularly targeted agents has provided numerous effective options for the treatment of cancer. However, at the same time, this has added a level of complexity in determining the most appropriate initial treatment plan for each individual patient [56].

In a phase I trial comprised of patients with BRAF V600 mutation-positive melanoma aimed at evaluating concurrent treatment with vemurafenib and ipilimumab, dose-limiting hepatotoxicity was observed, with further patient accrual to the study stopped [57]. Future studies aimed to optimize doses, timing, and other factors could result in lower, more manageable toxicity of these drugs. Several different approaches could be considered for evaluation. Results from an additional phase I study provided evidence of both clinical activity and a manageable safety profile for an anti-PD-L1 antibody used either in combination with dabrafenib and trametinib in BRAF mutation-positive melanoma patients, in combination with trametinib in BRAF wild-type melanoma patients, or following trametinib in BRAF wild-type melanoma patients [58]. While these data are encouraging, longer follow-up studies to include the duration of response data are necessary to properly assess these treatments. Information gained from clinical studies in melanoma patients may be translatable to gastric cancer patients.

Guidelines for treatment selection of patients with specific tumor types and clinical features are reconsidered routinely so that to accommodate the increasingly complex treatment landscapes.

12.9 Combination of Anti-angiogenic Drugs and Immunotherapy

Vascular endothelial growth factor (VEGF) is thought to suppress the immune system. In addition to promoting angiogenesis, it is known to both suppress dendritic cell maturation and modulate lymphocyte endothelial trafficking. It is thought that vascular normalization could be accompanied by decreased hypoxia. Because hypoxia could be associated with the development of immunosuppressive mechanisms, the suppression of hypoxia could function as a mechanism to modulate tumor-induced immunosuppression [59].

Preventing new vessel formation is yet another mechanism to impact the tumor microenvironment. This mechanism would increase hypoxia and induce apoptosis and necrosis. Indeed, a synergistic antitumor effect has been demonstrated using a combination of anti-angiogenic drugs and immunotherapy [60].

It should be noted that anti-angiogenic molecules do not act only on endothelial cells but also on immune cells. These molecules inhibit the development of certain immunosuppressive mechanisms developed by tumors, such as Tregs, myeloid-derived suppressor cells, and immunosuppressive cytokines [61]. The dual blockade of both PD-1 and VEGF receptor 2 was found to result in an increase in tumor growth inhibition as compared to when each monoclonal antibody treatment was used alone [62]. A significant increase in the expression of several potent pro-inflammatory cytokines and $CD4^+$, $CD8^+$ T cells was also reported.

Consequently, the combination of bevacizumab with ipilimumab treatment is currently being evaluated in a phase I clinical study in patients with advanced melanoma (NCT00790010). On-treatment tumor biopsies revealed activated vessel endothelium with extensive macrophage cell and $CD8^+$ infiltration. Peripheral blood analyses demonstrated increased numbers of CCR7(+/−)/CD45RO(+) cells and anti-galectin antibodies. Bevacizumab was found to cause alterations in tumor vasculature and immune responses with ipilimumab administration. A combination therapy with bevacizumab and ipilimumab can be safely administered and has been found to reveal VEGF-A blockade influences on inflammation, lymphocyte trafficking, and immune regulation [63]. Moreover, nivolumab treatment is currently being combined with sunitinib or pazopanib in patients with metastatic RCC in another phase I trial (NCT01472081).

The majority of other combinatorial immunotherapy and anti-angiogenic drug treatments are still in preclinical testing. However, it was found that not all anti-angiogenic drugs exhibited the same impact on the immune system, likely depending on their targets. The precise mechanisms involved in the influence of anti-angiogenic drugs on the immune system are not fully understood. Future work should address the immunomodulatory effects of these targeted therapies in anticancer strategies to better prescribe these drugs. Some of the anti-angiogenic effects could be successfully associated with immunotherapeutic strategies. Furthermore, the identification of immune biomarkers to predict an anti-angiogenic response would enable for a better selection of patients, avoiding unnecessary adverse events and undue cost.

12.10 Conclusion and Outlook

It is appropriate to state that, in the future, effective anti-GC immunotherapy strategies must be developed as combined approaches. These combined approaches should use both systemic radio-/chemotherapy and molecule-targeted treatment to diminish the tumor burden or to remove immune-suppressive cells, along a tailored immunotherapy strategy customized to each individual patient.

The key question remaining is how best to determine which patients need combination strategies and which combination strategies would prove most effective in any given patient. Some patients have been shown to achieve a durable benefit with monotherapy alone and may not need combinational immunotherapy. Thus, there remains an urgent need to develop biomarkers to identify patients that should be preselected for monotherapy treatment, in order to avoid exposure to unnecessary toxicities associated with combination immunotherapy. In addition, for those patients that do require combinational therapy, it is vital that biomarkers be developed in order to determine the optimal combination therapies appropriate for specific patients. Identification of such predictive biomarkers could lead to personalized cancer immunotherapy strategies that could in turn improve treatment efficacy, reduce toxicity associated with treatment, and reduce treatment costs.

Another issue that must be addressed when moving combinational treatments to the clinic is the potential for increased toxicity and adverse immune-related adverse events (irAEs). Importantly, patients that received a combination of immunotherapy were more likely to experience Grade 3 or 4 irAEs (53%). However, it should be noted that this combination yielded a substantially higher objective response rate than observed with either monotherapy. Overall, ongoing clinical results suggest that the modulation of dosages and clinically managing irAEs could be an effective strategy to alleviate symptoms and maintain patients on treatment [64].

In conclusion, emerging data have shown encouraging efficacy of combination treatments in gastric cancer patients. However, many questions remain unanswered. Results of ongoing clinical trials will enable us to evaluate the potential value of combining immunotherapy with other treatments.

References

1. Khalil DN, Smith EL, Brentjens RJ, Wolchok JD. The future of cancer treatment: immunomodulation, CARs and combination immunotherapy. Nat Rev Clin Oncol. 2016;13(5):273–90.
2. Macdonald JS, Smalley SR, Benedetti J, Hundahl SA, Estes NC, Stemmermann GN, et al. Chemoradiotherapy after surgery compared with surgery alone for adenocarcinoma of the stomach or gastroesophageal junction. N Engl J Med. 2001;345(10):725–30.
3. Niccolai E, Taddei A, Prisco D, Amedei A. Gastric cancer and the epoch of immunotherapy approaches. World J Gastroenterol. 2015;21(19):5778.
4. Larkin J, Chiarion-Sileni V, Gonzalez R, Grob JJ, Cowey CL, Lao CD, et al. Combined nivolumab and ipilimumab or monotherapy in untreated melanoma. N Engl J Med. 2015;373(1):23–34.
5. Gilboa E. How tumors escape immune destruction and what we can do about it. Cancer Immunol Immunother. 1999;48(7):382–5.
6. Kershaw MH, Devaud C, John LB, Westwood JA, Darcy PK. Enhancing immunotherapy using chemotherapy and radiation to modify the tumor microenvironment. Oncoimmunology. 2013;2(9):e25962.
7. Lake RA, Robinson BW. Immunotherapy and chemotherapy—a practical partnership. Nat Rev Cancer. 2005;5(5):397–405.
8. Kang TH, Mao C-P, Lee SY, Chen A, Lee J-H, Kim TW, et al. Chemotherapy acts as an adjuvant to convert the tumor microenvironment into a highly permissive state for vaccination-induced antitumor immunity. Cancer Res. 2013;73(8):2493–504.
9. Kroemer G, Galluzzi L, Kepp O, Zitvogel L. Immunogenic cell death in cancer therapy. Annu Rev Immunol. 2013;31:51–72.
10. Ma Y, Kepp O, Ghiringhelli F, Apetoh L, Aymeric L, Locher C, et al. Chemotherapy and radiotherapy: cryptic anticancer vaccines. Semin Immunol. 2010;22(3):113–24.
11. Vacchelli E, Senovilla L, Eggermont A, Fridman W, Galon J, Zitvogel L, et al. Trial watch: chemotherapy with immunogenic cell death inducers. Oncoimmunology. 2013;2:e23510.
12. Kolstad A, Kumari S, Walczak M, Madsbu U, Hagtvedt T, Bogsrud TV, et al. Sequential intranodal immunotherapy induces antitumor immunity and correlated regression of disseminated follicular lymphoma. Blood. 2015;125(1):82–9.
13. Michaud M, Martins I, Sukkurwala AQ, Adjemian S, Ma Y, Pellegatti P, et al. Autophagy-dependent anticancer immune responses induced by chemotherapeutic agents in mice. Science. 2011;334(6062):1573–7.
14. Arlen PM, Gulley JL, Parker C, Skarupa L, Pazdur M, Panicali D, et al. A randomized phase II study of concurrent docetaxel plus vaccine versus vaccine alone in metastatic androgen-independent prostate cancer. Clin Cancer Res. 2006;12(4):1260–9.
15. Apetoh L, Ghiringhelli F, Tesniere A, Obeid M, Ortiz C, Criollo A, et al. Toll-like receptor 4-dependent contribution of the immune system to anticancer chemotherapy and radiotherapy. Nat Med. 2007;13(9):1050–9.
16. Sharabi A, Haran-Ghera N. Immune recovery after cyclophosphamide treatment in multiple myeloma: implication for maintenance immunotherapy. Bone Marrow Res. 2011;2011:269519.
17. Heylmann D, Bauer M, Becker H, Van Gool S, Bacher N, Steinbrink K, et al. Human $CD4^+$ $CD25^+$ regulatory T cells are sensitive to low dose cyclophosphamide: implications for the immune response. PLoS One. 2013;8(12):e83384.
18. Ma Y, Adjemian S, Mattarollo SR, Yamazaki T, Aymeric L, Yang H, et al. Anticancer chemotherapy-induced intratumoral recruitment and differentiation of antigen-presenting cells. Immunity. 2013;38(4):729–41.
19. Ko H-J, Kim Y-J, Kim Y-S, Chang W-S, Ko S-Y, Chang S-Y, et al. A combination of chemoimmunotherapies can efficiently break self-tolerance and induce antitumor immunity in a tolerogenic murine tumor model. Cancer Res. 2007;67(15):7477–86.

20. Nowak AK, Robinson BW, Lake RA. Synergy between chemotherapy and immunotherapy in the treatment of established murine solid tumors. Cancer Res. 2003;63(15):4490–6.
21. Zheng Y, Dou Y, Duan L, Cong C, Gao A, Lai Q, et al. Using chemo-drugs or irradiation to break immune tolerance and facilitate immunotherapy in solid cancer. Cell Immunol. 2015;294(1):54–9.
22. Hsu F-T, Chen T-C, Chuang H-Y, Chang Y-F, Hwang J-J. Enhancement of adoptive T cell transfer with single low dose pretreatment of doxorubicin or paclitaxel in mice. Oncotarget. 2015;6(42):44134–50.
23. Tesniere A, Schlemmer F, Boige V, Kepp O, Martins I, Ghiringhelli F, et al. Immunogenic death of colon cancer cells treated with oxaliplatin. Oncogene. 2010;29(4):482–91.
24. Gonzalez-Aparicio M, Alzuguren P, Mauleon I, Medina-Echeverz J, Hervas-Stubbs S, Mancheno U, et al. Oxaliplatin in combination with liver-specific expression of interleukin 12 reduces the immunosuppressive microenvironment of tumours and eradicates metastatic colorectal cancer in mice. Gut. 2011;60(3):341–9.
25. Correale P, Cusi MG, Tsang KY, Del Vecchio MT, Marsili S, La Placa M, et al. Chemo-immunotherapy of metastatic colorectal carcinoma with gemcitabine plus FOLFOX 4 followed by subcutaneous granulocyte macrophage colony-stimulating factor and interleukin-2 induces strong immunologic and antitumor activity in metastatic colon cancer patients. J Clin Oncol. 2005;23(35):8950–8.
26. Masuzawa T, Fujiwara Y, Okada K, Nakamura A, Takiguchi S, Nakajima K, et al. Phase I/II study of S-1 plus cisplatin combined with peptide vaccines for human vascular endothelial growth factor receptor 1 and 2 in patients with advanced gastric cancer. Int J Oncol. 2012;41(4):1297–304.
27. Noguchi M, Moriya F, Koga N, Matsueda S, Sasada T, Yamada A, et al. A randomized phase II clinical trial of personalized peptide vaccination with metronomic low-dose cyclophosphamide in patients with metastatic castration-resistant prostate cancer. Cancer Immunol Immunother. 2016;65:151–60.
28. Cui J, Li L, Wang C, Jin H, Yao C, Wang Y, et al. Combined cellular immunotherapy and chemotherapy improves clinical outcome in patients with gastric carcinoma. Cytotherapy. 2015;17(7):979–88.
29. Kalbasi A, June CH, Haas N, Vapiwala N. Radiation and immunotherapy: a synergistic combination. J Clin Invest. 2013;123(7):2756–63.
30. Cui J, Wang N, Zhao H, Jin H, Wang G, Niu C, et al. Combination of radiofrequency ablation and sequential cellular immunotherapy improves progression-free survival for patients with hepatocellular carcinoma. Int J Cancer. 2014;134(2):342–51.
31. Mole R. Whole body irradiation—radiobiology or medicine? Br J Radiol. 1953;26(305):234–41.
32. Lee Y, Auh SL, Wang Y, Burnette B, Wang Y, Meng Y, et al. Therapeutic effects of ablative radiation on local tumor require CD8+ T cells: changing strategies for cancer treatment. Blood. 2009;114(3):589–95.
33. Dewan MZ, Galloway AE, Kawashima N, Dewyngaert JK, Babb JS, Formenti SC, et al. Fractionated but not single-dose radiotherapy induces an immune-mediated abscopal effect when combined with anti-CTLA-4 antibody. Clin Cancer Res. 2009;15(17):5379–88.
34. Liu LL, Smith MJ, Sun BS, Wang GJ, Redmond HP, Wang JH. Combined IFN-γ-endostatin gene therapy and radiotherapy attenuates primary breast tumor growth and lung metastases via enhanced CTL and NK cell activation and attenuated tumor angiogenesis in a murine model. Ann Surg Oncol. 2009;16(5):1403–11.
35. Postow MA, Chesney J, Pavlick AC, Robert C, Grossmann K, McDermott D, et al. Nivolumab and ipilimumab versus ipilimumab in untreated melanoma. N Engl J Med. 2015;372(21):2006–17.
36. Matsumura S, Wang B, Kawashima N, Braunstein S, Badura M, Cameron TO, et al. Radiation-induced CXCL16 release by breast cancer cells attracts effector T cells. J Immunol. 2008;181(5):3099–107.
37. Ganss R, Ryschich E, Klar E, Arnold B, Hämmerling GJ. Combination of T-cell therapy and trigger of inflammation induces remodeling of the vasculature and tumor eradication. Cancer Res. 2002;62(5):1462–70.
38. Kleponis J, Skelton R, Zheng L. Fueling the engine and releasing the break: combinational therapy of cancer vaccines and immune checkpoint inhibitors. Cancer Biol Med. 2015;12(3):201.
39. Taube JM, Klein A, Brahmer JR, Xu H, Pan X, Kim JH, et al. Association of PD-1, PD-1 ligands, and other features of the tumor immune microenvironment with response to anti-PD-1 therapy. Clin Cancer Res. 2014;20(19):5064–74.
40. Lipson EJ, Sharfman WH, Drake CG, Wollner I, Taube JM, Anders RA, et al. Durable cancer regression off-treatment and effective reinduction therapy with an anti-PD-1 antibody. Clin Cancer Res. 2013;19(2):462–8.
41. Lutz ER, Wu AA, Bigelow E, Sharma R, Mo G, Soares K, et al. Immunotherapy converts nonimmunogenic pancreatic tumors into immunogenic foci of immune regulation. Cancer Immunol Res. 2014;2(7):616–31.
42. Pardoll DM. The blockade of immune checkpoints in cancer immunotherapy. Nat Rev Cancer. 2012;12(4):252–64.
43. Zheng L. Does vaccine-primed pancreatic cancer offer better candidates for immune-based therapies? Immunotherapy. 2014;6(10):1017–20.
44. Karyampudi L, Lamichhane P, Scheid AD, Kalli KR, Shreeder B, Krempski JW, et al. Accumulation of memory precursor CD8 T cells in regressing tumors following combination therapy with vaccine and anti-PD-1 antibody. Cancer Res. 2014;74(11):2974–85.
45. Soares KC, Rucki AA, Wu AA, Olino K, Xiao Q, Chai Y, et al. PD-1/PD-L1 blockade together with vaccine therapy facilitates effector T cell infiltration into pancreatic tumors. J Immunother. 2015;38(1):1–11.
46. Le DT, Lutz E, Uram JN, Sugar EA, Onners B, Solt S, et al. Evaluation of ipilimumab in combination with allogeneic pancreatic tumor cells transfected with a

GM-CSF gene in previously treated pancreatic cancer. J Immunother. 2013;36(7):382–9.
47. Wada S, Jackson CM, Yoshimura K, Yen H-R, Getnet D, Harris TJ, et al. Sequencing CTLA-4 blockade with cell-based immunotherapy for prostate cancer. J Transl Med. 2013;11(1):1–89.
48. John LB, Devaud C, Duong CP, Yong CS, Beavis PA, Haynes NM, et al. Anti-PD-1 antibody therapy potently enhances the eradication of established tumors by gene-modified T cells. Clin Cancer Res. 2013;19(20):5636–46.
49. Peng W, Liu C, Xu C, Lou Y, Chen J, Yang Y, et al. PD-1 blockade enhances T-cell migration to tumors by elevating IFN-γ inducible chemokines. Cancer Res. 2012;72(20):5209–18.
50. Larkin J, Chiarion-Sileni V, Gonzalez R, Grob JJ, Cowey CL, Lao CD, et al. Combined nivolumab and ipilimumab or monotherapy in untreated melanoma. N Engl J Med. 2015;2015(373):23–34.
51. Linch SN, McNamara MJ, Redmond WL. OX40 agonists and combination immunotherapy: putting the pedal to the metal. Front Oncol. 2015;5:34.
52. Redmond WL, Linch SN, Kasiewicz MJ. Combined targeting of costimulatory (OX40) and coinhibitory (CTLA-4) pathways elicits potent effector T cells capable of driving robust antitumor immunity. Cancer Immunol Res. 2014;2(2):142–53.
53. Marabelle A, Kohrt H, Sagiv-Barfi I, Ajami B, Axtell RC, Zhou G, et al. Depleting tumor-specific Tregs at a single site eradicates disseminated tumors. J Clin Invest. 2013;123(6):2447–63.
54. Guo Z, Wang X, Cheng D, Xia Z, Luan M, Zhang S. PD-1 blockade and OX40 triggering synergistically protects against tumor growth in a murine model of ovarian cancer. PLoS One. 2014;9(2):e89350.
55. Melero I, Grimaldi AM, Perez-Gracia JL, Ascierto PA. Clinical development of immunostimulatory monoclonal antibodies and opportunities for combination. Clin Cancer Res. 2013;19(5):997–1008.
56. Atkins MB, Larkin J. Immunotherapy combined or sequenced with targeted therapy in the treatment of solid tumors: current perspectives. J Natl Cancer Inst. 2016;108(6):djv414.
57. Ribas A, Hodi FS, Callahan M, Konto C, Wolchok J. Hepatotoxicity with combination of vemurafenib and ipilimumab. N Engl J Med. 2013;368(14):1365–6.
58. Ribas A, Butler M, Lutzky J, Lawrence DP, Robert C, Miller W, et al. Phase I study combining anti-PD-L1 (MEDI4736) with BRAF (dabrafenib) and/or MEK (trametinib) inhibitors in advanced melanoma. ASCO Annual Meeting Proceedings; 2015.
59. Huang Y, Yuan J, Righi E, Kamoun WS, Ancukiewicz M, Nezivar J, et al. Vascular normalizing doses of antiangiogenic treatment reprogram the immunosuppressive tumor microenvironment and enhance immunotherapy. Proc Natl Acad Sci. 2012;109(43):17561–6.
60. Garber K. Promising early results for immunotherapy-antiangiogenesis combination. J Natl Cancer Inst. 2014;106(11):dju392.
61. Terme M, Colussi O, Marcheteau E, Tanchot C, Tartour E, Taieb J. Modulation of immunity by antiangiogenic molecules in cancer. Clin Dev Immunol. 2012;2012:492920.
62. Yasuda S, Sho M, Yamato I, Yoshiji H, Wakatsuki K, Nishiwada S, et al. Simultaneous blockade of programmed death 1 and vascular endothelial growth factor receptor 2 (VEGFR2) induces synergistic anti-tumour effect in vivo. Clin Exp Immunol. 2013;172(3):500–6.
63. Hodi FS, Lawrence D, Lezcano C, Wu X, Zhou J, Sasada T, et al. Bevacizumab plus ipilimumab in patients with metastatic melanoma. Cancer Immunol Res. 2014;2(7):632–42.
64. Weber JS, Kähler KC, Hauschild A. Management of immune-related adverse events and kinetics of response with ipilimumab. J Clin Oncol. 2012;30(21):2691–7.

Part IV

Use of Nanomedicine in the Diagnosis and Treatment of Gastric Cancer

13 Use of Nanomedicine in the Diagnosis of Gastric Cancer

Rutian Li and Xiaoping Qian

Gastric cancer is one of most common cancers and is a leading global cause of cancer-related deaths [1]. This is particularly true in the eastern regions of China [2, 3]. Unfortunately, gastric cancer is difficult to cure, in large part because most patients are diagnosed at advanced stages of the disease. Apart from the need for early diagnosis, clinically important practices are also the diagnosis for tumor staging, planning for surgical resection, and determining prognosis. It should be noted that gastric cancer is considered as a more "localized tumor," which is slightly different from the "systemic tumors" such as breast and lung cancers. With this in mind, locoregional metastasis is the most important negative prognostic factor of gastric cancer [4–6]. As a result, the diagnosis of gastric cancer includes (1) its early detection; (2) its systemic imaging; (3) its local imaging, especially that of regional lymphatic imaging; and (4) detection of its circulating tumor cells (CTC).

Thanks to its unique, nanoscale material composition, nanomedicine provides many benefits for the diagnosis and treatment of cancer. To this end, a number of nano-drugs have been clinically used, including liposomal doxorubicin (Doxil) [7–9], pegylated liposomal doxorubicin [10–12], liposomal daunorubicin (DaunoXome) [13–15], liposomal paclitaxel [16], liposomal cytarabine (DepoCyt) [17, 18], and albumin-bound paclitaxel (Abraxane) [19–21]], etc. Collectively, such nano-drugs promote the efficacy and reduce side effects of the chemotherapeutics with which they are loaded. Ultimately, these benefits act to increase their effectiveness in gastric cancer treatment.

Nanomedicine also has a promising role in cancer diagnosis [22–25], with some having gotten as far as clinical trials [26]. However, nanodiagnostics are only currently used in a limited number of situations [23]. Beginning with tumor imaging contrast, nanotechnology has also been applied to lymphatic imaging, circulating tumor cell (CTC) detection, and early cancer diagnosis. Moreover, theranostic based on nanomedicine have also attracted increasing attention, due to their construction as multifunctional, nanosystems with integrated diagnostic and therapeutic capabilities in a single nanoparticle [27–29]. With this in mind, in the following section, we will focus on the interface between gastric cancer and nano-diagnosis.

13.1 Nanomedicine in the Early Diagnosis of Gastric Cancer

Apart from occult blood test of stools, endoscopy is the most important and effective diagnostic method for the early detection of gastric cancer. That being said, conventional white-light

R. Li (✉) • X. Qian
The Comprehensive Cancer Center of Drum-Tower Hospital, Medical School of Nanjing University & Clinical Cancer Institute of Nanjing University, Nanjing 210008, China
e-mail: li_rutian@163.com

J. Wei, B. Liu (eds.), *Personalized Management of Gastric Cancer*, DOI 10.1007/978-981-10-3978-2_13

endoscopy offers only structural information of the gastrointestinal tract without any attendant biochemical data. To enhance the sensitivity of endoscopy, a non-contact, fiber optic-based Raman spectroscopy device was reported by Zavaleta et al. [30]. This device has the potential to provide real-time, multiplexed functional information during routine endoscopy and thus is ideally suited for the detection of functionalized, surface-enhanced Raman scattering (SERS) nanoparticles as molecular imaging contrast agents. As a result, certain cellular subgroups (e.g., cancer cells) are able to be identified. A good case of this is the work of Wang et al. [31, 32], who applied monoclonal antibodies against epidermal growth factor receptor (anti-EGFR mAb) and human epidermal growth factor receptor-2 (anti-HER-2 mAb) SERS NPs to the lumenal surface of the rat esophagus. Their results showed that EGFR- and HER-2-expressing tumor cells were not only precisely located, but that biomarker visualization and expression quantification were in agreement with both immunohistochemistry and flow cytometry data. Obviously, this technique is based on the idea that one or more molecules are highly and specifically expressed on the surface of cancer cells. For gastric cancer, such molecules include carcinoembryonic antigen (CEA), cancer-related antigen 19-9 (CA19-9), cancer-related antigen 72-4 (CA72-4), HER-2, and EGFR. Although none of the aforementioned markers are 100% sensitive and specific, the combination of routine optical endoscopy and SERS nanoparticles would still provide a more sensitive and specific means for early gastric cancer detection than is currently available.

The detection of gastric cancer-related biomarkers is also an important part of early diagnosis. Due to their specific properties, the development of nanostructured biosensors with high analytical performance has continuously increased [33, 34]. The use of nanoparticles may increase the sensitivity of a given biosensor and generate higher accuracies, speed, and precision [33]. Nanoparticles can be applied into optical-based nanosensors [35–38], fluorescence-based nanosensors [39], electrical-/electrochemical-based nanosensors [33, 40–43], and magnetism-based nanosensors [44–46], to name a few. Among those nanoparticles used in nanosensors, gold and magnetic nanoparticles-based biosensors as well as quantum dots are the predominant types [34, 35, 47–52]. These nanoparticles have been reported to be used in nanosensors designed to detect CEA [53–56], CA125 [35, 57–59], CA724 [60], and HER-2 [61]. As these nanoparticle-enhanced nanosensors are of greater sensitivity and accuracy, they may also be used to the exploration of new biomarkers for early gastric cancer detection [62].

Some other nanostructures have also been applied to gastric cancer-related biomarkers. For instance, Chen et al. [55] reported an immunosensor for CEA that was based on nanosilver-coated magnetic beads and gold-graphene nanolabels. This nano-biosensor could detect CEA at a concentration as low as 1.0 pg/mL. In another instance, Jokerst et al. [63] integrated semiconductor nanoparticle quantum dots (QDs) into a modular, microfluidic biosensor for the multiplexed quantification of CEA, CA125, and HER-2/Neu. They found that using QD probes in a miniaturized biosensor format leads to signal amplification that was 30 times that of standard molecular fluorophores. Moreover, they also saw a reduction in observed limits of detection by nearly two orders of magnitude relative to an enzyme-linked immunosorbent assay (ELISA).

13.2 Nanomedicine in the Systemic Imaging of Gastric Cancer

The methods used for whole body scanning include computed tomography (CT), magnetic resonance imaging (MRI), positron emission computed tomography (PET), single-photon emission computed tomography (SPECT), and PET-CT. For organ-specific examinations, a fast and low-cost method is ultrasound [23]. The current imaging and therapeutic agents suffer from nonspecific body distribution, not to mention rapid clearance, poor pharmacokinetics, and undesirable side effects [64–68]. Therefore, the development of cancer nanomedicine provides new pathways for enhanced cancer imaging using new types of nanomaterials. A variety of nanoparticles have recently emerged as promising strategies for cancer diagnosis owing to their nanoscale sizes, high agent loading capability, tailorable surface properties, controllable release patterns, and enhanced permeability and retention (EPR) [65, 67, 68]. Although successfully developing safe and effective nanoparticle-based imaging modalities for in vivo gastric cancer targeting imaging remains a large challenge, some studies have made progress in the right direction.

Superparamagnetic iron oxide (SPIO) MRI contrast agents are the first agents to have been clinically approved and include ferumoxides (Feridex in the USA, Endorem in Europe) and ferucarbotran (Resovist). However, both Feridex and Resovist are approved only for MRI of the liver. Nevertheless, magnetic nanoparticles are still the most frequently used in gastric cancer imaging.

Wang et al. [69] reported on SPIO nanoparticles (SPION) coated with SiO_2 as core-shell nanoparticles. Nanoparticles were labeled with a near-infrared fluorescence (NIRF) dye in addition to an anti-CD146 monoclonal antibody [70] for magnetic resonance MR/NIRF imaging. The MKN45 xenograft tumor model was easily identifiable in as little time as 30 min postinjection.

BRCAA1 monoclonal antibodies that were conjugated to fluorescent, magnetic nanoparticles for in vivo, targeted gastric cancer imaging were also reported by Wang et al [71]. The nanoparticles could target in vivo gastric cancer tissues in the xenograft of mice and could then be used for gastric cancer imaging using either fluorescence imaging or magnetic resonance imaging.

Zhou et al. [72] reported using folic acid (FA)-conjugated silica-capped gold nanoclusters for gastric cancer imaging. This type of nanoprobe exhibited good biocompatibility and was able to actively target both FA(+) MGC-803 cells and in vivo gastric cancer tissue (5 mm in diameter) in a nude mice model. Importantly, these nanoclusters allowed for excellent red-emitting fluorescence and CT imaging.

Trastuzumab (Herceptin) is a humanized monoclonal antibody targeted to the extracellular domain of HER-2, a tyrosine kinase receptor. Trastuzumab was approved by the Food and Drug Administration (FDA) of the USA for the treatment of HER-2-overexpressing metastatic gastric cancer [73–75]. Several trastuzumab-conjugated, inorganic nanoparticles have been reported for purposes of imaging and diagnosis [73]. These include dextran iron oxide nanoparticles [76], mesoporous silica nanoparticles [77], PLGA nanoparticles [78], and liposome-coated fluorescent magnetic nanoparticles [79]. Although the aforementioned nanoparticles were used in breast cancer, these systems can also be applied to HER-2-overexpressing gastric cancers [73, 80, 81].

Nanomaterials were also used in the area of ultrasound. For instance, Fan et al. [82] reported on nanobubbles, which were used as an ultrasound contrast agent. The nanobubbles exhibited a superior contrast imaging effect over SonoVue® microbubbles in gastric cancer xenografts. Additional studies showed that the nanobubbles could pass through the gaps between the endothelial cells into the tumor vascular system in order to enter the tissue space. Taken together, these findings provide morphological evidence for the applications of nanoparticles in ultrasound imaging of tumors.

Moreover, nanomaterials have been used into nuclear imaging of gastric cancer. To this end, increased expression of cellular membrane bound glucose-regulated protein 78 (GRP78) is considered to be a gastric cancer biomarker. Cheng et al. synthesized glucose-regulated protein 78 binding peptide (GRP78BP) guide^{111} in labeled polymeric micelles [83]. In vivo studies in murine gastric xenograft revealed that the radioactive intensity measured in subjects treated with GRP78BP-guided^{111}, labeled micelles was statistically higher than in animals receiving only labeled micelles. These results indicated that GRP78 is a useful probing target that can be used for nuclear imaging and gastric cancer diagnosis.

13.3 Nanomedicine in Local Gastric Cancer Imaging

Lymphatic metastasis is one of the most important in dependent prognostic factor for gastric cancer [84, 85]. Consequently, it is undoubtedly helpful for treatment planning to know pretreatment status of lymph nodes of gastric cancer patients. Furthermore, intraoperative diagnosis of lymph node metastasis in patients with gastric cancer is vital for the extent of lymph node dissection [86]. However, to date, no imaging modality has been shown to be capable of effectively detecting gastric cancer lymphatic metastasis [87].

Ferumoxtran-10 (Combidex) is an MRI lymphotropic contrast agent for the detection of metastatic lymph nodes in various types of cancers. For instance, Tatsumi et al. [88] investigated the efficacy of ferumoxtran-10-enhanced MRI for the detection of metastases to lymph nodes in gastric cancer. The parameters for predictive accuracy were far superior to those evaluated by either CT or ultrasound alone. Nodes in the retroperitoneal and paraaortic regions were more readily identified on the MR images than those in the perigastric region. Therefore, the use of this modality shows promise in treatment planning and decision-making for gastric cancer patients.

Recently, Qiao et al. [87] reported on a new kind of molecular imaging probe that was based on upconversion nanoparticles with highly sensitive detection of lymphatic metastasis in gastric cancer. The core-shell, structured upconversion nanoparticles were coated with polyethylene glycol (PEG). In vivo studies in an orthotopic mouse model of human gastric cancer were then conducted, with the primary tumor and adjacent lymphatic metastatic sites being clearly differentiated. Moreover, lymphatic metastases that were smaller than 1 mm were successfully detected. These results show the promise that this nanoparticle has a highly effective approach to gastric cancer diagnosis.

Using photosensitive nanoparticles loaded with the indocyanine green (ICG) derivative ICG-loaded lactosome (ICGm), Tsujimoto et al. [86] detected metastatic lymph nodes in the ICGm-, but not ICG-, treated mice. PDT using ICGm was able to induce apoptosis and inhibited the growth of metastatic lymph nodes significantly. These results indicate that ICGm is a promising theranostic modality for lymph node metastasis in gastric cancer.

Image-guided surgery (IGS) has the potential to substantially impact patient treatment. Clinical trials of IGS using the FDA-approved fluorophores indocyanine green (ICG) and methylene blue have already exhibited preliminary successes. Moreover, incorporation of fluorescent nanoparticles will likely improve detection by providing a higher signal-to-noise ratio and reducing false-positive rates by means of active targeting [89]. Several types of fluorescent nanoparticles have been reported, such as liposome-embedded ICG [90, 91], SPIO-phospholipid-PEG-ICG [92], and hyaluronic acid (HLA)-derived nanoparticles loading ICG [93].

13.4 Using Nanomedicine to Detect Circulating Tumor Cells (CTCs) in Gastric Cancer

Circulating tumor cells (CTCs) are cancer cells that break away from either a primary tumor or a metastatic site and circulate in the peripheral blood. Crucially, they are supposed to serve as the cellular origin of metastasis [94]. Blood CTCs have been widely studied as a potential biomarker for diagnosis, prognosis, and molecular testing of metastatic gastric cancer [95, 96]. It is also vital for the real-time diagnosis, treatment planning, and evaluation of patients, leading to its classification as a "liquid biopsy." However, due to their rarity and heterogeneity, it remains challenging to develop a CTC detection method with clinically significant sensitivity and specificity. This difficulty remains even with the commercialization of some devices such as CellSearch [97, 98] (it should be noted that CellSearch has not been approved for use in gastric cancer). With the recent advances in nanotechnology, a series of new and promising nanomaterials have been reported to enhance CTC detection [95, 99].

These include microfluidic chips [99, 100], nanoroughened structures [99], NanoVelcro chips [94], nanofibers [101], as well as nanoparticles [95, 102].

Microfluidics integrates physical, chemical, and biological technologies at the micro- and nanoscale levels, thus providing a miniaturized and portable tool for efficient CTCs separation [103]. In the latest decade, a great number of microfluidic chips have been shown to be capable of separating CTCs of prostate [104], breast [105–107], esophageal [107], and lung cancers [108] in addition to melanoma [109].

To this end, Galletti et al. [106] reported a novel HER-2 (human epidermal receptor-2)-based microfluidic device for the isolation of CTCs from the peripheral blood of patients with HER-2-expressing gastric cancers. They applied the HER-2 microfluidic device into the detection of CTCs from blood of metastatic gastric cancer patients and found that circulating tumor cells were detected not only in HER-2 high-expressing cancer patients but also in HER-2 low-expressing patients. As HER-2 is expressed in 67% of gastric cancer patients and overexpressed in 13–30% of the cases [106, 110, 111], the microfluidic device based on HER-2 is quite promising for the detection of CTCs in gastric cancer patients.

Based on a negative enrichment technique, Hyun et al. [105] reported a geometrically activated surface interaction (GASI) chip with an asymmetric herringbone structure designed to generate enhanced mixing flows. CD45 antibodies were immobilized inside the channel to capture leukocytes and release CTCs to the outlet. Blood samples from four patients with gastric cancer were then analyzed. CTCs were detected from all four samples, and the number of isolated CTCs varied from 1 to 5 in 1 mL of blood.

The materials used in nanoparticles designed for the detection of CTC have included gold [112], magnetic [113, 114], quantum dots [115], graphenes/graphene oxides [116], dendrimers, and stimuli-responsive polymers [117, 118]. That being said, previous studies focused on CTC detection and isolation using nanoparticles have mostly concentrated on breast, prostate, lung, and colon cancers. Reports on the detection of gastric CTCs using nanoparticles are comparatively little. For instance, He et al. [119] reported CTC isolation from gastric cancer patients' peripheral blood samples with a biocompatible nano-film composed of TiO_2 nanoparticles. Furthermore, 50% of the captured cells could be detached from the substrate and were expected to be of future clinical use.

It is also important to note that some nanoparticles have emerged that are able to detect special gastric cancer or gastric cancer stem cell markers, such as CD [102, 120], HER-2 [79], CD44 [121], and CD146 [69, 70]. These nanoparticles are expected to be promising candidates for gastric CTC detection.

Conclusions

Due to the high morbidity and mortality of gastric cancer, the exploration of more effective modalities for its diagnosis and treatment is critically important. Nanomedicine has shown great potential for increasing the sensitivity and specificity with regard to gastric cancer—not just with early detection. It has also shown promise with systemic and local imaging for the evaluation and treatment determination of gastric cancer, image-guided surgery, and the detection and isolation of CTCs. However, there are also several limitations that must be considered. First, most of the studies currently in the literature are either preclinical or in vitro. As a result, the safety and clinical applicability of most nanomaterials remain unclear. Second, most studies for gastric cancer diagnosis have been based on specific markers or ligands expressed by gastric cancer. However, the specificity of these molecules is usually limited, which restricts nanoparticle applications. Finally, a large proportion of the studies were derived from similar studies about breast, lung, and colorectal cancers. Studies based solely and specifically on the clinical characteristics of gastric cancer are comparatively rare. Therefore, to further promote the development of nanomedicine in the diagnosis of gastric cancer, more in-depth studies and increased interdisciplinary collaboration and information exchange between scientists will be needed [23].

References

1. Ferlay J, Soerjomataram I, Dikshit R, Eser S, Mathers C, Rebelo M, et al. Cancer incidence and mortality worldwide: sources, methods and major patterns in GLOBOCAN 2012. Int J Cancer. 2015;136(5):E359–86.
2. Yang L. Incidence and mortality of gastric cancer in China. World J Gastroenterol. 2006;12(1):17–20.
3. Zhou M, Wang H, Zhu J, Chen W, Wang L, Liu S, et al. Cause-specific mortality for 240 causes in China during 1990–2013: a systematic subnational analysis for the Global Burden of Disease Study 2013. Lancet. 2016;387(10015):251–72.
4. Imano M, Yasuda A, Itoh T, Satou T, Peng YF, Kato H, et al. Phase II study of single intraperitoneal chemotherapy followed by systemic chemotherapy for gastric cancer with peritoneal metastasis. J Gastrointest Surg. 2012;16(12):2190–6.
5. Ishigami H, Kitayama J, Kaisaki S, Hidemura A, Kato M, Otani K, et al. Phase II study of weekly intravenous and intraperitoneal paclitaxel combined with S-1 for advanced gastric cancer with peritoneal metastasis. Ann Oncol. 2010;21(1):67–70.
6. Ishigami H, Kitayama J, Kaisaki S, Yamaguchi H, Yamashita H, Emoto S, et al. Phase I study of biweekly intravenous paclitaxel plus intraperitoneal cisplatin and paclitaxel for gastric cancer with peritoneal metastasis. Oncology. 2010;79(3-4):269–72.
7. Yamaguchi N, Fujii T, Aoi S, Kozuch PS, Hortobagyi GN, Blum RH. Comparison of cardiac events associated with liposomal doxorubicin, epirubicin and doxorubicin in breast cancer: a Bayesian network meta-analysis. Eur J Cancer. 2015;51(16):2314–20.
8. Khan DR, Webb MN, Cadotte TH, Gavette MN. Use of targeted liposome-based chemotherapeutics to treat breast cancer. Breast Cancer (Auckl). 2015;9(Suppl 2):1–5.
9. Rivankar S. An overview of doxorubicin formulations in cancer therapy. J Cancer Res Ther. 2014;10(4):853–8.
10. Arias JL. Advanced methodologies to formulate nanotheragnostic agents for combined drug delivery and imaging. Expert Opin Drug Deliv. 2011;8(12):1589–608.
11. Poveda AM, Selle F, Hilpert F, Reuss A, Savarese A, Vergote I, et al. Bevacizumab combined with weekly paclitaxel, pegylated liposomal doxorubicin, or topotecan in platinum-resistant recurrent ovarian cancer: analysis by chemotherapy cohort of the randomized phase III AURELIA trial. J Clin Oncol. 2015;33(32):3836–8.
12. Mahner S, Meier W, du Bois A, Brown C, Lorusso D, Dell'Anna T, et al. Carboplatin and pegylated liposomal doxorubicin versus carboplatin and paclitaxel in very platinum-sensitive ovarian cancer patients: results from a subset analysis of the CALYPSO phase III trial. Eur J Cancer. 2015;51(3):352–8.
13. Clavio M, Venturino C, Pierri I, Garrone A, Miglino M, Canepa L, et al. Combination of liposomal daunorubicin (DaunoXome), fludarabine, and cytarabine (FLAD) in patients with poor-risk acute leukemia. Ann Hematol. 2004;83(11):696–703.
14. Sedki M, Vannier JP, Leverger G, Yakouben K, Adjaoud D, Vilmer E, et al. Liposomal daunorubicin (Daunoxome) and polyethylated glycol conjugated asparaginase (PEG-ASPA) in children with relapsed and refractory acute lymphoblastic leukemia treated on compassionate basis. J Egypt Natl Canc Inst. 2008;20(1):55–62.
15. Camera A, Rinaldi CR, Palmieri S, Cantore N, Mele G, Mettivier V, et al. Sequential continuous infusion of fludarabine and cytarabine associated with liposomal daunorubicin (DaunoXome) (FLAD) in primary refractory or relapsed adult acute myeloid leukemia patients. Ann Hematol. 2009;88(2):151–8.
16. Hu L, Liang G, Yuliang W, Bingjing Z, Xiangdong Z, Rufu X. Assessing the effectiveness and safety of liposomal paclitaxel in combination with cisplatin as first-line chemotherapy for patients with advanced NSCLC with regional lymph-node metastasis: study protocol for a randomized controlled trial (PLC-GC trial). Trials. 2013;14:45.
17. Phuphanich S, Maria B, Braeckman R, Chamberlain M. A pharmacokinetic study of intra-CSF administered encapsulated cytarabine (DepoCyt) for the treatment of neoplastic meningitis in patients with leukemia, lymphoma, or solid tumors as part of a phase III study. J Neurooncol. 2007;81(2):201–8.
18. Beauchesne P, Blonski M, Brissart H. Response to intrathecal infusions of Depocyt(R) in secondary diffuse leptomeningeal gliomatosis. A case report. In Vivo. 2011;25(6):991–3.
19. Kundranda MN, Niu J. Albumin-bound paclitaxel in solid tumors: clinical development and future directions. Drug Des Devel Ther. 2015;9:3767–77.
20. Nehate C, Jain S, Saneja A, Khare V, Alam N, Dubey RD, et al. Paclitaxel formulations: challenges and novel delivery options. Curr Drug Deliv. 2014;11(6):666–86.
21. Cecco S, Aliberti M, Baldo P, Giacomin E, Leone R. Safety and efficacy evaluation of albumin-bound paclitaxel. Expert Opin Drug Saf. 2014;13(4):511–20.
22. Zhang L, Zhao D. Applications of nanoparticles for brain cancer imaging and therapy. J Biomed Nanotechnol. 2014;10(9):1713–31.
23. Baetke SC, Lammers T, Kiessling F. Applications of nanoparticles for diagnosis and therapy of cancer. Br J Radiol. 2015;88(1054):20150207.
24. Ho D. Nanodiamond-based chemotherapy and imaging. Cancer Treat Res. 2015;166:85–102.
25. Ryu JH, Koo H, Sun IC, Yuk SH, Choi K, Kim K, et al. Tumor-targeting multi-functional nanoparticles for theragnosis: new paradigm for cancer therapy. Adv Drug Deliv Rev. 2012;64(13):1447–58.
26. Wang YX. Superparamagnetic iron oxide based MRI contrast agents: current status of clinical application. Quant Imaging Med Surg. 2011;1(1):35–40.

27. Chen F, Ehlerding EB, Cai W. Theranostic nanoparticles. J Nucl Med. 2014;55(12):1919–22.
28. Muthu MS, Leong DT, Mei L, Feng SS. Nanotheranostics—application and further development of nanomedicine strategies for advanced theranostics. Theranostics. 2014;4(6):660–77.
29. Wang L, Wang Y, Li Z. Nanoparticle-based tumor theranostics with molecular imaging. Curr Pharm Biotechnol. 2013;14(7):683–92.
30. Zavaleta CL, Garai E, Liu JT, Sensarn S, Mandella MJ, Van de Sompel D, et al. A Raman-based endoscopic strategy for multiplexed molecular imaging. Proc Natl Acad Sci USA. 2013;110(25):E2288–97.
31. Wang YW, Kang S, Khan A, Bao PQ, Liu JT. In vivo multiplexed molecular imaging of esophageal cancer via spectral endoscopy of topically applied SERS nanoparticles. Biomed Opt Express. 2015;6(10):3714–23.
32. Wang YW, Khan A, Leigh SY, Wang D, Chen Y, Meza D, et al. Comprehensive spectral endoscopy of topically applied SERS nanoparticles in the rat esophagus. Biomed Opt Express. 2014;5(9):2883–95.
33. Perfezou M, Turner A, Merkoci A. Cancer detection using nanoparticle-based sensors. Chem Soc Rev. 2012;41(7):2606–22.
34. Ravalli A, Marrazza G. Gold and magnetic nanoparticles-based electrochemical biosensors for cancer biomarker determination. J Nanosci Nanotechnol. 2015;15(5):3307–19.
35. Vilela D, Gonzalez MC, Escarpa A. Sensing colorimetric approaches based on gold and silver nanoparticles aggregation: chemical creativity behind the assay. A review. Anal Chim Acta. 2012;751:24–43.
36. Baker GA, Moore DS. Progress in plasmonic engineering of surface-enhanced Raman-scattering substrates toward ultra-trace analysis. Anal Bioanal Chem. 2005;382(8):1751–70.
37. Salvati E, Stellacci F, Krol S. Nanosensors for early cancer detection and for therapeutic drug monitoring. Nanomedicine (Lond). 2015;10(23):3495–512.
38. Tothill IE. Biosensors for cancer markers diagnosis. Semin Cell Dev Biol. 2009;20(1):55–62.
39. Huang S, Zhu F, Qiu H, Xiao Q, Zhou Q, Su W, et al. A sensitive quantum dots-based "OFF-ON" fluorescent sensor for ruthenium anticancer drugs and ctDNA. Colloids Surf B Biointerfaces. 2014;117: 240–7.
40. Hayat A, Catanante G, Marty JL. Current trends in nanomaterial-based amperometric biosensors. Sensors (Basel). 2014;14(12):23439–61.
41. Swierczewska M, Liu G, Lee S, Chen X. High-sensitivity nanosensors for biomarker detection. Chem Soc Rev. 2012;41(7):2641–55.
42. Shiddiky MJ, Rauf S, Kithva PH, Trau M. Graphene/quantum dot bionanoconjugates as signal amplifiers in stripping voltammetric detection of EpCAM biomarkers. Biosens Bioelectron. 2012;35(1):251–7.
43. Afreen S, Muthoosamy K, Manickam S, Hashim U. Functionalized fullerene (C(6)(0)) as a potential nanomediator in the fabrication of highly sensitive biosensors. Biosens Bioelectron. 2015;63:354–64.
44. Shao H, Chung J, Lee K, Balaj L, Min C, Carter BS, et al. Chip-based analysis of exosomal mRNA mediating drug resistance in glioblastoma. Nat Commun. 2015;6:6999.
45. Muluneh M, Issadore D. Microchip-based detection of magnetically labeled cancer biomarkers. Adv Drug Deliv Rev. 2014;66:101–9.
46. Wittrup A, Zhang SH, Svensson KJ, Kucharzewska P, Johansson MC, Morgelin M, et al. Magnetic nanoparticle-based isolation of endocytic vesicles reveals a role of the heat shock protein GRP75 in macromolecular delivery. Proc Natl Acad Sci USA. 2010;107(30):13342–7.
47. Nie L, Liu F, Ma P, Xiao X. Applications of gold nanoparticles in optical biosensors. J Biomed Nanotechnol. 2014;10(10):2700–21.
48. Jena BK, Ghosh S, Bera R, Dey RS, Das AK, Raj CR. Bioanalytical applications of au nanoparticles. Recent Pat Nanotechnol. 2010;4(1):41–52.
49. Devi RV, Doble M, Verma RS. Nanomaterials for early detection of cancer biomarker with special emphasis on gold nanoparticles in immunoassays/sensors. Biosens Bioelectron. 2015;68:688–98.
50. Chan WC, Maxwell DJ, Gao X, Bailey RE, Han M, Nie S. Luminescent quantum dots for multiplexed biological detection and imaging. Curr Opin Biotechnol. 2002;13(1):40–6.
51. Kim S, Bawendi MG. Oligomeric ligands for luminescent and stable nanocrystal quantum dots. J Am Chem Soc. 2003;125(48):14652–3.
52. Zhang Y, Zhou D. Magnetic particle-based ultrasensitive biosensors for diagnostics. Expert Rev Mol Diagn. 2012;12(6):565–71.
53. Zhong Z, Wu W, Wang D, Shan J, Qing Y, Zhang Z. Nanogold-enwrapped graphene nanocomposites as trace labels for sensitivity enhancement of electrochemical immunosensors in clinical immunoassays: carcinoembryonic antigen as a model. Biosens Bioelectron. 2010;25(10):2379–83.
54. Shu H, Wen W, Xiong H, Zhang X, Wang S. Novel electrochemical aptamer biosensor based on gold nanoparticles signal amplification for the detection of carcinoembryonic antigen. Electrochem Commun. 2013;37:15–9.
55. Chen H, Tang D, Zhang B, Liu B, Cui Y, Chen G. Electrochemical immunosensor for carcinoembryonic antigen based on nanosilver-coated magnetic beads and gold-graphene nanolabels. Talanta. 2012;91:95–102.
56. Ling S, Yuan R, Chai Y, Zhang T. Study on immunosensor based on gold nanoparticles/chitosan and MnO2 nanoparticles composite membrane/Prussian blue modified gold electrode. Bioprocess Biosyst Eng. 2009;32(3):407–14.
57. Ravalli A, Dos Santos GP, Ferroni M, Faglia G, Yamanaka H, Marrazza G. New label free CA125 detection based on gold nanostructured screen-printed electrode. Sens Actuators B. 2013;179:194–200.
58. Das J, Kelley SO. Protein detection using arrayed microsensor chips: tuning sensor footprint to achieve

ultrasensitive readout of CA-125 in serum and whole blood. Anal Chem. 2011;83(4):1167–72.
59. Tang D, Su B, Tang J, Ren J, Chen G. Nanoparticle-based sandwich electrochemical immunoassay for carbohydrate antigen 125 with signal enhancement using enzyme-coated nanometer-sized enzyme-doped silica beads. Anal Chem. 2010;82(4):1527–34.
60. Wu D, Guo Z, Liu Y, Guo A, Lou W, Fan D, et al. Sandwich-type electrochemical immunosensor using dumbbell-like nanoparticles for the determination of gastric cancer biomarker CA72-4. Talanta. 2015;134:305–9.
61. Chun L, Kim S-E, Cho M, Choe W-S, Nam J, Lee DW, et al. Electrochemical detection of HER2 using single stranded DNA aptamer modified gold nanoparticles electrode. Sens Actuators B Chem. 2013;186:446–50.
62. Cainap C, Nagy V, Gherman A, Cetean S, Laszlo I, Constantin AM, et al. Classic tumor markers in gastric cancer. current standards and limitations. Clujul Med. 2015;88(2):111–5.
63. Jokerst JV, Raamanathan A, Christodoulides N, Floriano PN, Pollard AA, Simmons GW, et al. Nano-bio-chips for high performance multiplexed protein detection: determinations of cancer biomarkers in serum and saliva using quantum dot bioconjugate labels. Biosens Bioelectron. 2009;24(12):3622–9.
64. Li R, Li X, Xie L, Ding D, Hu Y, Qian X, et al. Preparation and evaluation of PEG-PCL nanoparticles for local tetradrine delivery. Int J Pharm. 2009;379(1):158–66.
65. Li R, Wu W, Liu Q, Wu P, Xie L, Zhu Z, et al. Intelligently targeted drug delivery and enhanced antitumor effect by gelatinase-responsive nanoparticles. PLoS One. 2013;8(7):e69643.
66. Li R, Xie L, Zhu Z, Liu Q, Hu Y, Jiang X, et al. Reversion of pH-induced physiological drug resistance: a novel function of copolymeric nanoparticles. PLoS One. 2011;6(9):e24172.
67. Davis ME, Chen ZG, Shin DM. Nanoparticle therapeutics: an emerging treatment modality for cancer. Nat Rev Drug Discov. 2008;7(9):771–82.
68. Mirkin C, Meade TJ, Petrosko SH, Stegh AH. Nanotechnology based precision tools for the detection and treatment of cancer. New York: Springer; 2015. p. 322.
69. Wang P, Qu Y, Li C, Yin L, Shen C, Chen W, et al. Bio-functionalized dense-silica nanoparticles for MR/NIRF imaging of CD146 in gastric cancer. Int J Nanomedicine. 2015;10:749–63.
70. Liu WF, Ji SR, Sun JJ, Zhang Y, Liu ZY, Liang AB, et al. CD146 expression correlates with epithelial-mesenchymal transition markers and a poor prognosis in gastric cancer. Int J Mol Sci. 2012;13(5):6399–406.
71. Wang K, Ruan J, Qian Q, Song H, Bao C, Zhang X, et al. BRCAA1 monoclonal antibody conjugated fluorescent magnetic nanoparticles for in vivo targeted magnetofluorescent imaging of gastric cancer. J Nanobiotechnology. 2011;9:23.
72. Zhou Z, Zhang C, Qian Q, Ma J, Huang P, Zhang X, et al. Folic acid-conjugated silica capped gold nanoclusters for targeted fluorescence/X-ray computed tomography imaging. J Nanobiotechnology. 2013;11:17.
73. Kulhari H, Pooja D, Rompicharla SV, Sistla R, Adams DJ. Biomedical applications of trastuzumab: as a therapeutic agent and a targeting ligand. Med Res Rev. 2015;35(4):849–76.
74. Kataoka H, Mori Y, Shimura T, Nishie H, Natsume M, Mochizuki H, et al. A phase II prospective study of the trastuzumab combined with 5-weekly S-1 and CDDP therapy for HER2-positive advanced gastric cancer. Cancer Chemother Pharmacol. 2016;77(5):957–62.
75. Fornaro L, Lucchesi M, Caparello C, Vasile E, Caponi S, Ginocchi L, et al. Anti-HER agents in gastric cancer: from bench to bedside. Nat Rev Gastroenterol Hepatol. 2011;8(7):369–83.
76. Chen TJ, Cheng TH, Chen CY, Hsu SC, Cheng TL, Liu GC, et al. Targeted Herceptin-dextran iron oxide nanoparticles for noninvasive imaging of HER2/neu receptors using MRI. J Biol Inorg Chem. 2009;14(2):253–60.
77. Tasi C-P, Chen C-Y, Hung Y, Chang F-H, Mou C-Y. Monoclonal antibody-functionalized mesoporous silica nanoparticles (MSN) for selective targeting breast cancer cells. J Mater Chem. 2009;19(7):5737–43.
78. Li K, Liu Y, Pu K-Y, Feng S-S, Zhna R, Liu B. Polyhedral oligomeric silsesquioxanes-containing conjugated polymer loaded PLGA nanoparticles with trastuzumab (herceptin) functionalization for HER2-positive cancer cell detection. Adv Funct Mater. 2011;21(2):287–94.
79. Jang M, Yoon YI, Kwon YS, Yoon TJ, Lee HJ, Hwang SI, et al. Trastuzumab-conjugated liposome-coated fluorescent magnetic nanoparticles to target breast cancer. Korean J Radiol. 2014;15(4):411–22.
80. Rajagopal I, Niveditha SR, Sahadev R, Nagappa PK, Rajendra SG. HER 2 expression in gastric and gastro-esophageal junction (GEJ) adenocarcinomas. J Clin Diagn Res. 2015;9(3):EC06–10.
81. De Carli DM, Rocha MP, Antunes LC, Fagundes RB. Immunohistochemical expression of HER2 in adenocarcinoma of the stomach. Arq Gastroenterol. 2015;52(2):152–5.
82. Fan X, Wang L, Guo Y, Tong H, Li L, Ding J, et al. Experimental investigation of the penetration of ultrasound nanobubbles in a gastric cancer xenograft. Nanotechnology. 2013;24(32):325102.
83. Cheng CC, Huang CF, Ho AS, Peng CL, Chang CC, Mai FD, et al. Novel targeted nuclear imaging agent for gastric cancer diagnosis: glucose-regulated protein 78 binding peptide-guided 111In-labeled polymeric micelles. Int J Nanomedicine. 2013;8:1385–91.

84. Jian-Hui C, Shi-Rong C, Hui W, Si-le C, Jian-Bo X, Er-Tao Z, et al. Prognostic value of three different lymph node staging systems in the survival of patients with gastric cancer following D2 lymphadenectomy. Tumour Biol. 2016;37(8):11105–13.
85. Kang WM, Meng QB, Yu JC, Ma ZQ, Li ZT. Factors associated with early recurrence after curative surgery for gastric cancer. World J Gastroenterol. 2015;21(19):5934–40.
86. Tsujimoto H, Morimoto Y, Takahata R, Nomura S, Yoshida K, Hiraki S, et al. Theranostic photosensitive nanoparticles for lymph node metastasis of gastric cancer. Ann Surg Oncol. 2015;22(Suppl 3):923–8.
87. Qiao R, Liu C, Liu M, Hu H, Hou Y, Wu K, et al. Ultrasensitive in vivo detection of primary gastric tumor and lymphatic metastasis using upconversion nanoparticles. ACS Nano. 2015;9(2):2120–9.
88. Tatsumi Y, Tanigawa N, Nishimura H, Nomura E, Mabuchi H, Matsuki M, et al. Preoperative diagnosis of lymph node metastases in gastric cancer by magnetic resonance imaging with ferumoxtran-10. Gastric Cancer. 2006;9(2):120–8.
89. Hill TK, Mohs AM. Image-guided tumor surgery: will there be a role for fluorescent nanoparticles? Wiley Interdiscip Rev Nanomed Nanobiotechnol. 2016;8(4):498–511.
90. Lozano N, Al-Ahmady ZS, Beziere NS, Ntziachristos V, Kostarelos K. Monoclonal antibody-targeted PEGylated liposome-ICG encapsulating doxorubicin as a potential theranostic agent. Int J Pharm. 2015;482(1–2):2–10.
91. Yaseen MA, Yu J, Jung B, Wong MS, Anvari B. Biodistribution of encapsulated indocyanine green in healthy mice. Mol Pharm. 2009;6(5):1321–32.
92. Ma Y, Tong S, Bao G, Gao C, Dai Z. Indocyanine green loaded SPIO nanoparticles with phospholipid-PEG coating for dual-modal imaging and photothermal therapy. Biomaterials. 2013;34(31):7706–14.
93. Hill TK, Abdulahad A, Kelkar SS, Marini FC, Long TE, Provenzale JM, et al. Indocyanine green-loaded nanoparticles for image-guided tumor surgery. Bioconjug Chem. 2015;26(2):294–303.
94. Lin M, Chen JF, Lu YT, Zhang Y, Song J, Hou S, et al. Nanostructure embedded microchips for detection, isolation, and characterization of circulating tumor cells. Acc Chem Res. 2014;47(10):2941–50.
95. Myung JH, Tam KA, Park SJ, Cha A, Hong S. Recent advances in nanotechnology-based detection and separation of circulating tumor cells. Wiley Interdiscip Rev Nanomed Nanobiotechnol. 2016;8(2):223–39.
96. Wang HY, Wei J, Zou ZY, Qian XP, Liu BR. Circulating tumour cells predict survival in gastric cancer patients: a meta-analysis. Contemp Oncol (Pozn). 2015;19(6):451–7.
97. Cristofanilli M, Budd GT, Ellis MJ, Stopeck A, Matera J, Miller MC, et al. Circulating tumor cells, disease progression, and survival in metastatic breast cancer. N Engl J Med. 2004;351(8):781–91.
98. Olmos D, Arkenau HT, Ang JE, Ledaki I, Attard G, Carden CP, et al. Circulating tumour cell (CTC) counts as intermediate end points in castration-resistant prostate cancer (CRPC): a single-centre experience. Ann Oncol. 2009;20(1):27–33.
99. Yoon HJ, Kozminsky M, Nagrath S. Emerging role of nanomaterials in circulating tumor cell isolation and analysis. ACS Nano. 2014;8(3):1995–2017.
100. Chen Z, Hong G, Wang H, Welsher K, Tabakman SM, Sherlock SP, et al. Graphite-coated magnetic nanoparticle microarray for few-cells enrichment and detection. ACS Nano. 2012;6(2):1094–101.
101. Hou S, Zhao L, Shen Q, Yu J, Ng C, Kong X, et al. Polymer nanofiber-embedded microchips for detection, isolation, and molecular analysis of single circulating melanoma cells. Angew Chem Int Ed Engl. 2013;52(12):3379–83.
102. Bhana S, Wang Y, Huang X. Nanotechnology for enrichment and detection of circulating tumor cells. Nanomedicine (Lond). 2015;10(12):1973–90.
103. Huang D, Xiang N, Tang W, Ni Z. Microfluidics-based circulating tumor cells separation. Prog Chem. 2015;7(27):882–912.
104. Nagrath S, Sequist LV, Maheswaran S, Bell DW, Irimia D, Ulkus L, et al. Isolation of rare circulating tumour cells in cancer patients by microchip technology. Nature. 2007;450(7173):1235–9.
105. Hyun KA, Lee TY, Jung HI. Negative enrichment of circulating tumor cells using a geometrically activated surface interaction chip. Anal Chem. 2013;85(9):4439–45.
106. Galletti G, Sung MS, Vahdat LT, Shah MA, Santana SM, Altavilla G, et al. Isolation of breast cancer and gastric cancer circulating tumor cells by use of an anti HER2-based microfluidic device. Lab Chip. 2014;14(1):147–56.
107. Ohnaga T, Shimada Y, Takata K, Obata T, Okumura T, Nagata T, et al. Capture of esophageal and breast cancer cells with polymeric microfluidic devices for CTC isolation. Mol Clin Oncol. 2016;4(4):599–602.
108. He W, Xu D, Wang Z, Xiang X, Tang B, Li S, et al. Detecting ALK-rearrangement of CTC enriched by nanovelcro chip in advanced NSCLC patients. Oncotarget. 2016; doi:10.18632/oncotarget.8305.
109. Sarioglu AF, Aceto N, Kojic N, Donaldson MC, Zeinali M, Hamza B, et al. A microfluidic device for label-free, physical capture of circulating tumor cell clusters. Nat Methods. 2015;12(7):685–91.
110. Hofmann M, Stoss O, Shi D, Buttner R, van de Vijver M, Kim W, et al. Assessment of a HER2 scoring system for gastric cancer: results from a validation study. Histopathology. 2008;52(7):797–805.
111. Janjigian YY, Werner D, Pauligk C, Steinmetz K, Kelsen DP, Jager E, et al. Prognosis of metastatic gastric and gastroesophageal junction cancer by HER2 status: a European and USA International collaborative analysis. Ann Oncol. 2012;23(10):2656–62.

112. Galanzha EI, Shashkov EV, Kelly T, Kim JW, Yang L, Zharov VP. In vivo magnetic enrichment and multiplex photoacoustic detection of circulating tumour cells. Nat Nanotechnol. 2009;4(12):855–60.
113. Xu H, Aguilar ZP, Yang L, Kuang M, Duan H, Xiong Y, et al. Antibody conjugated magnetic iron oxide nanoparticles for cancer cell separation in fresh whole blood. Biomaterials. 2011;32(36):9758–65.
114. Song EQ, Hu J, Wen CY, Tian ZQ, Yu X, Zhang ZL, et al. Fluorescent-magnetic-biotargeting multifunctional nanobioprobes for detecting and isolating multiple types of tumor cells. ACS Nano. 2011;5(2):761–70.
115. Lee HJ, Cho HY, Oh JH, Namkoong K, Lee JG, Park JM, et al. Simultaneous capture and in situ analysis of circulating tumor cells using multiple hybrid nanoparticles. Biosens Bioelectron. 2013;47: 508–14.
116. Viraka NBP, Kanchanapally R, Pramanik A, Sinha SS, Chavva SR, Hamme AN, et al. Aptamer-conjugated graphene oxide membranes for highly efficient capture and accurate identification of multiple types of circulating tumor cells. Bioconjug Chem. 2015;26(2):235–42.
117. Gaddes ER, Gydush G, Li S, Chen N, Dong C, Wang Y. Aptamer-based polyvalent ligands for regulated cell attachment on the hydrogel surface. Biomacromolecules. 2015;16(4):1382–9.
118. Zhao W, Cui CH, Bose S, Guo D, Shen C, Wong WP, et al. Bioinspired multivalent DNA network for capture and release of cells. Proc Natl Acad Sci USA. 2012;109(48):19626–31.
119. He R, Zhao L, Liu Y, Zhang N, Cheng B, He Z, et al. Biocompatible TiO2 nanoparticle-based cell immunoassay for circulating tumor cells capture and identification from cancer patients. Biomed Microdevices. 2013;15(4):617–26.
120. Chen YW, Liou GG, Pan HB, Tseng HH, Hung YT, Chou CP. Specific detection of CD133-positive tumor cells with iron oxide nanoparticles labeling using noninvasive molecular magnetic resonance imaging. Int J Nanomedicine. 2015;10:6997–7018.
121. Chen Y, Lian G, Liao C, Wang W, Zeng L, Qian C, et al. Characterization of polyethylene glycol-grafted polyethylenimine and superparamagnetic iron oxide nanoparticles (PEG-g-PEI-SPION) as an MRI-visible vector for siRNA delivery in gastric cancer in vitro and in vivo. J Gastroenterol. 2013;48(7):809–21.

Systemic Drug Delivery in Gastric Cancer

14

Rutian Li and Mi Yang

14.1 Physiological Drug Resistance (PDR) and the Role of Copolymeric Nanoparticles in Its Reversion

Copolymeric nanoparticles (NPs) have been proven to be effective carriers for the delivery of antitumor agents with some of them have come into clinical use [1–3]. The effectiveness of NPs resides in their enhanced permeability and retention (EPR) effects, rather than on an active targeting strategy [4, 5]. Ultimately, this results in sustained release of drugs from their NP vectors [6]. In this section, we will introduce another important mechanism inherent to copolymeric NPs: their ability to reverse physiological drug resistance (PDR).

Although genetic and epigenetic changes in cancer cells have been a major research focus, the tumor microenvironment is also a vital factor that has attracted increasing attention in recent years. This is because solid tumors are three-dimensional structures composed of both cancer and stromal cells in addition to matrix and vascular network [7]. The physicochemical factors in the tumor microenvironment are quite different from those found in normal tissue. These altered physicochemical factors are significant for the treatment of cancer because they can influence the efficacy of anticancer agents; for instance, the pH of tumor tissue is classic example. The extracellular pH of cancer cells is more acidic than that of normal tissue, whereas the intracellular pH of tumor is nearly equivalent [8]. As to the weakly basic agents that have an acid dissociation constant (Pka) in the range of 7.5–9.5, this unusual intracellular-extracellular pH gradient can influence the effect of these agents. In this scenario, such drugs would be protonated at the extracellular tumor pH value [7]. Since the protonated forms of these agents become much less membrane permeable, they would accumulate predominantly outside of the cell. As such, the intracellular environment would have a low concentration of such weakly basic drugs, leading to a markedly reduced ability to kill cancer cells. Raghunand et al. has defined this phenomenon as "physiological drug resistance", which is different from the "biochemical drug resistance" (e.g. MDR or drug resistance) that is caused by the changes of signaling pathways and/or protein expression [9].

However, pH is not the solely physiochemical factor influencing drug distribution in tumor tissue. The disorganized vascular network and the absence of a functional lymphatic system of

R. Li • M. Yang (✉)
The Comprehensive Cancer Center of Drum-Tower Hospital, Medical School of Nanjing University & Clinical Cancer Institute of Nanjing University, Nanjing 210008, People's Republic of China

J. Wei, B. Liu (eds.), *Personalized Management of Gastric Cancer*,
DOI 10.1007/978-981-10-3978-2_14

tumor tissue causes increased interstitial fluid pressure (IFP). Moreover, the composition and structure of the extracellular matrix (ECM) can passively influence the movement of molecules within the tumor [10, 11]. Given these additional features of the tumor microenvironment, the delivery of anticancer drugs often fails to reach cells that are distal from functioning blood vessels [12].

With this in mind, the following section will define "physiological drug resistance" (PDR) as any and all kinds of tumor resistance to anticancer drugs that are caused by the physiochemical factors of the tumor itself. This kind of drug resistance is usually composed of two subtypes: [1] "pH-induced physiological drug resistance" (PIPDR), which is caused by the unusual tumor intracellular-extracellular pH gradient and [2] "penetration-defect related physiological drug resistance" (PDPDR), which is caused by the impaired penetration of drugs into the tumor tissue (Fig. 14.1).

PDR plays a significant role in chemotherapy and targeted therapy failure since it is a phenomenon that occurs in most tumors [13]. These different physicochemical factors exist widely in most tumor types, irrelevant to their genetic background. As such, they can influence the effectiveness of a large number of drugs regardless of their mechanism of action. Given this, reversion of PDR would certainly improve drug effectiveness in nearly all kinds of tumors. Unfortunately, very little attention has been paid to this kind of drug resistance. In the following section, we will discuss the two kinds of PDR—PIPDR and PDPDR—in addition to the role copolymeric nanoparticles can play in the reversion of PDR.

14.1.1 PIPDR

Among the various micro environmental factors, pH is of the greatest importance. This is for two reasons: firstly, the lower extracellular pH values are detected in most tumor tissues [13]; secondly, most of the present-day chemotherapeutics for gastric cancer are weakly basic drugs such as doxorubicin, epirubicin, paclitaxel, and docetaxel [14]. Several studies have proven that the cytotoxicity of these drugs is hindered at lower extracellular tumor pH values [9, 14–16].

Raghunand et al. [8, 9, 15, 16] have demonstrated the existence of PIPDR in chemotherapeutics more than 10 years ago. Since its discovery, several attempts have been made to overcome PIPDR. For instance, Lee et al. [17] treated cancer cells with the combination of doxorubicin and either chloroquine (a competing base) or omeprazole (an H^+-pump inhibitor). In the study reported by Raghunand et al. [16], the in vivo effectiveness of doxorubicin was enhanced by adding sodium bicarbonate to the drinking water of mice. However, these methods rely on the use of additional agents, or they alter normal homeostasis. Either way, severe side effects may result. Accordingly, most of these treatments failed to attain clinical use because of their inherent or potential toxicity or the likelihood of side effects [17, 18]. The only in vivo study on the reversion of PIPDR was reported by Raghunand et al. [16] in which bicarbonate-induced extracellular alkalinization led to significantly improve the therapeutic effectiveness of doxorubicin against MCF-7 xenografts. However, the potential for side effects is significant since the increase in extracellular pH occurs nonspecifically.

Polymeric NPs are better candidates to overcome PIPDR than other approaches since they

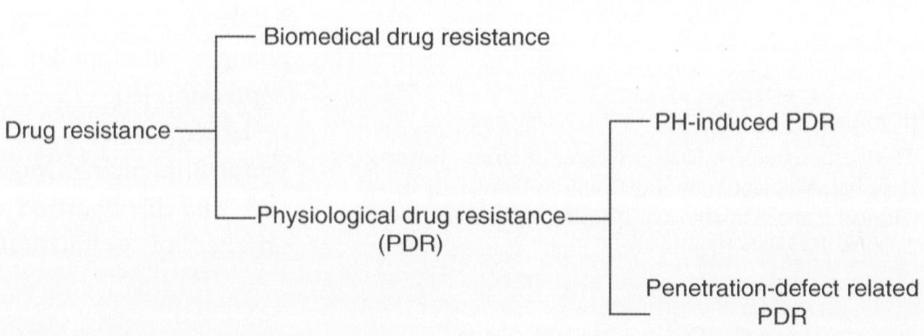

Fig. 14.1 Types of drug resistance caused by tumors

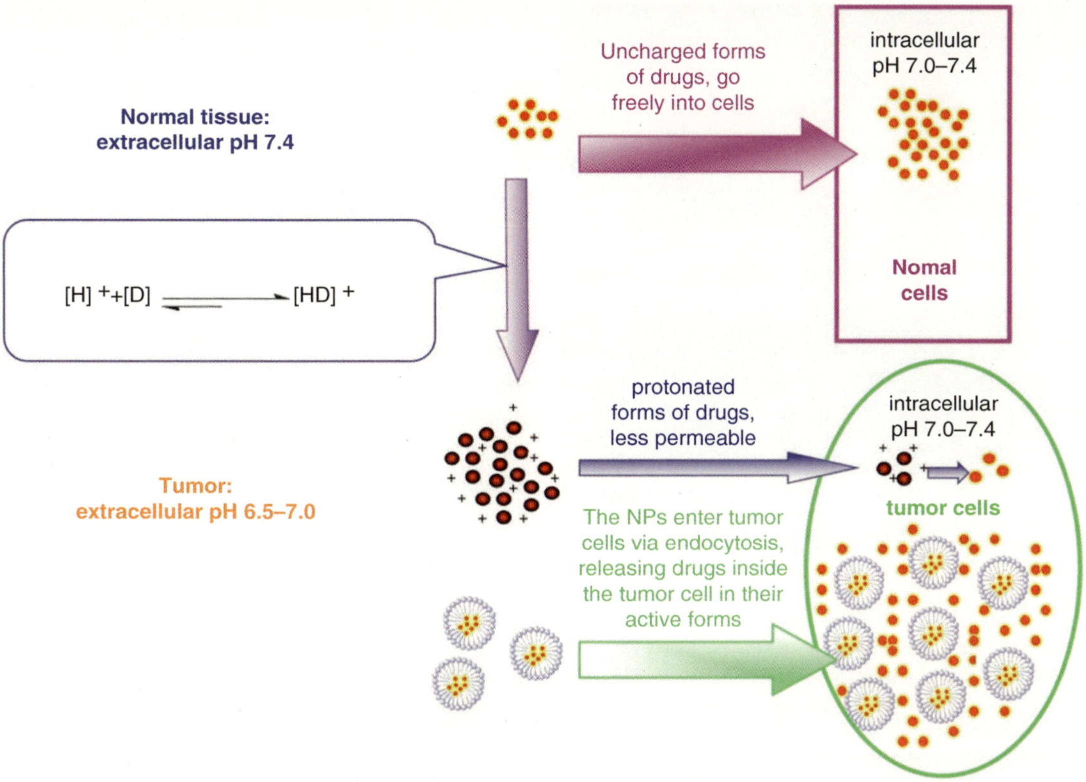

Fig. 14.2 Mechanism for nanoparticle-driven reversion of PIPDR [21]

are more effective and present with fewer inherent toxicities. NPs enter cells via endocytic uptake, thereby allowing for the intracellular release of their drug cargo [19, 20]. When weakly basic drugs are incorporated into NPs, the drug will be able to effectively enter the cancer cell via endocytosis. The intracellular pH is physiologically normal (around 7. 4), meaning that the basic drugs released in the cytoplasm would keep their active, uncharged forms. Thus, this approach would lead to more effective termination of cancer cells (Fig. 14.2).

Previous work [21] from our lab used a murine model for the study of NP-driven reversion of PIPDR. In this model, tetrandrine (Tet, Pka 7.80), an alkaloid isolated from traditional Chinese medicine, was incorporated into the diblock copolymer methoxy poly(ethylene glycol)-polycaprolactone (mPEG-PCL). In vitro cytotoxicity studies showed that the cytotoxicity of free Tet was significantly decreased ($p < 0.05$) when the extracellular pH decreased from 7.4 to 6.8. Importantly, the cytotoxicity of Tet-loaded nanoparticles (Tet-NPs) was not significantly influenced by this same change in pH. Our evaluation of the antitumor effects of free Tet versus Tet-NPs in a murine model confirmed the successful reversion of PIPDR by Tet-NPs. Moreover, the NPs reversed in vivo PIPDR more efficiently than other existing methods with meaningfully fewer side effects. Collectively, these results revealed a new mechanism for copolymeric NPs and expanded our understanding of copolymeric drug carriers into an area where cancer microenvironmental factors must be considered.

14.1.2 PDPDR

PDPDR is caused by increased interstitial fluid pressure (IFP) and altered composition and structure of the extracellular matrix (ECM). Taken

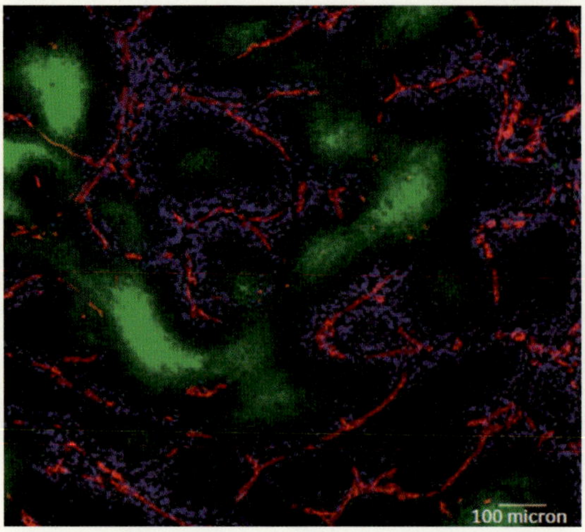

Fig. 14.3 In vivo distribution of doxorubicin. A section from a mouse mammary tumor showing the distribution of doxorubicin (*blue*) in relation to tumor blood vessels (*red*) and regions of hypoxia (*green*). It is obvious that doxorubicin is distributed around the tumor blood vessels but far away from the hypoxic region of tumors. Bar = 100 μm. Reproduced with permission from Ref. [22]

together, these changes slow down the movement of molecules within the tumor. Many anticancer drugs—including chemotherapeutics and molecular-targeted agents—have limited distribution from blood vessels into solid tumors, which limits their effectiveness [7, 11, 12] (Fig. 14.3).

Traditional methods used to enhance drug penetration into tumor tissue are limited and most have remained at the preclinical stage. These approaches will be described in more detail below.

14.1.2.1 Angiogenesis Inhibitors

Anti-angiogenesis agents (e.g. bevacizumab) directly inhibit vascular endothelial growth factor (VEGF). They have been shown to enhance the clinical effects of chemotherapeutics in several kinds of tumors. This result may appear paradoxical, since the inhibition of angiogenesis would lead to decreases in blood vessel density, thus impairing drug penetration and delivery to cancer cells. However, recent studies have revealed that the mechanisms of angiogenesis therapy act to normalize tumor vascular architecture, thereby improving blood flow to cancer cells and reducing IFP [23–25]. As a result, drug penetration would be improved. It is possible that this is a neglected mechanism for the synergistic effect between chemotherapeutics and angiogenetic agents [26].

14.1.2.2 ECM Modification

The ECM in the tumor microenvironment comprises a diverse network of structural and instructional molecules that is closely linked to the tumor cells [27]. An abnormal extracellular matrix (ECM) is a major factor leading to impaired drug penetration in solid tumors. To this end, a series of approaches have been reported to partially degrade or downregulate the expression of ECM proteins in order to improve drug penetration [28]. The agents used to degrade ECM include collagenase [29, 30], hyaluronidase [29, 31], and matrix metalloproteinase-8 (MMP-8) [32], to name a few. However, these strategies will likely present a double-edged sword, as both MMPs and proteinases play an important role in promoting tumor invasion and metastasis.

Numerous studies have shown that nanoparticles enhance the penetration of their loaded drug agents [33–36], whether alone or in combination with other treatments such as hyperthermia [37], anti-angiogenic agents, or tumor-penetrating peptides. However, nanoparticle penetration is still influenced by the particle size and tumor environment, meaning that multiple biobarriers will need to be overcome before nanomedicines are clinically capable of being delivered to the target site.

Local administration of a nanoparticle-based delivery system results in high drug concentrations and retention times at the tumor site. The clinical benefits of intraperitoneal chemotherapy in advanced stage cancer patients was verified in work that showed local regional chemotherapy improved their clinical outcomes. However, chemotherapeutic efficacy also depends on the accessibility and retention of the delivered drug to tumor tissue. To this end, Saltzman et al. [38] studied the pharmacokinetic and tissue distribution of local polymer implants in the rat brain. They showed that at the end of the first day, therapeutic agent penetration was

5 mm from the site of implantation. From days 3 to 14, therapeutic penetration was reduced to 1 mm. According to rapid in vitro release kinetics, 84% of the drug was cumulatively released from this delivery system during the first 24 h. In the first few days after implantation, the penetration distance of the polymeric drug was reduced since the drug diffusion gradient was significantly diminished. It is possible that intraoperative administration could cause acute injury and enhance drug penetration via convection of interstitial fluid. This phenomenon might also be the reason for the rapid drug elimination seen after day three. It should be noted that the authors did not take into account the effect of interstitial fluid convection to tissue penetration.

After reaching the target site, the cell membrane is an additional barrier to cross in order for efficient delivery of the loaded drug in nanodrug delivery systems (NDDSs) into specific organelles within the cytoplasm of cancer cells. Various strategies have been tried to stabilize lysosomal membrane and prevent lysosomal, such as targeting ligands, antibodies, as well as cell-penetrating peptides (CPPs). Suitable nanoparticle size also influences the penetration property of nanomedicines and affects their cellular uptake. It was found that 30-nm nanoparticles could more easily extravasate and penetrate into tumor tissue when compared with larger size nanoparticles. Moreover, the penetration advantages of smaller nanoparticles exhibited distinct therapeutic effects.

Cell-penetrating peptides (CPPs) have been shown to help polymeric nanoparticles permeate cellular membranes and internalize into cancer cells. For instance, TATp, as a pegylated CPPs, has been used to modify liposomes. The prepared micelles could be efficiently taken up by cancer cells and provided for high transfection productivity in cell nuclei. As a result, TATp improved cytoplasmic drug levels and overcame drug resistance in tumor-bearing mice.

Finally, iRGD is a tumor-specific penetrating peptide that can significantly enhance IP doxorubicin penetration into disseminated peritoneal tumor nodules in mice [39]. Intraperitoneal coadministration of iRGD and doxorubicin specifically labeled suppressed peritoneal metastases in a mouse model. Importantly, iRGD improved intratumoral dextran and doxorubicin concentrations up to 3 and 2.5 times, respectively. When compared with administration of just intraperitoneal doxorubicin, a combination of iRGD and doxorubicin treatment significantly inhibited the growth of peritoneal metastatic tumors and reduced systemic drug toxicity. According to their study, intraperitoneal iRGD and nano drugs were a simple and effective strategy to improve the IP therapeutic index and reduce systemic cytotoxicity for peritoneal carcinomatosis.

14.2 Nanoparticle Applications in Gastric Cancer Treatment

Nanoparticles have inherently adjustable physical properties, which include multivalent targeting abilities, high loading abilities, scalability, easy dispersibility in water, and can pass through biological barriers. As such, further exploration of nanomedical technology could potentially allow for safer and more effective radiographic imaging and detection systems, in addition to more robust early diagnosis and individualized treatments for gastric cancer [40]. More specifically, nanoparticles composed of magnetic iron oxide, magnetic fluorescence, metal, semiconductors, quantum dots, nanodiamonds, nanowires, nanometer polymer, nanocarbon, and graphene have all been used in related medical research fields.

14.2.1 Albumin Nanoparticles

Human serum albumin (HAS) has many medical advantages: good biocompatibility, low toxicity, no immunogenicity, easy preparation, targeted and controlled release, and it can increase drug stability. Given this extensive list, it has drawn considerable attention. In particular, HAS nanoparticles are good drug carriers with the ability to localize within tumor tissues. This would therefore increase the antitumor effects of the loaded drug [41, 42].

Some scholars have used disulfide-PDPH (3-(2-pyridyldithio) propionyl hydrazide) to combine hydrophobic adriamycin (ADR) with HAS. The result has been an amphiphilic adriamycin-human serum albumin nano-micelle ADR-HAS [43] with redox sensitivity. In a nude mouse transplanted tumor models established by NCI-N87 cells, the tumor inhibition rate of ADR-HSA nanoparticles was as high as 69.98%.

14.2.2 NK105

Since paclitaxel (PTX) is hydrophobic, its clinical application depends on its addition to polyoxyethylene castor oil EL. However, this combination will likely lead to allergic reactions [44]. To this end, NK105 is a type of "core-shell" poly-micelle nanoparticle that can "wrap" PTX. It can be directly used for intravenous administration without the addition of further solvents. Therefore, NK105 has a greater clinical advantage than PTX alone [45]. Importantly, Phase clinical study results have shown that the recommended dose of NK105 was 150 mg every 3 weeks, which was equivalent to PTX/m^2 [46].

A Phase II clinical study was conducted to assess the efficacy and safety of NK105 in patients with advanced gastric cancer who had failed first-line chemotherapy [47]. All patients included in the study had to have measurable lesions and had to have also undergone chemotherapy without paclitaxel at least once. Every 3 weeks, patients received a 30-min NK105 intravenous infusion (150 mg equivalent to PTX/m^2), without allergy-free pretreatment. These infusions occurred until a given patient's condition improved, until he/she could no longer tolerate the side effects, or he/she refused. The primary end point event was overall response rate (ORR) after baseline. The secondary end point events were progression-free survival (PFS), time to treatment failure (TTF), and overall survival (OS).

From November 2007 to July 2009, 57 patients were included in the study, and 56 of them were evaluated. Two of them achieved complete remission, 12 achieved partial, and the ORR was 25%. The meso-position PFS was 3.0 months, meso-position TTF 2.8 months, and meso-position OS 14.4 months. Drug-associated toxicity went from light to severe, with the following percent of patients reporting the following: neutropenia (64.0%), leukopenia (17.5%), lymphopenia (8.8%), abnormal nerve sensory (1.8%), fatigue (3.5%), and oral cavity inflammation (1.8%). There were no treatment-related deaths.

14.2.3 Chitosan Nanoparticles

Chitosan is a type of natural, linear polysaccharide polymer obtained from a deacetylation chitin reaction. Chitosan has unique properties, including being a biological adhesive, having good biocompatibility and biodegradability, being nontoxic, and having low immunogenicity. As such, it has been widely used in pharmacological and biomedical domains. The existence in amidogen and carboxyl groups in the chitosan molecule makes it easy for chemical modification to occur. Importantly, such modifications can imbue chitosan with amphipathy. The resulting amphiphilic molecules can form self-assembled nanoparticles, which can carry and bring drugs to specific locations. They can then achieve good drug targeting by conjugating specific targeting molecules into the drug-loaded nanoparticles.

N-trimethyl chitosan (TMC) is a type of water-soluble, cationic polyelectrolyte that can be used for oral and intravenous administration of PTX. TMC has biocompatibility and biodegradability properties, and it can form nanoparticles with diameters of 150–200 nm using an ion gelation method [48]. Embedding PTC into TMC can effectively solve the problem of the poor water solubility exhibited by PTX and lead to more controlled release and a prolonged drug half-life. For instance, Song et al. [49] prepared spherical, paclitaxel-loaded, n-trimethyl chitosan chloride TMC-PTX nanoparticles. The loaded amount of PTX in this particle was approximately 30%. TMC-PTX treatment inhibited proliferation and induced apoptosis in NCI-N87 and SGC-7901, two strains of human gastric carcinoma cells. In addition, comparison of TMC-PTX with PTX alone revealed that the former had enhanced therapeutic effects in both NCI-N87 and SGC-7901 types of nude mouse transplanted tumor models. Importantly, there were no evident side effects.

Polyethylene glycol (PEG) is a type of nonionic, hydrophilic polymer that has beneficial characteristics including nontoxicity, no immunogenicity, long circulation times, and good biocompatibility. Therefore, PEG could be widely used in cross-linked polymer combinations. Epigallocatechin-3-gallate (EGCG) is the main component of tea polyphenols found in green tea and has both anti-inflammatory and antioxidant effects. Moreover, it can inhibit tumor growth through anti-angiogenetic effects in addition to inhibiting proliferation and inducing apoptosis [50–54]. Some researchers have made FCS/PCS/Gel/EGCG nanoparticles from fucose-chitosan (FCS), PEG-chitosan (PCS), EGCG, and gelatin [55]. It was found that oral administration of this nanoparticle could effectively reduce drug release in environments containing gastric acid. This led to significant decreases in gastric cancer activity and reductions in inflammatory reactions of the stomach and liver.

14.2.4 Calcium Carbonate Nanoparticles

Nanometer calcium carbonate is a new type of functional, inorganic, and nonmetallic mineral filler that was developed in the 1980s. It is also emerging as a viable gene transfection vector that can be medicated using inorganic nanoparticles. In addition to its easy preparation, good biocompatibility, and biodegradability, it also has a high transfection efficiency and good reproducibility. Furthermore, no buffered solution is needed during the preparative process to control pH [56].

He et al. [57] prepared calcium carbonate ($CaCO_3$) nanoparticles to deliver vascular endothelial growth factor (VEGF) C-siRNA. The diameter of this $CaCO_3$ nanoparticle was 58 mm, and the surface positive charge was +28.6 mV. When compared with lipidosome nanoparticles, the $CaCO_3$ nanoparticles did not show evidence of cytotoxicity to SGC-7901 cells. Additionally, SGC-7901 cells successfully inhibited VEGF-C expression when transfected with $CaCO_3$ nanoparticles loaded with VEGF-C siRNA. In a SGC-7901 cell subcutaneous transplantation tumor model, $CaCO_3$ nanoparticles were also able to effectively inhibit tumor lymphangion genesis and tumor cell growth. Taken together, these results demonstrate that $CaCO_3$ nanoparticles can effectively deliver siRNA nonviral vectors, highlighting their potential use in the genetic treatment of gastric cancer.

14.2.5 Gold Nanoparticles

Gold nanoparticles (GNPs) have very unique physical and chemical properties that are mainly manifested in the following three aspects: (1) gold nanoparticles are relatively safe, easy to prepare, and have good stability, (2) gold nanoparticles are basically inactive and completely nontoxic, and (3) their synthesis is relatively easy and the resulting diameter range controlled within a range of 1–150 nm. (4) They have the same small size, surface, quantum size, macroscopic quantum tunneling, and dielectric effects as those found in nanoparticles. (5) They have unique electrical catalytic, optical, magnetic, and biological affinity effects. Therefore, gold nanoparticles have wide, potential use in the biomedical field. To this end, Singh et al. prepared gold nanoparticles with stable electrical-biological properties. Gold nanoparticles to pH and demonstrated its anti-carcinoma effect inYCC-3 gastric cells [58].

14.2.6 Gelatinase-Targeted Nanoparticles

The matrix metalloproteinases (MMPs) family is an umbrella classification for endopeptidases related to extracellular matrix degradation [59]. Extensive study on MMPs has shown that they are highly expressed in all human tumors. MMP expression levels are related to tumor progression, lower patient survival rate, and tumor metastasis. Gelatinase (GEL), also known as MMP-2 and MMP-9, are components that have been studied the most. Whether in cell or animal models or in clinical observation, MMP-2 plays an important role in tumor growth as well as invading metastasis. Moreover, MMP-9 plays an important role in tumor growth [60], metastasis, and immune adjustment [61–64]. Gelatinase—especially MMP-9—is also an important factor in the tumor metastatic niche. Therefore, treatment strategies targeting MMPs like MMP-2 and MMP-9 are of great significance for the diagnosis and treatment of malignant tumors [65, 66]

To this end, miR-200c is a microRNA capable of inhibiting tumor stem cells. For instance, we [67] adopted a phthalein amine method and a twice-ring opening polymerization and synthesized the macromolecule targeted drug carrier PEG-Pep-PCL that contained a gelatinase substrate section [68]. We also prepared miR-200c single-drug nanoparticles and miR-200c/DOC enzyme-targeted double-drug nanoparticles by using a double-solvent evaporation technique. The transfection efficiency of miR-200c single-drug nanoparticles was found to be high, meaning this approach could improve long-term miR-200c cellular content, reduce TUBB3 expression, and increase sensibilization on DOC. These results showed that the antitumor effect of miR-200c/DOC double-drug nanoparticles was higher than that of DOC single-drug particles.

Work with miR-200c has shown that it can significantly increase the expression of E-cadherin and reduce the expression of the gastric cancer stem cell marker CD44. These findings led to the conclusion that the tumor's invasive and metastatic abilities were lower than that those of either single-drug particles or Taxotere. A near-infrared live imaging experiment indicated that nanoparticles can localize in the transplanted, subcutaneous sarcoma of human gastric cancer. Laser confocal microscopy also revealed that miR-200c marked by FAM and nanoparticles marked by rhodamine-B both localized around and entered tumor tissue. miR-200c/DOC double-drug nanoparticles have also been shown to effectively inhibit tumor growth. As a result, miR-200c and E-cadherin expression in tumor tissues increased, while TUBB3 and CD44 expression decreased. The proliferative activity of cells was significantly decreased, while apoptosis increased. When the remaining tumor cells were subcutaneously transplanted in a nude mouse model, the growth rate of the second transplanted tumor in the double-drug nanoparticle group had the slowest rate in addition to longest survival time.

Additional work of us [69] found that gelatinase-targeted PEG-Pep-PCL nanoparticles loaded with miR-200c had radiotherapy sensibilization in gastric cancer cells. Further work [70] found that in highly expressing gelatinase gastric cancer cell strains, gelatinase nanoparticles loaded with docetaxel had significantly more radiotherapy sensibilization than those treated with simple docetaxel.

Wu et al. from our group further [71] prepared gelatinase-targeted 5-fluorouridine (5-FU), 5-Aza-2-deoxycytidine (DAC), and double-loaded nanoparticles. These three kinds of particles were all successfully delivered to gastric cancer cells. Results revealed that these nanoparticles enhanced DAC stability, so as to reexpress TFAP2E. The demethylation effect of TFAP2E also increased5-Fu sensitivity. Therefore, these results showed that double-loaded nanoparticles could further inhibit gastric cancer proliferation and induce cellular apoptosis.

14.2.7 Silk Fibroin Microspheres

Silk fibroin is a natural, fibrous polymer protein, composed of 18 kinds of amino acids. Of these, glycine, alanine, and serine account for approximately 80% of the total amino acid content. The protein molecular chain is folded in indentation and is connected by hydrogen bonds, while the interlamination is linked by van der Waals forces. Each silk fibroin molecule is a complex composed of a proportion of 6:6:1 of heavy chain (H chain, ~350 kDa), light chain (L chain, ~26 kDa), and P25 glycoprotein (~30 kDa). The light and heavy chains are connected by disulfide bonds formed by cysteine residues at the carboxy ends. The glycoprotein P25 forms non-covalent bonds in the complex, leading to the formation of stable light-heavy chain complexes [72, 73]. The crystalline and noncrystalline regions of silk fibroin are distributed in an alternating fashion. The heavy chain alternatingly passes through the crystalline and noncrystalline regions, while the light chain only exists in the noncrystalline region.

When compared with other high polymer materials, silk fibroin has good biocompatibility, biodegradability, flexibility, and plasticity. It has also been widely used in tissue engineering and drug delivery systems. In addition, its characteristics of nontoxicity, non-stimulation, and sound stability provide favorable drug carrier conditions.

Wu et al. from our group [73] developed silk fibroin nanoparticles (PTX-SF-NPs) carrying Taxol through the self-assembly of silk fibroin. The resulting particle diameter was approximately 130 nm. In nanoparticles, the main conformation of silk fibroin is a silk I conformation without β-folded structure. In cellular uptake experiments, gastric cancer cells BGC-823 and SGC-7901 both took up silk fibroin nanoparticles carrying coumarin-6 in 2 hours. In vitro cytotoxicity experiments indicated that the silk fibroin carrier itself had no toxicity, even at 200 μg/ml. Importantly, Taxol carried in PTX-SF-NPs kept its pharmacological activity. Subsequent in vivo antitumor experiments featuring subcutaneous tumor, gastric carcinoma nude mice compared nude drug and PTX-SF-NPs systemic administration. Results indicated that the local administration of PTX-SF-NPs had better antitumor growth effects.

14.2.8 Nano-iodized Oil Emulsion

Sentinel lymph nodes (SLNs) refer to special lymph nodules that are the first to receive primary tumor lymphatic drainage and are also the first to have tumor metastases. To this end, sentinel lymph node biopsy (SLNB) is the most commonly used method to determine gastric cancer metastasis. Its basic approach is as follows: [1] inject a tracer around the tumor, and mark the metastasized lymph nodules by marking the extent of the tracer, and [2] determine the nature of the metastasized nodules through biopsy. This tracing approach can be divided into three types depending on the tracer materials used: dye method, nuclide method, and a combined dye-nuclide method. To this end, using nanomaterials as SLN tracers has received recent and extensive attention. More specifically, common nanocarriers, like liposomes, dendrimers, quantum dots, nanoparticles, and ultrasonic vesicles, have received wide attention and research [74].

Lim et al. [75] prepared nanometer-iodized oil emulsion particles with a size of 117 ± 6 nm. They then used this nanometer-iodized oil emulsion to conduct endoscopic submucosal injection with subsequent CT angiography on sentinel lymph nodes. The agreement rate of nanometer-iodized oil emulsion CT angiography with the indocyanine green method was shown to be 84% (16/19). The agreement rate with the dye method was 78.6% (11/14). These results show that the application of this technique could be of great significance for the early detection of gastric cancer.

14.2.9 Endosomal Nanoparticles

Endosomes are a new type of dendritic polymers. They are kind of spherical bubble of supramolecular materials and nucleic acid compounds that are embedded in a lipophilic shell [76].

Farnesiferol C (FC) is a natural compound with anticancer effects. Zohreh et al. [77] prepared dendrosomal farnesiferol C (DFC) and investigated its effects at the cellular level. They showed that at high concentrations (>50 μM), DFC was able to inhibit proliferation of human gastric cancer AGS cell strains. Moreover, this inhibitory effect was time-dose dependent.

14.2.10 Magnetic Nanoparticles

Magnetic nanoparticles typically refer to magnetic materials with particle sizes within the range of 1–100 nm. Not only do they have the surface, volume quantum size, and macroscopic quantum tunneling effects that ordinary nano-level materials have but also have special magnetic properties, which are mainly embodied in the following four aspects:

1. Superparamagnetism: superparamagnetism occurs when the particle diameter of a magnetic particle has reached a critical dimension such that it will have strong magnetism within an existing magnetic field. When the external magnetic field disappears, there is no residual magnetism in the material. Whether or not magnetic nanoparticles have superparamagnetism is a very important issue to a material's biomedical applications.
2. High coercivity: high coercivity is the magnetic field intensity that is needed for magnetism to return back to zero along the hysteresis loop. When the magnetic particle size reaches a critical size, a very large reverse magnetic field is needed for the permanent magnet to lose magnetism. Thus, the magnetic nanoparticles would show a high coercivity.
3. Magnetic susceptibility: magnetic susceptibility refers to the ratio of the magnetization intensity when a material is attracted into or repelled out of a magnetic field. Magnetic susceptibility is closely related to the parity of the total number of electrons contained in the particle's material(s). When the total electrons contained is an odd number, the magnetic susceptibility obeys Curie-Weiss law; when it is an even number, it does not obey Curie-Weiss law, but is in direct proportion to thermal motion energy.
4. Curie temperature: Curie temperature is also called the Curie point or magnetic transition point. It refers to the temperature at which magnetic materials change between ferromagnetic and paramagnetic materials.

The size of magnetic nanoparticles is controllable. When compared to the particle diameter of cells, viruses, proteins, and/or genes, it is of an equivalent or smaller size. This provides them with the possibility of combining with biological entities, thereby allowing for a controlled, marking strategy. Moreover, the magnetism of magnetic nanoparticles obeys Coulomb's law. This means that they can be controlled by an additional magnetic field, allowing for the delivery of anticancer drugs and/or radioactive atoms to the targeted (e.g., cancerous) location and achieving the desired treatment effect. In the biomedical field, magnetic nanomaterials have potentially broad applications in targeted drug delivery, biological magnetic separation, and magnetic heat treatment, to name a few.

Some researchers have used biosensor system based on giant magneto-impedance effect and superparamagnetic iron oxide particles (RGD-Fe3O4@chitosan) decorated by chitosan. This has allowed them to combine with the integrin present in gastric cancer cells, thus allowing for their specific targeting of gastric cancer cells [78].

BRCAA1 antigens are highly expressed in some gastric cancer cell lines, such as MKN-1, MKN-74, SGC-7901, KATO-III, and MGC803. Given this, some researchers have attempted to use BRCAA1 as the targeting molecule for gastric cancer cells. For instance, Wang [79] prepared BRCAA1 monoclonal antibody fluorescently labeled magnetic nanoparticles (BRCAA1-FMNPs). Later studies confirmed that this particle was not only able to target and enter gastric cancer cells but was also able to allow for magnetic fluorescence imaging.

There is also work that has constructed ferroferric oxide-carboxymethyl cellulose (CMC)-fluorouracil (5FU, fe3o4-cmc-5fu) nano drugs. This work found that when compared with 5-Fu, such nano drugs could improve the eradication of gastric cells [80]. Additional mechanistic research yielded results counter to previously held beliefs. In the past, it was generally thought that nano drugs killed gastric cells by damaging the DNA of tumor cells. Instead, this research found that at least this particular nano drug attacked gastric cancer cells by damaging mitochondria.

Finally, Chen et al. [81] prepared nanoparticles that could not only deliver siRNA but were (1) targeted to gastric cancer and had (2) magnetic resonance. These nanoparticles were termed polyethylene glycol-polyethyleneimine-superparamagnetic iron oxide nanoparticles, orscFvCD44v6,-PEG-g-PEI-SPION. In vivo work demonstrated its gastric cancer targeting properties through nuclear magnetic resonance (NMR) as well as immunohistochemistry.

References

1. Ibrahim NK, Samuels B, Page R, Doval D, Patel KM, Rao SC, et al. Multicenter phase II trial of ABI-007, an albumin-bound paclitaxel, in women with metastatic breast cancer. J Clin Oncol. 2005;23(25):6019–26.
2. Nishiyama N. Nanomedicine: nanocarriers shape up for long life. Nat Nanotechnol. 2007;2(4):203–4.
3. Sanhai WR, Sakamoto JH, Canady R, Ferrari M. Seven challenges for nanomedicine. Nat Nanotechnol. 2008;3(5):242–4.
4. Hoffman AS. The origins and evolution of "controlled" drug delivery systems. J Control Release. 2008;132(3):153–63.
5. Matsumura Y. Poly (amino acid) micelle nanocarriers in preclinical and clinical studies. Adv Drug Deliv Rev. 2008;60(8):899–914.
6. Jeong B, Bae YH, Lee DS, Kim SW. Biodegradable block copolymers as injectable drug-delivery systems. Nature. 1997;388(6645):860–2.
7. Tredan O, Galmarini CM, Patel K, Tannock IF. Drug resistance and the solid tumor microenvironment. J Natl Cancer Inst. 2007;99(19):1441–54.
8. Raghunand N, Altbach MI, van Sluis R, Baggett B, Taylor CW, Bhujwalla ZM, et al. Plasmalemmal pH-gradients in drug-sensitive and drug-resistant MCF-7 human breast carcinoma xenografts measured by 31P magnetic resonance spectroscopy. Biochem Pharmacol. 1999;57(3):309–12.
9. Raghunand N, Gillies RJ. pH and drug resistance in tumors. Drug Resis Updat. 2000;3(1):39–47.
10. Netti PA, Berk DA, Swartz MA, Grodzinsky AJ, Jain RK. Role of extracellular matrix assembly in interstitial transport in solid tumors. Cancer Res. 2000;60(9):2497–503.
11. Tannock IF, Lee CM, Tunggal JK, Cowan DS, Egorin MJ. Limited penetration of anticancer drugs through tumor tissue: a potential cause of resistance of solid tumors to chemotherapy. Clin Cancer Res. 2002;8(3):878–84.
12. Minchinton AI, Tannock IF. Drug penetration in solid tumours. Nat Rev Cancer. 2006;6(8):583–92.
13. Gerweck LE, Seetharaman K. Cellular pH gradient in tumor versus normal tissue: potential exploitation for the treatment of cancer. Cancer Res. 1996;56(6):1194–8.
14. Vukovic V, Tannock IF. Influence of low pH on cytotoxicity of paclitaxel, mitoxantrone and topotecan. Br J Cancer. 1997;75(8):1167–72.
15. Raghunand N, Gillies RJ. pH and chemotherapy. Novartis Found Symp. 2001;240:199–211. discussion 265–8
16. Raghunand N, He X, van Sluis R, Mahoney B, Baggett B, Taylor CW, et al. Enhancement of chemotherapy by manipulation of tumour pH. Br J Cancer. 1999;80(7):1005–11.
17. Lee CM, Tannock IF. Inhibition of endosomal sequestration of basic anticancer drugs: influence on cytotoxicity and tissue penetration. Br J Cancer. 2006;94(6):863–9.
18. Rotin D, Wan P, Grinstein S, Tannock I. Cytotoxicity of compounds that interfere with the regulation of intracellular pH: a potential new class of anticancer drugs. Cancer Res. 1987;47(6):1497–504.
19. Hillaireau H, Couvreur P. Nanocarriers' entry into the cell: relevance to drug delivery. Cell Mol Life Sci. 2009;66(17):2873–96.
20. Rosen H, Abribat T. The rise and rise of drug delivery. Nat Rev Drug Discov. 2005;4(5):381–5.
21. Li R, Xie L, Zhu Z, Liu Q, Hu Y, Jiang X, et al. Reversion of pH-induced physiological drug resistance: a novel function of copolymeric nanoparticles. PLoS One. 2011;6(9):e24172.
22. Primeau AJ, Rendon A, Hedley D, Lilge L, Tannock IF. The distribution of the anticancer drug Doxorubicin in relation to blood vessels in solid tumors. Clin Cancer Res. 2005;11(24 Pt 1):8782–8.
23. Brooks S, Takita H, Shin K, Fang Y, Vaughan M, Sharma S, et al. Intratumoral injection of GM-CSF in perspective—a review. J Med. 2003;34(1-6):149–53.
24. Datta M, Via LE, Kamoun WS, Liu C, Chen W, Seano G, et al. Anti-vascular endothelial growth factor treatment normalizes tuberculosis granuloma vasculature and improves small molecule delivery. Proc Natl Acad Sci U S A. 2015;112(6):1827–32.
25. Ma J, Chen CS, Blute T, Waxman DJ. Antiangiogenesis enhances intratumoral drug retention. Cancer Res. 2011;71(7):2675–85.
26. Tolaney SM, Boucher Y, Duda DG, Martin JD, Seano G, Ancukiewicz M, et al. Role of vascular density and normalization in response to neoadjuvant bevacizumab and chemotherapy in breast cancer patients. Proc Natl Acad Sci U S A. 2015;112(46):14325–30.
27. Schaefer L, Reinhardt DP. Special issue: Extracellular matrix: Therapeutic tools and targets in cancer treatment. Adv Drug Deliv Rev. 2016;97:1–3.
28. Choi IK, Strauss R, Richter M, Yun CO, Lieber A. Strategies to increase drug penetration in solid tumors. Front Oncol. 2013;3:193.
29. Ganesh S, Gonzalez-Edick M, Gibbons D, Van Roey M, Jooss K. Intratumoral coadministration of hyaluronidase enzyme and oncolytic adenoviruses enhances virus potency in metastatic tumor models. Clin Cancer Res. 2008;14(12):3933–41.
30. McKee TD, Grandi P, Mok W, Alexandrakis G, Insin N, Zimmer JP, et al. Degradation of fibrillar collagen in a human melanoma xenograft improves the efficacy of an oncolytic herpes simplex virus vector. Cancer Res. 2006;66(5):2509–13.
31. Eikenes L, Tufto I, Schnell EA, Bjorkoy A, De Lange Davies C. Effect of collagenase and hyaluronidase on free and anomalous diffusion in multicellular spheroids and xenografts. Anticancer Res. 2010;30(2): 359–68.
32. Mok W, Boucher Y, Jain RK. Matrix metalloproteinases-1 and -8 improve the distribution and efficacy of an oncolytic virus. Cancer Res. 2007;67(22):10664–8.
33. Ruoslahti E. Tumor penetrating peptides for improved drug delivery. Adv Drug Deliv Rev. 2016. Doi:10.1016/j.addr.2016.03.008.

34. Masood F. Polymeric nanoparticles for targeted drug delivery system for cancer therapy. Mater Sci Eng C Mater Biol Appl. 2016;60:569–78.
35. Cho H, Lai TC, Tomoda K, Kwon GS. Polymeric micelles for multi-drug delivery in cancer. AAPS PharmSciTech. 2015;16(1):10–20.
36. Grinberg S, Linder C, Heldman E. Progress in lipid-based nanoparticles for cancer therapy. Crit Rev Oncog. 2014;19(3-4):247–60.
37. Frazier N, Ghandehari H. Hyperthermia approaches for enhanced delivery of nanomedicines to solid tumors. Biotechnol Bioeng. 2015;112(10):1967–83.
38. Fung LK, Shin M, Tyler B, Brem H, Saltzman WM. Chemotherapeutic drugs released from polymers: distribution of 1,3-bis(2-chloroethyl)-1-nitrosourea in the rat brain. Pharm Res. 1996;13(5):671–82.
39. Sugahara KN, Scodeller P, Braun GB, de Mendoza TH, Yamazaki CM, Kluger MD, et al. A tumor-penetrating peptide enhances circulation-independent targeting of peritoneal carcinomatosis. J Control Release. 2015;212:59–69.
40. Torre LA, Bray F, Siegel RL, Ferlay J, Lortet-Tieulent J, Jemal A. Global cancer statistics, 2012. CA Cancer J Clin. 2015;65(2):33–64. 1
41. Langer K, Balthasar S, Vogel V, Dinauer N, Briesen HV, Schubert D. Optimization of the preparation process for human serum albumin (HSA) nanoparticles. Int J Pharm. 2003;257(1–2):169–80.
42. Dreis S, Rothweiler F, Michaelis M, Cinatl Jr J, Kreuter J, Langer K. Preparation, characterisation and maintenance of drug efficacy of doxorubicin-loaded human serum albumin (HSA) nanoparticles. Int J Pharm. 2007;341(1–2):207–14.
43. Chen L, Chen F, Zhao M, Zhu X, Ke C, Yu J, et al. A redox-sensitive Micelle-Like nanoparticle self-assembled from amphiphilic adriamycin-human serum albumin conjugates for tumor targeted therapy. Biomed Res Int. 2015;2015:1–10.
44. Kloover JS, Bakker MAD, Gelderblom H, Meerbeeck JPV. Fatal outcome of a hypersensitivity reaction to paclitaxel: a critical review of premedication regimens. Br J Cancer. 2004;90(2):304–5.
45. Hamaguchi T, Matsumura Y, Suzuki M, Shimizu K, Goda R, Nakamura I, et al. NK105, a paclitaxel-incorporating micellar nanoparticle formulation, can extend in vivo antitumour activity and reduce the neurotoxicity of paclitaxel. Br J Cancer. 2005;92(7):1240–6.
46. Hamaguchi T, Kato K, Yasui H, Morizane C, Ikeda M, Ueno H, et al. A phase I and pharmacokinetic study of NK105, a paclitaxel-incorporating micellar nanoparticle formulation. Br J Cancer. 2007;597(2–3):266–9.
47. Kato K, Chin K, Yoshikawa T, Yamaguchi K, Tsuji Y, Esaki T, et al. Phase II study of NK105, a paclitaxel-incorporating micellar nanoparticle, for previously treated advanced or recurrent gastric cancer. Investig New Drugs. 2012;30(4):1621–7.
48. Slütter B, Jiskoot W. Dual role of CpG as immune modulator and physical crosslinker in ovalbumin loaded N-trimethyl chitosan (TMC) nanoparticles for nasal vaccination. J Control Release. 2010;148(1):117–21.
49. Song RF, Li XJ, Cheng XL, Fu AR, Wang YH, Feng YJ, et al. Paclitaxel-loaded trimethyl chitosan-based polymeric nanoparticle for the effective treatment of gastroenteric tumors. Oncol Rep. 2014;32(4):1481–8.
50. Jung YD, Kim MS, Shin BA, Chay KO, Ahn BW, Liu W, et al. EGCG, major component of green tea, inhibits tumor growth by inhibiting VEGF production in human colon carcinoma cells. Br J Cancer. 2001;84(6):844–50.
51. Lee IT, Lin CC, Lee CY, Hsieh PW, Yang CM. Protective effects of (−)-epigallocatechin-3-gallate against TNF-α-induced lung inflammation via ROS-dependent ICAM-1 inhibition. J Nutr Biochem. 2013;24(1):124–36.
52. Ihara N, Schmitz S, Kurisawa M, Chung JE, Uyama H, Kobayashi S. Amplification of inhibitory activity of catechin against disease-related enzymes by conjugation on poly(epsilon-lysine). Biomacromolecules. 2004;5(5):1633–6.
53. Shankar S, Ganapathy S, Hingorani SR, Srivastava RK. EGCG inhibits growth, invasion, angiogenesis and metastasis of pancreatic cancer. Front Biosci. 2008;13(4):440–52.
54. Tipoe GL, Leung TM, Hung MW, Fung ML. Green tea polyphenols as an anti-oxidant and anti-inflammatory agent for cardiovascular protection. Cardiovasc Hematol Disord Drug Targets. 2007;7(2):135–44.
55. Lin YH, Chen ZR, Lai CH, Hsieh CH, Feng CL. Active targeted nanoparticles for oral administration of gastric cancer therapy. Biomacromolecules. 2015;16(9):3021–32.
56. Zhao D, Zhuo RX, Cheng SX. Modification of calcium carbonate based gene and drug delivery systems by a cell-penetrating peptide. Mol BioSyst. 2012;8(12):3288–94.
57. He XW, Liu T, Chen YX, Cheng DJ, Li XR, Xiao Y, et al. Calcium carbonate nanoparticle delivering vascular endothelial growth factor-C siRNA effectively inhibits lymphangiogenesis and growth of gastric cancer in vivo. Cancer Gene Ther. 2008;15(3):193–202.
58. Singh M, Chandrasekaran N, Mukherjee A, Kumar M, Kumaraguru AK. Cancerous cell targeting and destruction using pH stabilized amperometric bioconjugated gold nanoparticles from marine macroalgae. Bioprocess Biosyst Eng. 2014;37(9):1–11.
59. Klein G, Vellenga E, Fraaije MW, Kamps WA, de Bont ES. The possible role of matrix metalloproteinase (MMP)-2 and MMP-9 in cancer, e.g. acute leukemia. Crit Rev Oncol Hematol. 2004;50(2):87–100.
60. Bergers G, Brekken R, McMahon G, Vu TH, Itoh T, Tamaki K, et al. Matrix metalloproteinase-9 triggers the angiogenic switch during carcinogenesis. Nat Cell Biol. 2000;2(10):737–44.
61. Coussens LM, Tinkle CL, Hanahan D, Werb Z. MMP-9 supplied by bone marrow–derived cells contributes to skin carcinogenesis. Cell. 2000;103(3):481–90.
62. Deryugina EI, Luo GX, Reisfeld RA, Bourdon MA, Strongin A. Tumor cell invasion through matrigel is

regulated by activated matrix metalloproteinase-2. Anticancer Res. 1900;17(5A):3201–10.
63. Hua J, Muschel RJ. Inhibition of matrix metalloproteinase 9 expression by a ribozyme blocks metastasis in a rat sarcoma model system. Cancer Res. 1996;56(22):5279–84.
64. Mcquibban GA, Butler GS, Gong JH, Bendall L, Power C, Clark-Lewis I, et al. Matrix metalloproteinase activity inactivates the CXC chemokine stromal cell-derived factor-1. J Biol Chem. 2001;276(47):43503–8.
65. Nguyen DX, Bos PD, Massagué J. Metastasis: from dissemination to organ-specific colonization. Nat Rev Cancer. 2009;9(4):274–84.
66. Psaila B, Lyden D. The metastatic niche: adapting the foreign soil. Nat Rev Cancer. 2009;9(4):285–93.
67. Liu Q, Li RT, Qian HQ, Wei J, Xie L, Shen J, et al. Targeted delivery of miR-200c/DOC to inhibit cancer stem cells and cancer cells by the gelatinases-stimuli nanoparticles. Biomaterials. 2013;34(29):7191–203.
68. Li R, Wu W, Liu Q, Wu P, Xie L, Zhu Z, et al. Intelligently targeted drug delivery and enhanced antitumor effect by gelatinase-responsive nanoparticles. PLoS One. 2013;8(7):e69643.
69. Cui FB, Liu Q, Li RT, Shen J, Wu PY, Yu LX, et al. Enhancement of radiotherapy efficacy by miR-200c-loaded gelatinase-stimuli PEG-Pep-PCL nanoparticles in gastric cancer cells. Int J Nanomedicine. 2014;9(1):2345–58.
70. Cui FB, Li RT, Liu Q, Wu PY, Hu WJ, Yue GF, et al. Enhancement of radiotherapy efficacy by docetaxel-loaded gelatinase-stimuli PEG-Pep-PCL nanoparticles in gastric cancer. Cancer Lett. 2014;346(1):53–62.
71. Wu FL, Li RT, Yang M, Yue GF, Wang HY, Liu Q, et al. Gelatinases-stimuli nanoparticles encapsulating 5-fluorouridine and 5-aza-2′-deoxycytidine enhance the sensitivity of gastric cancer cells to chemical therapeutics. Cancer Lett. 2015;363(1):7–16.
72. Inoue S, Tanaka K, Arisaka F, Kimura S, Ohtomo K, Mizuno S. Silk fibroin of *Bombyx mori* is secreted, assembling a high molecular mass elementary unit consisting of H-chain, L-chain, and P25, with a 6:6:1 molar ratio. J Biol Chem. 2000;275(51):40517–28.
73. Wu P, Liu Q, Li R, Wang J, Zhen X, Yue G, et al. Facile preparation of paclitaxel loaded silk fibroin nanoparticles for enhanced antitumor efficacy by locoregional drug delivery. ACS Appl Mater Interfaces. 2013;5(23):12638–45.
74. Jain R, Dandekar P, Patravale V. Diagnostic nanocarriers for sentinel lymph node imaging. J Control Release. 2009;138(2):90–102.
75. Lim JS, Choi J, Song J, Yong EC, Lim SJ, Sang KL, et al. Nanoscale iodized oil emulsion: a useful tracer for pretreatment sentinel node detection using CT lymphography in a normal canine gastric model. Surg Endosc. 2012;26(8):2267–74.
76. Sarbolouki MN, Sadeghizadeh M, Yaghoobi MM, Karami A, Lohrasbi T. Dendrosomes: a novel family of vehicles for transfection and therapy. J Chem Technol Biotechnol. 2000;75(75):919–22.
77. Aas Z, Babaei E, Hosseinpour Feizi MA, Dehghan G. Anti-proliferative and apoptotic effects of Dendrosomal Farnesiferol C on gastric cancer cells. Asian Pac J Cancer Prev. 2014;16(13):5325–9.
78. Chen L, Bao CC, Yang H, Li D, Lei C, Wang T, et al. A prototype of giant magnetoimpedance-based biosensing system for targeted detection of gastric cancer cells. Biosens Bioelectron. 2011;26(7):3246–53.
79. Kan W, Jing R, Qian Q, Hua S, Bao C, Zhang X, et al. BRCAA1 monoclonal antibody conjugated fluorescent magnetic nanoparticles for in vivo targeted magnetofluorescent imaging of gastric cancer. J Nanobiotechnology. 2011;9(1):23.
80. Liu X, Deng X, Li X, Xue D, Zhang H, Liu T, et al. A visualized investigation at the atomic scale of the antitumor effect of magnetic nanomedicine on gastric cancer cells. Nanomedicine. 2016;9(9):1389–402.
81. Chen Y, Wang W, Lian G, Qian C, Wang L, Zeng L, et al. Development of an MRI-visible nonviral vector for siRNA delivery targeting gastric cancer. Int J Nanomedicine. 2012;7(9):359–68.

Local Drug Delivery Strategies for Gastric Cancer Treatment

15

Qin Liu and Baorui Liu

15.1 The Clinical Need for Localized Gastric Cancer Therapy

Gastric cancer is associated with poor patient prognosis and, as a result, is the leading cause of cancer-related death worldwide [1]. Systemic chemotherapy is the major treatment for locally advanced and metastatic gastric cancer, despite the fact that satisfactory clinical outcomes have not been reached with this approach. As such, exploring more effective modalities for gastric cancer management is necessary. Increasing evidence has shown that the most advanced gastric cancer patients ultimately die from local recurrence or metastasis. To this end, it has been reported that positive peritoneal washing cytology is a negative prognostic factor in patients with gastric cancer [2]. According to a phase II study, the 1-year survival rate after receiving treatment with modified FOLFOX-4 for 48 gastric cancer patients with malignant ascites was 27.2% [3]. Many advanced gastric cancer patients have died from local metastasis, especially peritoneum metastasis. Additionally, intraperitoneal chemotherapy has been proven to improve survival rates as well as decrease peritoneal recurrence in gastric cancer patients with peritoneal dissemination [4, 5].

Both systemic and local administrations of nanoparticles (NPs) have been shown to increase the sensitivity and effectiveness of gastric cancer management. Typically, NPs accumulate at the targeted solid tumor(s), either by passive diffusion via an enhanced permeability and retention (EPR) effect or through an active targeting moiety. Of these, actively targeted NPs are superior to those that are passively targeted NPs. This is due to their conjugation to the ligand of tumor cells overexpressed and/or a unique marker such as folic acid, a monoclonal antibody, and/or transferrin. These environment-responsive nanocarriers are then triggered to release the loaded drugs in response to tumor cell differences in pH and/or temperature. Generally, the ability of the nanomaterial to accumulate at the tumor site is the primary driving force behind the selected therapeutic drug concentrations, particularly for intravenous administration. That being said, the reticuloendothelial system can take up and remove most drug-loaded nanoparticles when given intravenously. Larger amounts of therapeutic drugs can also accumulate within several normal organs, especially the liver, spleen, and kidney. This limits the amount of drug that can actually accumulate at the tumoral sites. As

Q. Liu (✉) • B. Liu
The Comprehensive Cancer Center of Drum-Tower Hospital, Medical School of Nanjing University & Clinical Cancer Institute of Nanjing University, Zhongshan Road 321, Nanjing 210008, People's Republic of China
e-mail: liuqinxh@126.com

J. Wei, B. Liu (eds.), *Personalized Management of Gastric Cancer*, DOI 10.1007/978-981-10-3978-2_15

such, it is difficult to achieve sufficient chemotherapeutic drug concentrations within the targeted sites. Furthermore, satisfactory antitumor effects and reduced side effects are difficult to achieve due to the drug distribution and bioavailability. For example, when given intravenously, nearly 50% of paclitaxel is removed from the body 24 h post-administration with only 0.5% of the drug capable of accumulating at the targeted tumor. Importantly, intraperitoneal delivery of docetaxel has a pharmacokinetic advantage hundreds of times higher than when it is given intravenously [5].

The local administration of drug-loaded carriers is superior to systemic delivery in the following aspects: [1] easy loading of water-insoluble drugs and high loading efficiencies; [2] maintaining high local drug concentrations and allowing for controlled drug release; [3] prolonging drug retention and uptake into cancer cells; [4] decreasing administration times, thus improving patients' convenience; and [5] reducing side effects due to the less drug distribution in nontargeted organs. After intravenous administration, a large percentage of drug-loaded nanoparticles are taken up by several healthy organs, such as the liver, spleen, and kidney. Afterwards, only a small amount of drug will be distributed to the tumor site(s) themselves. However, the EPR effect can significantly influence the distribution of nanomedicine deposition in tumors and normal organs. Several other factors can influence the antitumor efficacy of nanodrugs, such as their inherent characteristics including size, shape, surface charge, hydrophilicity, and targeting functionality. The tumor microenvironment can also contribute to treatment toxicity and influence tumor blood vessels, interstitium penetration, and retention time at the site.

In order to minimize the systemic side effects posed by such drugs, it is necessary to allow for local delivery of the chemodrug. A series of studies have examined this issue, showing that such local delivery of drug carriers is highly effective at controlling recurrence or metastatic tumor growth in various local tumor recurrent animal models.

15.2 Intraperitoneal (IP) Delivery of Therapeutic Agents

Advanced gastric cancer patients usually die from peritoneal metastasis, which itself has a reported association with poorer patient prognosis. Given this, it is a pressing concern that systemic chemotherapy has only limited effectiveness on the control of gastric cancer metastasis. With this concern, intraperitoneal (IP) chemotherapy has emerged as a promising drug delivery approach, as it achieves high local drug concentrations for an extended period of time. Moreover, its route of delivery minimizes systemic exposure. Taxanes have a large molecular weight and high fat solubility. Noticeably, taxanes are absorbed through the openings of the lymphatic system, which are important locations for peritoneal dissemination formation. Given its promise for use in drug delivery, IP injections have been widely used in a variety of cancers. For instance, IP paclitaxel significantly increased local drug concentration 1000 times that than of systemic administration. For this reason, NCCN recommends that patients with metastatic cancer should receive intraperitoneal chemotherapy.

The peritoneal barrier includes blood capillary endothelium and cellular-interstitial matrix. Collectively, these barriers provide the major form of physical resistance to drug penetration. Several recent studies have confirmed that both the interstitium and capillary endothelium are major barriers in peritoneal carcinoma patients undergoing partial or total peritonectomy. Flessner et al. [6] explored peritoneal transport physiology in detail (Fig. 15.1). The residence time in the peritoneal cavity for systemically injected, small-molecular-weight agents is too short to allow for absorption through the peritoneal capillaries [7]. Therefore, this drug delivery approach does not allow for high or long-lasting therapeutic agent concentration at the targeted sites [8]. Thus, there has been a global research push to develop new techniques to overcome these biological limitations to yield efficient therapeutic results.

Keeping high and long-lasting local drug concentration is necessary for successful and efficient IP therapy [7]. Drugs with a small molecular weight (<20 kDa) enter circulation through peritoneal capillary absorption. The drug is then quickly removed

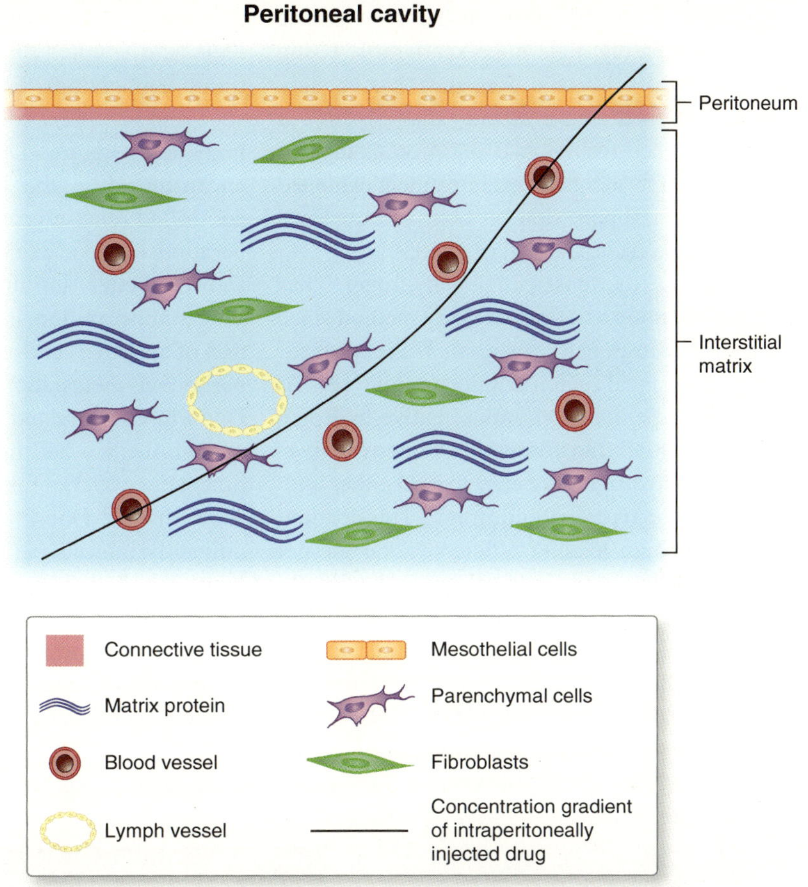

Fig. 15.1 The blood capillary endothelium and the cellular-interstitial matrix are major barriers to efficient drug transport. When compared with the mesothelium, the interstitium and capillary barriers play greater roles in possessing insignificant barrier properties (Adapted from Intraperitoneal delivery of nanoparticles for cancer gene therapy (2013), Hallaj-Nezhadi S et al. [6])

from circulation, and its residence time in the peritoneal cavity is not sufficient to get either high or long-lasting drug concentrations. In order to get satisfactory cytotoxicity, frequent or continuous dosing is required. However, this increased frequency can lead to catheter-related problems, increased risk of infection, and bowel complications in patients. Small molecular weight drugs do show systemic circulation. Pharmacokinetic studies in animals have shown that IP taxane (docetaxel or paclitaxel) was quickly cleared within 24 h from the peritoneal cavity. In addition, many free drugs are usually coupled with severe side effects. For example, Cremophor EL (Cr-EL) and dehydrated ethanol are usually used to increase paclitaxel solubility to get solvent-based PTX (Sb-PTX: Taxol®). Due to the large amount of Cr-EL added as well as the nonspecific drug biodistribution in other healthy organs, Sb-PTX has been reported to have moderated antitumor efficacy and severe side effects including hypersensitivity reactions, bone marrow suppression, and neurotoxicity.

With this in mind, nanoparticle albumin-bound paclitaxel (nab-paclitaxel, Abraxane®) [9] has been designed to address the aforementioned problems. Since it is an albumin-bound, 130-nm particle, neither ethanol nor Cr-EL is required. In animal models, Abraxane exhibited superior antitumor advantages and a more favorable safety profile when compared to free PTX. In the clinic, a randomized Phase II study investigated the overall response and the disease control rates for unresectable or recurrent gastric cancer patients treated with nab-paclitaxel. Results indicated responses of 27.8% and 59.3%, respectively [10]. Interestingly, one patient had a response rate of 100%. The median progression-free survival was 2.9 months, and overall survival time was 9.2 months. Recently, Kinoshita et al. [11] evaluated the therapeutic efficacy of nab-paclitaxel and free drug Sb-PTX on gastric cancer cell-bearing nude mice xenografts. Using this peritoneal metastatic xenograft model, nab-paclitaxel showed greater efficacy than Sb-PTX at equal doses when given as an IP injection. Compared with IP Sb-PTX, nab-paclitaxel treatment exhibited a better tumor suppression on both subcutaneous tumor size and ascites burden ($p < 0.05$).

Recently, thermosensitive hydrogel has attracted attention as a drug delivery method since it is a stimuli-responsive material. This is particularly true for local region administration [12]. At specified temperatures, thermosensitive hydrogel undergo a sol-gel transformation. Moreover, thermosensitive hydrogels are easy to load either with hydrophilic or hydrophobic drugs. This loading occurs with high loading efficiency, and the gel allows for controlled drug release behavior. In addition, thermosensitive hydrogels are easily acceptable to patients because they exist in one state when the temperature is lower than the sol-gel transition temperature [13] (Fig. 15.2).

In order to treat peritoneal dissemination of gastric cancer, Bae et al. [14] prepared a thermo-responsive hydrogel based on poloxamer and linoleic acid-coupled Pluronic F127 (Plu-CLA). At room temperature, Plu-CLA exists in a liquid state, but is rapidly converted to a gelatin state at body temperature. Docetaxel was successfully encapsulated in the Plu-CLA and exhibited a controlled release profile. Intraperitoneal administration of docetaxel-Plu-CLA (Doc-Plu-CLA) showed better antitumor advantages than free drug administration, as evidenced through induction of apoptosis and a reduction in the number of peritoneal metastatic nodules. In addition, the Doc-Plu-CLA-treated peritoneal gastric cancer xenograft mice had the longest median survival time (Fig. 15.3). Taken together, these results show that IP Doc-Plu-CLA administration significantly inhibits peritoneal metastasis and prolongs survival in a xenograft mouse model of gastric cancer.

As a local treatment option, photodynamic therapy (PDT) consists of activating a photosensitizing agent using a specific laser wavelength [15]. Since photosensitizing agents allow for accumulation specifically at tumor sites, PDT

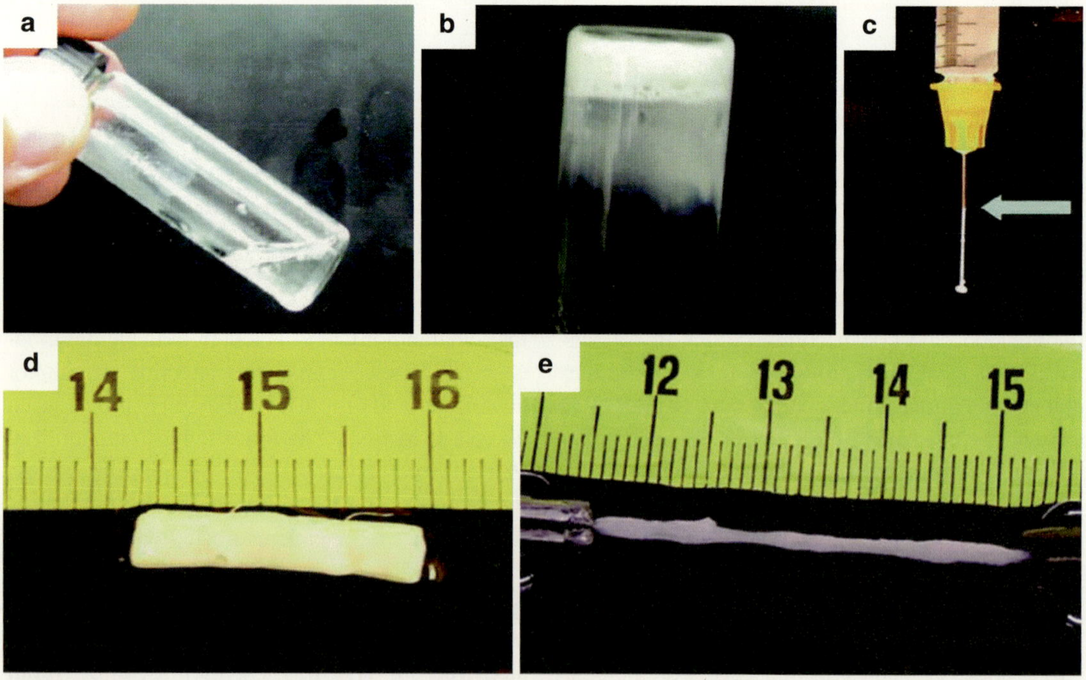

Fig. 15.2 (**a**) Thermosensitive gel is liquid at 4 °C. (**b**) Gelation at 37 °C. (**c**) Thermosensitive gel is easily injectable through a 26-gauge needle. (**d–e**) Thermosensitive gel is flexible at 37 °C. Reproduced with permission from Ref. [13]

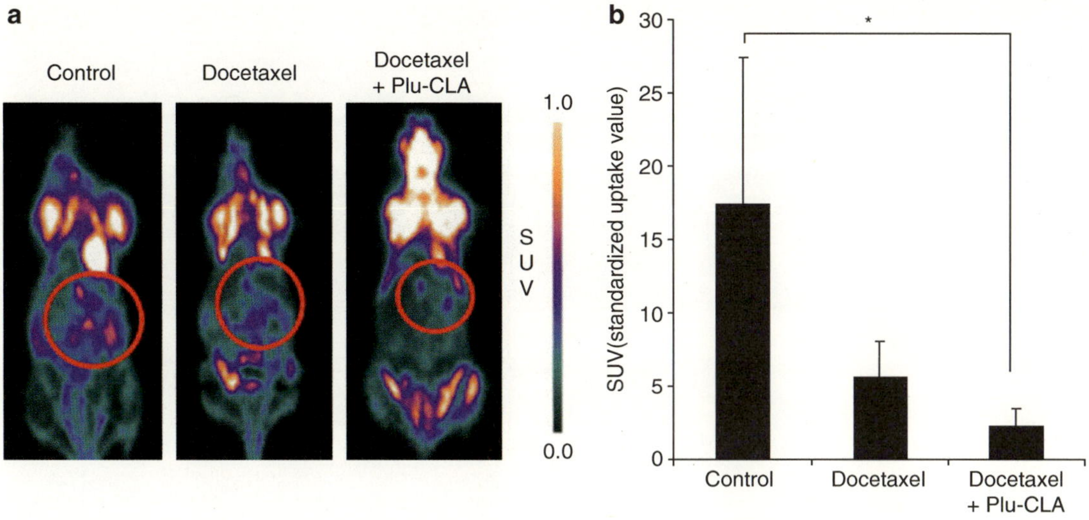

Fig. 15.3 ^{18}F-FDG PET image of mice with peritoneal metastases. (**a**) Tumoral ^{18}F-FDG uptake (*circle*) based on microPET images. (**b**) Comparison of ^{18}F-FDG SUV uptake in the control, docetaxel- and Doc-Plu-CLA-treated groups. *$p < 0.05$. Reproduced with permission from Ref. [14]

showed fewer side effects and reduced damage to normal tissue. When compared with either radiation or chemotherapy, PDT also rarely induced drug resistance. Due to the above advantages, PDT has been widely used to treat gastric, breast, and lung cancers, among other diseases. Tsujimoto et al. [16] prepared indocyanine green (ICG) derivatives-loaded nanoparticles and ICG-loaded lactosomes (ICGm) in order to investigate their PDT theranostic value in the mice model of experimental peritoneal dissemination of gastric cancer. After photodynamic therapy, the median survival time in ICGm- and ICG-treated mice was 32 days and 17 days, respectively. Moreover, body weight loss in ICG-treated group was significantly greater than that in ICGm-treated mice ($p < 0.05$). This result was taken as an indication of the safety of ICGm treatment.

15.3 Intratumoral Delivery of Therapeutic Agents

Local intratumoral delivery of chemotherapeutic agents is likely to provide better drug localization within the targeted tumor, thereby reducing systemic exposure to healthy organs. This would lead to increased efficacy and lower toxicity than treatment with aqueous, free drug solutions. To this end, Al-Abd et al. [17] prepared an injectable, thermosensitive hydrogel to deliver the anticancer drug doxorubicin (DOX). During their experiment, 0.6% of DOX was loaded into a 10% reversible thermal poly(organophosphazene) (PPZ) hydrogel that was capable of body temperature-dependent transformation. An in vitro release study showed that a initial burst drug release in the first few hours after administration. However, DOX was released in vivo in a controlled and sustained manner over a 5-week period. The hydrogel mass was not completely degraded over 7 weeks (Fig. 15.4). It should be noted that an initial burst effect is beneficial for fast control over tumor growth, with the subsequent sustained release ensuring long-lasting tumor control. The PPZ hydrogel was then given intratumorally in a human gastric tumor xenograft mice model. In this case, the tumor T1/T2 for locally and systemically administered DOX was 2.6 days to 4.6 days, respectively, showing successful increase in local drug retention. Moreover, the data suggest that the hydrogel decreased systemic exposure and cardiac toxicity. The longer tumor DOX exposure levels obtained in the hydrogel delivery system mean better antitumor

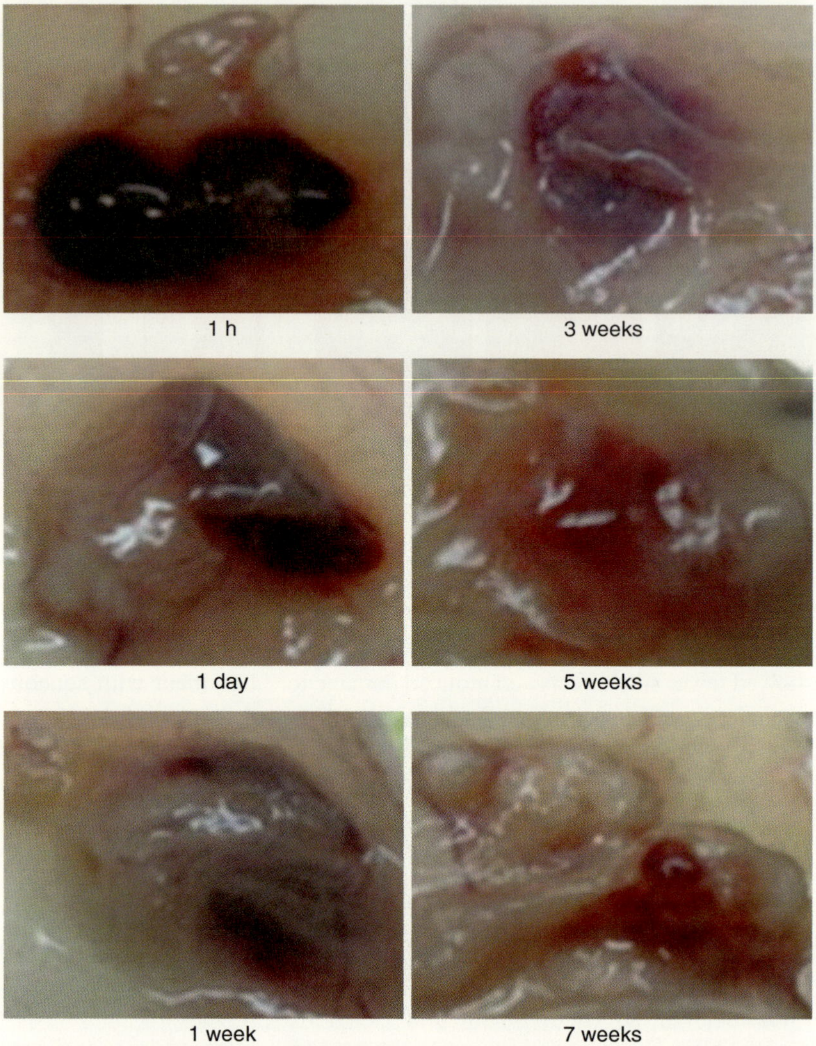

Fig. 15.4 DOX-loaded hydrogel contacted the tumor as a mass with a well-defined margin. Reproduced with permission from Ref. [17]

efficacy. After a single intratumoral administration, the DOX hydrogel formulation controlled gastric cancer size for up to 49 days without significant signs of toxicity.

Combination chemotherapy has become an important option for advanced gastric cancer treatment. Coadministration of DOX and PTX formulations using PPZ thermosensitive hydrogel has been assessed for the in vivo antitumor efficacy in local tumor management in human gastric cancer cell-xenografted mice [18]. Following intratumoral injection of PPZ into human SNU-601 gastric cancer cell-bearing mice, the combined DOX (15 mg/kg) and PTX (30 mg/kg) containing hydrogel resulted in the highest tumor inhibition in the tested experimental groups. The PTX-DOX hydrogel was injected intratumorally and gelated within the tumor site. PPZ hydrogel treatment exhibited no drug-related adverse effects and no mortality for 97 days. In comparison, the mortality rates in the PTX-DOX solution intratumoral and intravenous groups are 5/8 and 4/9, respectively. These results demonstrate that sustained release of a combined DOX and PTX treatment yielded a reduction in drug-induced toxicity.

Liposomes have been reported to successfully delivery a wide range of drugs. A large amount of evidence has shown that drug-loaded liposomes are more advantageous than free drug in regard to cytotoxic and safety considerations. To this end, the antitumor effects of intratumoral docetaxel-loaded immuno-(trastuzumab)-liposomes (IDL) were evaluated in a local, clinical application of trastuzumab against NCI-N87 Her2/neu-overexpressing gastric cancer xenograft mouse model [19]. In this study, the liposome diameter was approximately 100 nm, as it has been reported that this size is more favorable for tumor uptake and retention time [20]. They also suggested that smaller liposomes may have greater surface-to-surface contact with the cell membrane. The NCI-N87 gastric cancer xenograft mice were treated with either IDL or docetaxel-loaded liposomes. When compared with docetaxel treatment alone, docetaxel-loaded liposomes, or the combined docetaxel/trastuzumab treatment, the intratumoral IDL-treated group exhibited higher drug concentration at the tumor site. Moreover, this treatment group also had far better antitumor efficacy in the N87 xenograft model. Intratumoral administration of either free trastuzumab or IDL significantly suppressed tumor cell growth without evidence of severe side effects. According to their study, intratumoral IDL administration resulted in a high docetaxel concentration in the tumor region and has great potential for use as a safe and effective local cancer therapy. It was also noted that the liposome delivery formations prolonged therapeutic retention time. Collectively, the docetaxel-loaded liposomes conjugated with trastuzumab exhibited several antitumor advantages, including [1] prolonged liposome-docetaxel retention time within tumor sites and [2] liposome promote trastuzumab to accumulation in tumors with no sign of decline. Furthermore nanoparticle formations could decrease the severe skin ulcerations resulting from docetaxel treatment. In this study, percutaneous injection of free docetaxel into the tumor sites resulted in severe skin ulceration in one-third (2/6) of mice. On the contrary, treatment with either DL or IDL did not result in any skin ulcerations. Thus, it is shown that docetaxel-loaded liposome formations may reduce the occurrence rate and severity of normal docetaxel side effects.

Nanoparticles have been explored to deliver their payloads at the local tumoral site and minimize systemic exposure. Previously, we prepared the paclitaxel (PTX) and berbamine (BA) co-deliver nanoparticles using methoxy poly (ethylene glycol)-polycaprolactone (mPEG-PCL) to [21]. This formulation allowed for both high encapsulation efficiency and controlled release at the tumor site. Intratumoral administration showed that when compared to free drug administration, PTX/BA-NP exhibited superior antitumor effects when delivered intratumorally in a human gastric cancer mouse model. This was evidenced by inhibition of tumor growth.

In addition to "passively" targeted nanocarriers, more and more "actively" targeted nanomedicines have been developed to improve therapeutic properties. Among them, stimulus-responsive drug delivery systems have significant benefits. These delivery systems are triggered upon exposure to a specific environmental condition, such as temperature, magnetic field, presence of tumor matrix metalloproteinases (MMPs), or low pH. Such stimulus-responsive nanomedicines accumulate within tumors via EPR effects, are transformed, and release their payloads under the influence of external impacts or conditions of the tumor microenvironment. Such a triggering mechanism might overcome transport barriers, decrease drug resistance, and allow for more controlled drug release. MMPs are highly expressed in various types of tumor tissues and play an important role in tumor invasion, metastasis, cancer stem cells, and drug resistance. The conjugation of polyethylene glycol (PEG) to nanoparticles, polymeric micelles, or liposomes can improve biocompatibility and prolong their time in blood circulation. However, it has been shown that PEGylation severely reduces their cellular uptake. To overcome this limitation, Park et al. developed a PEG-peptide-quantum dot (QD) that contained an MMP-2 cleavable peptide sequence. With this formulation, they showed that tumoral enzymatic dePEGylation effects improved intracellular drug delivery.

In a separate study, an antigen-binding fragment of an anti-MMP antibody was conjugated to doxorubicin-loaded liposomes via a PEG spacer. This approach showed enhanced tumor cell uptake and greater suppression of tumor growth in a cancer mouse model. In our previous studies, we have successfully synthesized PEG-PCL nanoparticles containing gelatinase-sensitive peptide. In the gelatinase (MMP2/9)-rich environment presented by gastric cancer tissue, nanoparticles have been shown to accumulate in both a targeted and effective manner. Moreover, nanoparticles provide a preferable platform for the co-delivery of different hydrophilic/hydrophobic agents including chemotherapeutics, nucleic acids, and small molecules of anti-gastric cancer activities, such as docetaxel [22], miR-200c [23], salinomycin, 5-aza-2'-deoxycytidine, and tetrandrine. Consequently, this kind of nanoparticles may also be used as a platform for local and regional delivery of therapeutic agents for the goal of tumor inhibition. We have also used this intelligent carrier to deliver a traditional medicine monomer evodiamine (EVO) [24]. These EVO-NPs were then intratumorally injected into tumor-bearing mice. Subsequent in vitro cellular uptake studies revealed gelatinase-stimuli nanoparticles could more easily enter the cytoplasm due to their hydrophobicity. Moreover, real-time in vivo nanoparticle biodistribution demonstrated that intelligent EVO-NPs could both efficiently accumulate and retain in the local tumor regions. Therefore, EVO-NPs showed higher tumor suppression and reduced side effects when compared to freely administered EVO ($p < 0.01$).

15.4 Peritumoral Delivery of Therapeutic Agents

Despite these advances, limitations still exist in achieving optimal intratumoral administration. For instance, it is difficult for drug-loaded nanoparticles to penetrate deep into the tumor mass and exert their growth inhibitory effects on cancer cells that are distant from the injection site. Tumor-induced lymphangiogenesis is directly correlated with tumor metastasis and progression. It has been found that peritumoral lymphatic vessel density (P-LVD) plays an important role in lymph node metastasis, while intratumoral lymphatic vessel density (I-LVD) is more associated with the depth of tumor invasion. Although P-LVD and I-LVD both contribute to gastric cancer progression and prognosis, peritumoral administration is superior to intratumoral injection [25]. This is because there is great improvement in the diffusion of the loaded drug throughout the tumor, resulting in improved tumor growth inhibition. Peritumoral administration is characterized by prolonged tumor exposure, enhanced drug concentration, and reduced systemic toxicity. Li et al. [26] developed a physically cross-linked gelatin hydrogel to encapsulate co-delivery of paclitaxel (PTX) and tetrandrine (TET) mPEG-PCL nanoparticles (P/T-NPs). This prepared nanoparticle/gelatin system (P/T-NPs-Gelatin) was locally implanted on the tumor site to allow for continuous drug release. Results showed that implanting P/T-NPs-Gelatin on the tumor surface led to a gradual melting at body temperature into a viscous sol. Gelatin has a phase shift that is below body temperature, but above its melting temperature. The phase of gelatin hydrogel shifts from solid to liquid as the temperature increases. Directly implanting the gel onto the tumor will greatly increase the contact area between the gel and the tumor, thereby accelerating the diffusion and penetration of the drug-loaded nanoparticles inside the tumor through tumor vessels. Their results showed the controlled release of drug-loaded nanoparticles from the gelatin during the melting process contributed most to the sustained loaded drug release and enabled continuous exposure of the tumor to the encapsulated drugs.

Previously, we reported a natural polymer novel silk fibroin (SF) nanoparticle for paclitaxel (PTX) delivery without adding any toxic organic solvents and surfactants [27]. The PTX-loaded silk fibroin nanoparticles (PTX-SF-NPs) had a 130-nm diameter and were efficiently taken up by human gastric cancer cells. An in vivo antitumor study showed that when compared to systemic administration, peritumoral delivery of PTX-SF-NPs [1] more effectively suppressed tumor growth and [2] decreased tumor weight in a gastric cancer

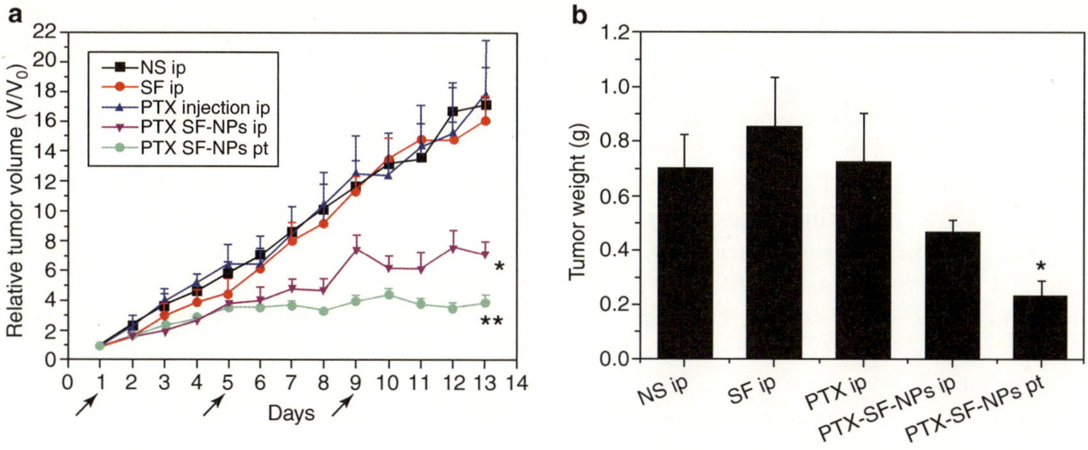

Fig. 15.5 (**a**) Relative tumor volumes for intraperitoneal (IP) PTX, intraperitoneal PTX-SF-NPs, and peritumoral (PT) injection of PTX-SF-NPs in a human gastric cancer xenograft mouse model (PTX concentration, 10 mg/kg). $*p < 0.05$, $**p < 0.01$. (**b**) Tumor weights in the group receiving IP PTX, IP PTX-SF-NPs, and PT on day 14 after administration of the first dose. $*p < 0.05$ when compared with PTX injection and PTX-SF-NPs IP groups. Reproduced with permission from Ref. [27]

nude mice xenograft model (Fig. 15.5). Furthermore, subsequent organ pathological examination clearly demonstrated that there were no obvious toxic side effects in the PTX-SF-NPs-treated groups, indicating the safety of in vivo nanoparticle use. Our results indicated that a peritumoral silk fibroin-based drug delivery system provides a promising strategy for reducing current treatment side effects and leading to overall improvements in future clinical cancer therapies.

15.5 Drug Penetration Concerns

Local administration of a nanoparticle-based delivery system results in high drug concentrations and retention times at the tumor site. The clinical benefits of intraperitoneal chemotherapy in advanced stage cancer patients were verified in work that showed local regional chemotherapy improved their clinical outcomes. However, chemotherapeutic efficacy also depends on the accessibility and retention of the delivered drug to tumor tissue. To this end, Saltzman et al. [28] studied the pharmacokinetic and tissue distribution of local polymer implants in the rat brain. They showed that at the end of the first day, therapeutic agent penetration was 5 mm from the site of implantation. From days 3 to 14, therapeutic penetration was reduced to 1 mm. According to rapid in vitro release kinetics, 84% of the drug was cumulatively released from this delivery system during the first 24 h. In the first few days after implantation, the penetration distance of the polymeric drug was reduced since the drug diffusion gradient was significantly diminished. It is possible that intraoperative administration could cause acute injury and enhance drug penetration via convection of interstitial fluid. This phenomenon might also be the reason for the rapid drug elimination seen after day 3. It should be noted that the authors did not take into account the effect of interstitial fluid convection to tissue penetration.

After reaching the target site, the cell membrane is an additional barrier to cross in order for efficient delivery of the loaded drug in nanodrug delivery systems (NDDSs) into specific organelles within the cytoplasm of cancer cells. Various strategies have been tried to stabilize lysosomal membrane and prevent lysosomes, such as targeting ligands, antibodies, as well as cell-penetrating peptides (CPPs). Suitable nanoparticle size also influences the penetration property of nanomedicines and affects their cellular uptake. It was found that 30-nm nanoparticles could more easily extravasate and penetrate into tumor tissue when compared with lager size nanoparticles. Moreover, the penetration advantages of smaller nanoparticles exhibited distinct therapeutic effects.

Cell-penetrating peptides (CPPs) have been shown to help polymeric nanoparticles permeate cellular membranes and internalize into cancer cells. For instance, TATP, as a PEGylated CPPs, has been used to modify liposomes. The prepared micelles could be efficiently taken up by cancer cells and provided for high transfection productivity in cell nuclei. As a result, TATP improved cytoplasmic drug levels and overcame drug resistance in tumor-bearing mice.

Finally, iRGD is a tumor-specific penetrating peptide that can significantly enhance IP doxorubicin penetration into disseminated peritoneal tumor nodules in mice [29]. Intraperitoneally, coadministration of iRGD and doxorubicin specifically labeled suppressed peritoneal metastases in a mouse model. Importantly, iRGD improved intratumoral dextran and doxorubicin concentrations up to 3 and 2.5 times, respectively. When compared with administration of just intraperitoneal doxorubicin, a combination of iRGD and doxorubicin treatment significantly inhibited the growth of peritoneal metastatic tumors and reduced systemic drug toxicity. According to their study, intraperitoneal iRGD and nanodrugs were a simple and effective strategy to improve the IP therapeutic index and reduce systemic cytotoxicity for peritoneal carcinomatosis.

15.6 Future Prospects

Many cancer patients, particularly those suffering from gastric and lung cancers, die from locoregional recurrence. In order to enhance antitumor efficacy and reduce the severe side effects with systemic chemotherapy, localized delivery has been used to achieve high intratumoral drug distribution and cellular uptake in order to prevent such local recurrence. In most cases, localized chemotherapy is usually used as a supplement to surgery and/or radiotherapy and has been shown to play an important part in controlling disease progression, improving curative effects, and lowering patient morbidity due to disseminated metastatic disease. Compared with systemic chemotherapy, local delivery can sterilize the local, higher drug concentration to reduce the incidence of locoregional tumor recurrence.

However, there are also limitations with drug delivery systems that are based on local strategies. First, most studies are preclinical or in vitro, which currently restricts our understanding of their clinical applications. Second, the role of local chemotherapy in preventing locoregional or distal metastasis is still unclear. It is both desirable and difficult to eliminate all residual malignant tumor cells. Once a single residual cancer cell enters systemic circulation, distal metastasis forms and becomes an immediate life-threatening condition. This scenario has been reported in many gastric patients, and many of those at an advanced stage have died of distal metastasis. In this situation, local therapy is likely to be ineffective in prolonging a patient's life and at preventing the formation of secondary tumor. Therefore, more work is needed to explore the role of local treatment in preventing metastasis due to the suppression of primary tumors. Third, a large proportion of the studies were derived from similar studies about breast, lung, and colorectal cancers. Studies based on the clinical characteristics of gastric cancer are comparatively few.

A locoregional drug delivery system for gastric cancer treatment can reduce systemic drug exposure of normal organs and provide high drug concentration at the tumor site. To further promote the development of polymer-based delivery systems in the local treatment of gastric cancer, more in-depth studies and increased interdisciplinary collaboration will be required. It is believed that more intelligent local delivery systems will be extremely beneficial to extending patients' lives, improving the convenience of treatment, and reducing the systemic toxicity of treatment.

References

1. Wadhwa R, Song S, Lee JS, Yao Y, Wei Q, Ajani JA. Gastric cancer-molecular and clinical dimensions. Nat Rev Clin Oncol. 2013;10(11):643–55.
2. Lee SD, Ryu KW, Eom BW, Lee JH, Kook MC, Kim YW. Prognostic significance of peritoneal washing

cytology in patients with gastric cancer. Br J Surg. 2012;99(3):397–403.
3. Oh SY, Kwon HC, Lee S, Lee DM, Yoo HS, Kim SH, Jang JS, Kim MC, Jeong JS, Kim HJ. A Phase II study of oxaliplatin with low-dose leucovorin and bolus and continuous infusion 5-fluorouracil (modified FOLFOX-4) for gastric cancer patients with malignant ascites. Jpn J Clin Oncol. 2007;37(12):930–5.
4. Kim JY, Bae HS. A controlled clinical study of serosa-invasive gastric carcinoma patients who underwent surgery plus intraperitoneal hyperthermo-chemo-perfusion (IHCP). Gastric Cancer. 2001;4(1):27–33.
5. Fushida S, Kinoshita J, Kaji M, Hirono Y, Goda F, Yagi Y, Oyama K, Sudo Y, Watanabe Y, Fujimura T. Phase I/II study of intraperitoneal docetaxel plus S-1 for the gastric cancer patients with peritoneal carcinomatosis. Cancer Chemother Pharmacol. 2013;71(5):1265–72.
6. Hallaj-Nezhadi S, Dass CR, Lotfipour F. Intraperitoneal delivery of nanoparticles for cancer gene therapy. Future Oncol. 2013;9(1):59–68.
7. Bajaj G, Yeo Y. Drug delivery systems for intraperitoneal therapy. Pharm Res. 2010;27(5):735–8.
8. Poveda A, Salazar R, del Campo JM, Mendiola C, Cassinello J, Ojeda B, Arranz JA, Oaknin A, Garcia-Foncillas J, Rubio MJ, Gonzalez MA. Update in the management of ovarian and cervical carcinoma. Clin Transl Oncol. 2007;9(7):443–51.
9. Gradishar WJ, Tjulandin S, Davidson N, Shaw H, Desai N, Bhar P, Hawkins M, O'Shaughnessy J. Phase III trial of nanoparticle albumin-bound paclitaxel compared with polyethylated castor oil-based paclitaxel in women with breast cancer. J Clin Oncol. 2005;23(31):7794–803.
10. Rugo HS, Barry WT, Moreno-Aspitia A, Lyss AP, Cirrincione C, Leung E, Mayer EL, Naughton M, Toppmeyer D, Carey LA, Perez EA, Hudis C, Winer EP. Randomized phase iii trial of paclitaxel once per week compared with nanoparticle albumin-bound nab-paclitaxel once per week or ixabepilone with bevacizumab as first-line chemotherapy for locally recurrent or metastatic breast cancer: CALGB 40502/NCCTG N063H (alliance). J Clin Oncol. 2015;33(21):2361–9.
11. Kinoshita J, Fushida S, Tsukada T, Oyama K, Watanabe T, Shoji M, Okamoto K, Nakanuma S, Sakai S, Makino I, Furukawa H, Hayashi H, Nakamura K, Inokuchi M, Nakagawara H, Miyashita T, Tajima H, Takamura H, Ninomiya I, Fujimura T, Masakazu Y, Hirakawa K, Ohta T. Comparative study of the antitumor activity of Nab-paclitaxel and intraperitoneal solvent-based paclitaxel regarding peritoneal metastasis in gastric cancer. Oncol Rep. 2014;32(1):89–96.
12. Gong C, Qi T, Wei X, Qu Y, Wu Q, Luo F, Qian Z. Thermosensitive polymeric hydrogels as drug delivery systems. Curr Med Chem. 2013;20(1):79–94.
13. Li Z, Wang F, Roy S, Sen CK, Guan J. Injectable, highly flexible, and thermosensitive hydrogels capable of delivering superoxide dismutase. Biomacromolecules. 2009;10(12):3306–16.
14. Bae WK, Park MS, Lee JH, Hwang JE, Shim HJ, Cho SH, Kim DE, Ko HM, Cho CS, Park IK, Chung IJ. Docetaxel-loaded thermoresponsive conjugated linoleic acid-incorporated poloxamer hydrogel for the suppression of peritoneal metastasis of gastric cancer. Biomaterials. 2013;34(4):1433–41.
15. Wang X, Sun K, Tan Y, Wu S, Zhang J. Efficacy and safety of selenium nanoparticles administered intraperitoneally for the prevention of growth of cancer cells in the peritoneal cavity. Free Radic Biol Med. 2014;72:1–10.
16. Tsujimoto H, Morimoto Y, Takahata R, Nomura S, Yoshida K, Horiguchi H, Hiraki S, Ono S, Miyazaki H, Saito D, Hara I, Ozeki E, Yamamoto J, Hase K. Photodynamic therapy using nanoparticle loaded with indocyanine green for experimental peritoneal dissemination of gastric cancer. Cancer Sci. 2014;105(12):1626–30.
17. Al-Abd AM, Hong KY, Song SC, Kuh HJ. Pharmacokinetics of doxorubicin after intratumoral injection using a thermosensitive hydrogel in tumor-bearing mice. J Control Release. 2010;142(1):101–7.
18. Cho JK, Kuh HJ, Song SC. Injectable poly(organophosphazene) hydrogel system for effective paclitaxel and doxorubicin combination therapy. J Drug Target. 2014;22(8):761–7.
19. Yamamoto Y, Yoshida M, Sato M, Sato K, Kikuchi S, Sugishita H, Kuwabara J, Matsuno Y, Kojima Y, Morimoto M, Horiuchi A, Watanabe Y. Feasibility of tailored, selective and effective anticancer chemotherapy by direct injection of docetaxel-loaded immunoliposomes into Her2/neu positive gastric tumor xenografts. Int J Oncol. 2011;38(1):33–9.
20. Wang SX, Bao A, Phillips WT, Goins B, Herrera SJ, Santoyo C, Miller FR, Otto RA. Intraoperative therapy with liposomal drug delivery: retention and distribution in human head and neck squamous cell carcinoma xenograft model. Int J Pharm. 2009;373(1–2):156–64.
21. Zhu L, Zhang B, Lu X, Shu Y, Liu B. Delivery of paclitaxel and berbamine by polymeric carriers to cure gastric cancer. Oncol Res. 2013;20(7):265–74.
22. Liu Q, Li RT, Qian HQ, Yang M, Zhu ZS, Wu W, Qian XP, Yu LX, Jiang XQ, Liu BR. Gelatinase-stimuli strategy enhances the tumor delivery and therapeutic efficacy of docetaxel-loaded poly(ethylene glycol)-poly(varepsilon-caprolactone) nanoparticles. Int J Nanomedicine. 2012;7:281–95.
23. Liu Q, Li RT, Qian HQ, Wei J, Xie L, Shen J, Yang M, Qian XP, Yu LX, Jiang XQ, Liu BR. Targeted delivery of miR-200c/DOC to inhibit cancer stem cells and cancer cells by the gelatinases-stimuli nanoparticles. Biomaterials. 2013;34(29):7191–203.
24. Zhang Q, Liu Q, Shen J, Chen H, Liu B. Tumor delivery efficiency and apoptosis enhancement by EVO nanoparticles on murie hepatic carcinoma cell line H22. J Biomed Nanotechnol. 2013;9(8):1354–61.
25. Pak KH, Jo A, Choi HJ, Choi Y, Kim H, Cheong JH. The different role of intratumoral and peritumoral lymphangiogenesis in gastric cancer progression and prognosis. BMC Cancer. 2015;15:498.

26. Zhang H, Tian Y, Zhu Z, Xu H, Li X, Zheng D, Sun W. Efficient antitumor effect of co-drug-loaded nanoparticles with gelatin hydrogel by local implantation. Sci Rep. 2016;6:26546.
27. Wu P, Liu Q, Li R, Wang J, Zhen X, Yue G, Wang H, Cui F, Wu F, Yang M, Qian X, Yu L, Jiang X, Liu B. Facile preparation of paclitaxel loaded silk fibroin nanoparticles for enhanced antitumor efficacy by locoregional drug delivery. ACS Appl Mater Interfaces. 2013;5(23):12638–45.
28. Fung LK, Shin M, Tyler B, Brem H, Saltzman WM. Chemotherapeutic drugs released from polymers: distribution of 1,3-bis(2-chloroethyl)-1-nitrosourea in the rat brain. Pharm Res. 1996;13(5):671–82.
29. Sugahara KN, Scodeller P, Braun GB, de Mendoza TH, Yamazaki CM, Kluger MD, Kitayama J, Alvarez E, Howell SB, Teesalu T, Ruoslahti E, Lowy AM. A tumor-penetrating peptide enhances circulation-independent targeting of peritoneal carcinomatosis. J Control Release. 2015;212:59–69.

Drug Delivery in Synergistic Combination with Other Treatments

16

Hanqing Qian and Baorui Liu

16.1 Introduction

"Combined therapy" is a term referring to either the coadministration of two or more pharmacotherapies or to the combination of different types of therapy methods. Combined therapy has played an important role in the treatment of gastric cancer, with the routine use of combination chemotherapy in the clinic. The FOLFOX, XELOX, and ECF have been adopted as important regimens for the treatment of gastric cancer [1, 2]. Combination chemotherapy has also been used as an adjuvant/neoadjuvant treatment both pre- and post-surgery [3]. Collectively, there has been wide use of chemotherapy and radiotherapy (RT) combinations which has led to enhanced response and survival rates in gastric cancer patients [4].

Recently, a great deal of interest has been focused on the application of combinational therapies in drug delivery systems [5]. As shown in Fig. 16.1, nanoparticle-based combination strategies include more than just the co-encapsulation of different chemotherapeutic agents in nanoparticles:

1. Combination of chemotherapeutics with other drugs (e.g., chemosensitizing agents, molecular targeting and nucleic acid-based drugs)
2. Combination of chemotherapeutics with other treatments (e.g., radiotherapy, photodynamic therapy, thermotherapy, and immunotherapy)
3. Combination of drug delivery with diagnoses

Due to the different pharmocokinetics of drugs administered in combinatorial regimens, the therapeutic effect of combination chemotherapy is often suboptimal. However, when drugs are co-encapsulated into one nanoparticle, they are simultaneously delivered to the tumor site and modulate tumor cells via different pathways. This allows for the synergistic effect to be maximized, thereby improving target selectivity, overcoming drug resistance, and reducing side effects.

It should be noted that since a lower drug dosage is required for combination therapies [6], their side effects are often reduced as well. When combining drug delivery systems with other therapies, therapeutic efficacy could also be enhanced by this synergistic effect. Drug-loaded nanoparticles themselves also act as sensitizers for other treatments due to their exceptional physical and chemical properties. In this chapter, we will summarize the current state of nanoparticle-based combination strategies for use in gastric cancer treatment. These will include both in vitro and in vivo approaches and will also

H. Qian (✉) • B. Liu
The Comprehensive Cancer Center of Drum Tower Hospital, Medical School of Nanjing University and Clinical Cancer Institute of Nanjing University, Nanjing 210008, China
e-mail: qianhanqing1986@163.com

J. Wei, B. Liu (eds.), *Personalized Management of Gastric Cancer*,
DOI 10.1007/978-981-10-3978-2_16

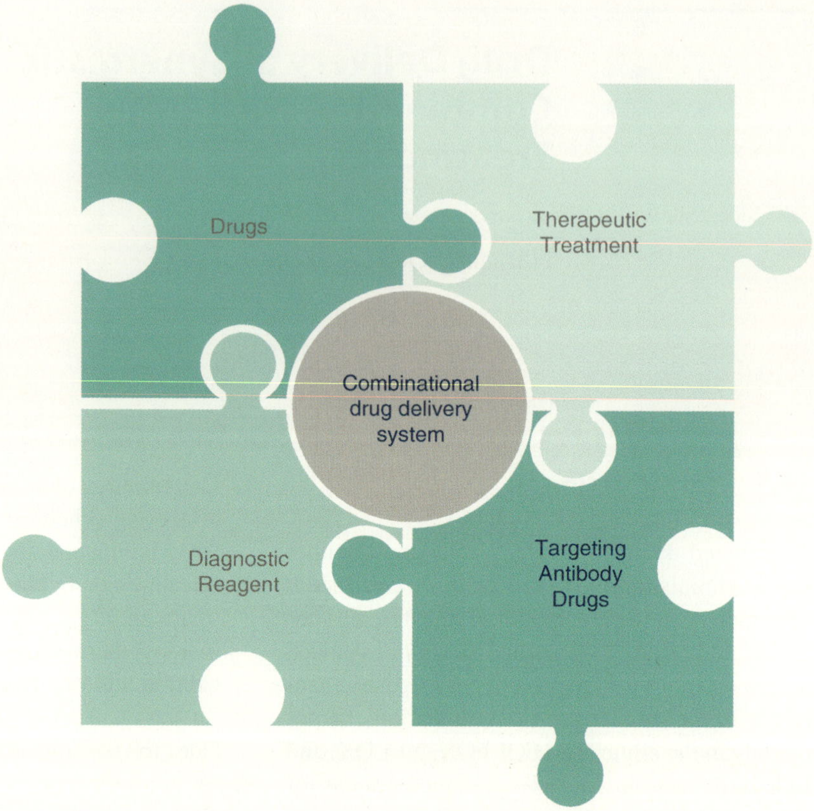

Fig. 16.1 Various strategies for nanoparticle-based combinational drug delivery systems

attempt to highlight their benefits, potential applications, and remaining challenges to their use in clinical translational research.

16.2 Combination of Chemotherapeutics with Other Drugs

Anticancer drugs are often used in combination so as to achieve the maximum synergistic therapeutic effect, itself greater than the sum of each drug's individual effects. This provides a marked advantage: When only one signal pathway is blocked by a single drug, tumor cells can compensate by either regulating relative protein expression or mutations, resulting in resistance, which is considered as the major reason for many anticancer treatment failures [7]. Alternatively, using two or more drugs that target different cellular pathways can overcome developed chemotherapeutic resistance. However, obtaining the optimal parameters for both the drug cocktail ratio and the treatment sequence is one of the major challenges facing combination drug therapy [6]. This is due in large part to the fact that different drugs have different pharmacokinetic and pharmacodynamic characteristics, biodistribution behavior, and bioavailability when used in combination with each other.

Given this, simultaneous encapsulation of different drugs into one nanoparticle is designed to take advantage of combination therapy as well as the nano-drug delivery system. In addition to using traditional anticancer chemotherapeutics, chemosensitizer agents, molecular targeting drugs, and gene and/or protein therapeutics are often adopted within the sphere of "combinational nanotherapy." We will now discuss each of these in turn.

16.2.1 Chemosensitizing Agents

Multidrug resistance (MDR) is a major obstacle to the effectiveness of chemotherapy. Tumor cells often increase the efflux of drugs through

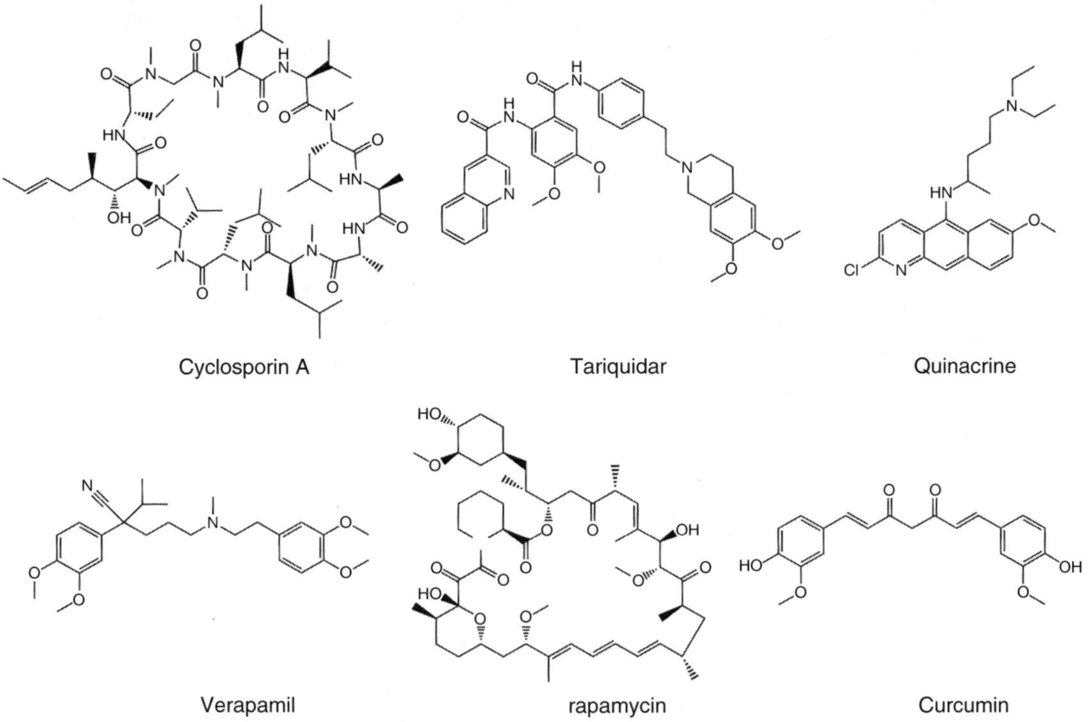

Fig. 16.2 Chemosensitizing agents used in combination with traditional chemotherapeutics

upregulation of P-glycoprotein (P-gp) or multidrug resistance protein 1 (MRP1), resulting in enhanced chemotherapy resistance. In particular, P-gp has been shown to be overexpressed in many types of cancer, including gastrointestinal, ovarian, and liver cancers [8, 9]. To combat this problem, cyclosporin A, verapamil, tariquidar, and quinacrine (Fig. 16.2) are all capable of inhibiting efflux pump activity. As such, they are the main chemosensitizing agents used to overcome multidrug resistance and enhance the therapy effectiveness [10, 11].

The response rate of 5-fluorouridine (5-FU) in gastric cancer is only about 11% [12]. The chemoresistance to 5-FU in many cancers is associated with the hypermethylation of transcription factor AP-2 epsilon (TFAP2E) [13]. Therefore, it is reasonable to suppose that a combination of DNA methyltransferase inhibitors and 5-FU could promote the sensitivity of many kinds of tumors to chemotherapy, further improving its therapeutic response. To this end, 5-Aza-2'-deoxycytidine (DAC) is one of the most widely investigated demethylating agents and is able to increase the expression of TFAP2E through its demethylating activity [14]. However, the efficacy of DAC in cancer treatment is inhibited by the drug's inherent instability [15]. When DAC and 5-FU were co-delivered using nanoparticles (NPs-5-FU-DAC) into a single gastric cancer cell, not only was DAC stability enhanced, but targeted cellular uptake was also achieved [16]. Importantly, the synergistic effect of NPs-5-FU-DAC could be detected 72 h after treatment in MKN-45 cells with high TFAP2E methylation levels. In contrast, this synergistic effect was not present in MKN28 cells after any length of incubation [16].

Paclitaxel (PTX) chemoresistance in tumor cells is proportional to total cellular antioxidant capacity. Importantly, PTX cytotoxicity is enhanced when the cell's endogenous antioxidant capacity is also inhibited by agents that can induce the formation of intracellular reactive oxygen species (ROS) [17]. Tetrandrine (Tet, an alkaloid isolated from Hang-Fang-Chi) is one such compound that can effectively increase the generation of intracellular ROS by enhancing cellular oxidative stress [18]. To illustrate this effect, Li et al. co-encapsulated PTX and Tet in PEG-PCL nanoparticles [19]. The synergistic antitumor effects of co-loaded Tet and PTX (PTX/Tet) were then shown in vitro in a gastric cancer cell line (BGC-823) [11]. Specifically, the viability of BGC-823 cells treated with PTX/Tet nanoparticles was significantly lower than cells treated singly with either nanoparticles containing PTX or Tet. In this study, the combination index (CI) [20] was below 1 when fraction affected (FA, fractional cell growth inhibition) was below 0.75, which indicated a synergistic therapeutic effect for nanoparticles co-loaded with PTX and Tet. Further research investigating the mechanism behind this synergistic antitumor effect when using combinational nanoparticles revealed that it acted to increase ROS production in tumor cells. Moreover, such co-loading also engendered its effect via suppression of the downstream Akt pathway, including Bcl2, Bax, and Caspase 3. Collectively, this resulted in the activation of tumor cells apoptosis [19].

Nanomedicine enables clinicians to precisely modulate the pharmacological properties of multidrug cocktails with cell-specific targeting. Accordingly, delivery of chemotherapeutics in combination with chemosensitizing agents using either passive or active targeting nanoparticles is a powerful approach to overcoming tumor.

16.2.2 Monoclonal Antibody Drugs

Monoclonal antibodies (mAbs) have been harnessed as a type of targeted therapeutic drug and have been primarily in the development for cancer treatment and immunological disorders. For instance, trastuzumab (Herceptin) was approved by the US Food and Drug Administration in combination with 5-fluorouracil and cisplatin for the treatment of HER2-overexpressing metastatic gastric cancer [21]. In the context of nanomedicine, mAbs have typically been used as conjugates on the surface of drug-loaded nanoparticles. In this way, specific tumor targeting can increase drug accumulation to the tumor site as well as resulting in enhanced intracellular uptake [22]. To this end, Li et al. covalently decorated an anti-HER2 Fab onto doxorubicin (Dox)-loaded, thermosensitive, polymeric micelles, which are self-assembled from poly(*N*-isopropylacrylomide-co-*N*,*N*-dimethylacrylamide)$_{118}$-b-poly(D,L-Lactide)$_{71}$ (PID$_{118}$-b-PLA$_{71}$) [23]. The resulting Fab-conjugated immunomicelles (FCIMs) have dual-targeting properties. Accordingly, it is expected that the tumor accumulation and cellular uptake of Dox would be enhanced by both of these properties—specific recognition and temperature. For the latter, the nanoparticle shell undergoes a hydrophilic-to-hydrophobic transition when the temperature is above the volume phase transition temperature (VPTT). This results in increased antibody-antigen interactions between the nanoparticles and the cell membrane. When incubated with N87 (HER2-overexpressing human gastric cancer cells), the IC$_{50}$ of FCIM was 9 times lower than that of Doxil. It was also half that of non-targeting micelles. After injection, FCIMs accumulated at the tumor site through passive targeting (EPR effect) and active targeting (HER2). Moreover, a hydrophilic-to-hydrophobic transition was also expected to occur, since solid tumor temperatures are often slightly higher than the VPTT of FCIMs. Based on an in vivo anticancer experiment, the relative tumor volume of the FCIMs group was <2. This is markedly lower than the volumes seen for the non-targeting micelle and Doxil groups 3 and 4, respectively. Thus, the antitumor activity was promoted both in vitro and in vivo by the combined effect of temperature and active targeting.

Similarly, epidermal growth factor receptor (EGFR) is overexpressed in many solid tumors. Synergistic effects have been observed when an EGFR inhibitor is combined with chemotherapeutics, such as PTX, irinotecan, and pemetrexed [24, 25]. Moreover, tumor-penetrating iRGD peptide is often used in drug delivery systems to enhance the accumulation of drug-loaded nanoparticles at the tumor site. This is done by increasing the vascular as well as tissue permeability. To this end, Bian et al. incorporated a recombinant protein—iRGD-fused EGFR single-domain antibody (anti-EGFR-iRGD)—to PTX-loaded silk fibroin nanoparticles (A-PTX-SF-NPs) by way of a carbodiimide-mediated coupling procedure [26]. This combined active tumor-targeting drug delivery system showed superior in vitro antitumor efficacy in a highly expressing EGFR cancer cell line (Hela) than in the low expressing line (MKN-45). These results were also corroborated in vivo.

16.3 Genetic-Based Therapeutics (DNA, siRNA, and miRNA)

Cancer gene therapy is the delivery of therapeutic nucleic acids at the tumor site. This treatment can eliminate tumors by (1) substituting in for mutated genes, (2) downregulating or silencing oncogenic pathways, (3) expressing pro-apoptotic proteins, and/or (4) activating the immune system. Co-delivery of a chemotherapeutic agent and genetic therapeutics against one or more targets could induce cancer cell apoptosis synergistically. Due to their different physicochemical properties, there are great challenges in effectively engineering encapsulation of macromolecular nucleic acids and small-molecule drugs to yield a combined gene and chemotherapy delivery system. Plasmid DNA, siRNA, and miRNA are the most widely used nucleic acid therapeutics that can be delivered using nanoparticles. Among them, micro-RNA (miRNA) is a type of small noncoding RNA molecule that contains about 22 nucleotides. They can act as oncogenes or tumor suppressors during the process of cancer initiation and progression [27]. The advantages of miRNA/small-molecule anticancer drugs combination are numerous, including the promotion of apoptosis and autophagy, downregulating adenosine triphosphate (ATP)-binding cassette (ABC) transporters, suppressing tumor angiogenesis, and reverting the epithelial-to-mesenchymal transition (EMT) [28]. However, owing to their relatively small molecular weight, miRNA are quickly eliminated from circulation and rapidly cleared via renal excretion [28]. In addition, the oligonucleotides are not stable in the acidic environment presented by endosomes/lysosomes and are thus susceptible to degradation before even reaching their cytosolic targets. Therefore, co-delivery of miRNA and anticancer drugs in the same nanovehicles could not only overcome the above miRNA delivery hurdles but also afford a synergistic antitumor effect through simultaneous cargo delivery to the same cancer cells.

To investigate this option, Liu et al. fabricated poly(ethylene glycol)-peptide-poly(ε-caprolactone) (PEG-PEP-PCL) nanoparticles for co-delivery of miR-200c and docetaxel (Doc). With this system, nanoparticles accumulated in the tumor region by EPR effect and the PEG corona was subsequently shed under gelatinase stimuli, resulting in enhanced delivery efficiency [29]. The miR-200c/DOC nanoparticles exhibited a significantly superior antitumor effect than either DOC or DOC-loaded nanoparticles alone. Collectively, their results demonstrated the miR-200c/DOC nanoparticles remarkably inhibited tumor growth in a synergistic manner. This combinational delivery system increased E-cadherin expression levels and decreased CD44 mRNA expression to simultaneously inhibit both cancer stem cells (CSC) and EMT cells. In addition, miR-200c also downregulated TUBB3 expression levels and restored the chemosensitivity of gastric cancer BGC-823 cells to DOC both in vitro and in vivo [17].

Special AT-rich binding protein (SATB1) is a critical regulator of cancer progression that regulates the expression of E-cadherin, ABL1, MMP2, and ERRB2 [30]. It has been reported that inhibiting SATB1 expression can induce the apoptosis of many tumor cells as well as inhibit their proliferation and invasion [31]. To investigate SATB1-focused therapies, Peng et al. fabricated a doxorubicin and SATB1 shRNA co-loaded thermosensitive magnetic cationic liposome. This magnetic-targeting delivery system had a phase transition temperature of 40.8 °C, thereby allowing its use for hyperthermic-response release of therapeutic agents [32]. Additionally, gene delivery efficiency could also be improved by the magnetic targeting properties of the delivery system. Collectively, their results showed that the combined delivery of DOX and SATB1 shRNA not only led to tumor cell apoptosis but also to in vitro as well as in vivo synergistic antitumor effects. Thus, this approach and delivery system resulted in improved tumor inhibition than other previously used formulations.

16.4 Combination of Chemotherapeutics with Other Treatments

In addition to chemotherapy, radiotherapy, photothermal therapy (PTT), and immunotherapy have all been used in the clinic as important cancer treatment options. Standard treatment plans in select European and American guidelines recommend that gastric cancer patients receive concurrent chemo- and radiotherapy (chemoradiotherapy) after surgery [4]. Physical therapies have the advantage of irreversibly destroying tumors. They also offer a synergistic treatment to eradicating cancer by generating a variety of therapeutic outcomes. Overall, the clinical efficacy in cancer patients would benefit from a specific combination of novel drug delivery system and some—or all—of these therapeutic treatments. A deeper discussion of each is provided below:

16.4.1 Radiotherapy

Radiotherapy (RT) is one of the dominant cancer treatment strategies. DNA double-strand breaks and induced tumor cell apoptosis are the key mechanisms through which radiotherapy kills cancer cells. It has been reported that this localized radiation effect can be enhanced by high-Z-containing material. To harness this effect, nanoparticles that are made of noble metals may be useful in increasing the radiation energy absorption due to their unique physical and chemical properties. The mechanisms involved in this synergistic anticancer effect have been attributed to increased ROS, oxidative stress, as well as vascular damage, resulting in apoptosis, necrosis, and autophagy of tumor cells [33, 34].

Many chemotherapeutics are often applied in the clinic with the goal of augmenting radiotherapy tumor effects, termed "radiosensitization." Docetaxel and concurrent radiotherapy are commonly used for a variety of cancers, including head and neck cancer, non-small cell lung cancer, and gastric cancer [35–37]. However, owing to the nonspecific distribution and side effects caused by docetaxel itself, further insights into effective sensitizer delivery of this combination treatment are needed to improve the therapeutic approach. Doxorubicin-, paclitaxel-, and etanidazole-loaded nanoparticles have been investigated and show better radiosensitizing effects than their free drug formulations [38, 39]. For instance, Cui et al. constructed a docetaxel-loaded nanoparticle (DOC-NPs) using the abovementioned gelatinase-responsive polymer, PEG-PEP-PCL. This was done to selectively enhance the radiation-induced cell death efficacy at the tumor site in addition to reducing the toxicity to normal tissue [40]. When compared with free docetaxel, the nanoparticle formulation exhibited higher drug concentrations and longer time acting in the tumor tissue. Given these results, it is quite possible that nanoparticles have the potential to support the radiation process in fewer doses. Sensitization enhancement ratios of DOC-NPs were 1.09-, 1.18-, and 1.24-fold higher than free docetaxel, respectively, in three gelatinase overexpressing GC cell lines. This is compared to only a 1.02-fold increase in normal, gelatinase-deficient gastric mucosa cells. In a subcutaneous transplant tumor model, DOC-NPs were more effective radiosensitizers than docetaxel and also had a superior ability to delay tumor growth in vivo. Mechanistic research revealed that $79.7 \pm 4.9\%$ cells arrested at the G2/M phase when treated with DOC-NPs, which is significantly higher than both the docetaxel and control groups. Since cells in the G2/M phase are more radiosensitive, this might be a major factor behind the enhanced radiosensitization observed in DOC-NPs. Furthermore, the improved radiosensitization efficacy of DOC-NPs was also associated with increased generation of ROS, promotion of cellular apoptosis, and more effective DNA double-strand breaks.

16.4.2 Photothermal Therapy

Tumor cells appear to be more sensitive to heat-induced destruction than normal cells, and treatment approaches have been developed to take advantage of this fact [41]. Photothermal therapy (PTT) refers to treatment utilizing (typically) near-infrared wavelengths of laser-generated heat for the treatment of cancer. Accordingly, tumor tissue can be hyperthermically eradicated through various mechanisms, including protein structural changes and/or tissue carbonization. To this end, several kinds of nanomaterials with the ability to convert light into hyperthermia have been exploited for minimally invasive tumor ablation [42]. Among them, gold-based nanomaterials and carbon materials exhibit unique photothermal properties have been widely investigated as therapeutic agents in photothermal therapy. Furthermore, combinations of photothermal and chemotherapies have also been shown to be a useful approach for cancer treatment [43]. During laser irradiation, the encapsulated drugs can be released under a controllable manner. Importantly, the permeability of tumor cells is increased due to the laser-induced hyperthermia, leading to overall more effective permeation of drugs across cancer cell membranes.

Furthermore, combining tumor imaging and targeted therapy in one nanoparticle holds great promise for the treatment of cancer. This would include all stages of cancer, from diagnosis to evaluation to treatment. Recently, a folic acid (FA)-modified gold nanorods/silica hybrid nanodelivery system (GNR-SiO_2-FA) was developed and investigated as a multifunctional nanoprobe for X-ray/CT imaging-guided targeting dual-mode radio- and photothermal therapies [44]. The weight of the conjugated FA on the surface of the prepared nanoparticles was approximately 15.21%, thus ensuring a highly selective targeting ability. The GNR-SiO_2-FA nanoparticles also showed enhanced RT and PTT effects in vitro, which depended on the targeted uptake efficiency of gold by MGC-803 gastric cancer cells. Therefore, these nanoparticles are a good candidate for in vivo X-ray/CT imaging due to their strong X-ray attenuation.

16.5 Combination of Therapy and Diagnoses

When combining therapeutic drugs with imaging agents, the integrated nanoparticles are referred to as a "theranostic system." This multifunctional and integrated system combines different properties, including the tumor targeting, imaging, selective cancer therapy, and response monitoring in an all-in-one system, thereby providing more useful multimodal methods for cancer treatment. Coupling therapeutic effects and contrast properties in combinational delivery system shows great potential in applications such as targeted primary/metastasis tumor diagnosis, simultaneous therapy, and in vivo tracking. Nanoparticles are good alternatives to realize theranostic function, thanks to its particular properties [45, 46]. There are generally two categories of theranostic nanoparticles: (1) the nanoparticles themselves can be detected by imaging modalities, such as gold-, magnetic- and other inorganic nanoparticles [47, 48] and (2) targeted co-delivery of diagnostic and therapeutic agents by nanoparticles. Up till now, a number of various nanoparticle-based theranostic modalities have been reported in the simultaneous diagnosis and treatment of gastric cancer.

16.5.1 Primary Tumor Imaging

Quantum dots (QDs) are a kind of photoluminescence material with strong fluorescent intensity and a tunable emission spectrum. QDs have begun to be widely used in live-cell imaging, immunoassays, and other biological application. For example, Jing et al. synthesized a targeting quantum dot nanoprobe (HER2-RQDs) by conjugating an HER2 monoclonal antibody to the surface of RNase A-associated CdTe quantum dot clusters [49]. The prepared HER2-RQDs were 40 nm in diameter and had an emission peak at 600 nm. Results showed that HER2-RQDs nanoprobes could perform in situ targeted imaging of a gastric cancer-bearing mouse model a mere 6 h after intravenous injection. In addition, this RNase A-loaded nanoprobe could selectively kill HER2 overexpressed gastric cancer MGC803 cells in vitro, inhibit tumor growth, and extend survival time in an in situ gastric cancer-bearing mouse model. This effect was caused by the degradation of total cytoplasmic RNA, inhibition of mRNA translation, and protein synthesis, which ultimately led to the induction of cellular apoptosis [49].

Cancer stem cells are cancer cells that possess the ability of self-renewal and the capacity to initiate tumor formation. They are also considered the responsible members of tumor invasion, metastasis, and resistance to anticancer treatment such as chemotherapy and radiotherapy [50]. Specifically, the $CD44^+$ subpopulation of gastric cancer cells within tumor tissue is endowed with stem cell properties [51]. Given this, CD44 has been taken as a gastric cancer stem cell (GCSC) surface marker. To harness this property of CD44, Liang et al. prepared PEGylated gold nanostars conjugated with CD44v6 monoclonal antibodies (CD44v6-GNS) [52]. These multifunctional nanoprobes were used for photoacoustic, infrared microscopic imaging, as well as photothermal therapy of GCSCs. $CD44^+$ cells were sorted from the MKN-45 GC cell line and then incubated with CD44v6-GNS. After the 24 h incubation, 83% of the CD44v6-GNS was either internalized or bound to $CD44^+$ spherical cells, thereby demonstrating a highly affinity with the stem cell-like $CD44^+$ subset of cells.

As shown in Fig. 16.3, photoacoustic imaging has revealed that the CD44v6-GNS is capable of targeting the tumor vascular system at 4 h postinjection in both orthotopic and subcutaneous xenografted tumor models in vivo [52]. In the subcutaneous xenografted model, photoacoustic imaging enhancements of CD44v6-GNS were 4.7-fold higher at 4 h postinjection. Comparatively, non-targeting gold nanostars were 1.75-fold higher at the same time point. The orthotopic xenografted model featured a deeper location of the orthotopic tumor and disturbance of the dermal vasculature. As a result, only slight enhancements were observed. However, with increasing time, a localized enhancement of the photoacoustic signal could be detected in the stomach area, indicating the accumulation of the nanoprobe in the tumors.

Owing to the plasmon absorption band in the near-infrared region, gold nanostars generate heat upon laser irradiation and could also be used in photothermal therapy. The high-affinity binding to GCSC sphere cells by CD44v6-GNS means that tumor ablation could occur with low-power density upon NIR laser radiation. Cell viability was only 0.7% when $CD44^+$ spheroid colonies had been incubated for 24 h with CD44v6-GNS, which were then exposed to NIR laser treatment (790 nm, 1.5 W/cm^2). The photothermal therapeutic effect of CD44v6-GNS was also investigated in vivo. Four hours after injection of CD44v6-GNS, photothermal therapy was performed at a density of 0.8 W/cm^2 for 5 min. After this, necrotic areas could be observed in the treatment center of the tumorous tissue. The tumor volume in the CD44v6-GNS group was reduced within 2 weeks after photothermal therapy and showed a significant difference when compared with controls. Taken together, these results showed that the multifunctional CD44v6-GNS nanoprobes displayed a great potential for GCSC-targeted combinational therapy of photoacoustic imaging and photothermal therapy, overcoming the resistance of CSCs to anticancer treatment [52].

Similarly, CD44v6 single-chain variable fragment ($scFv_{CD44v6}$) was utilized by Chen et al. to fabricate gastric cancer-targeting multifunctional nanoparticles [53]. These nanoparticles combined an siRNA delivery system and magnetic resonance imaging (MRI) that consisted of superparamagnetic iron oxide nanoparticles (SPION) and polyethylene glycol-grafted polyethylenimine (PEG-g-PEI). The content of $scFv_{CD44v6}$ attached to the nanoparticle surface was shown to be 16.7%. MRI revealed that the targeting $scFv_{CD44v6}$-PEG-PEI-SPION nanoparticles preferentially accumulated at the SGC-7901 tumor site of mice simultaneously bearing SGC-7901 (high CD44v6 expression) and A375 (low CD44v6 expression) tumors, demonstrating specific, in vivo gastric cancer targeting properties. In a follow-up study, the condensed siCD44v6 transferred by PEG-g-PEI-SPION downregulated the CD44v6 expression of gastric carcinoma cell line SGC-7901 in vitro and knocked

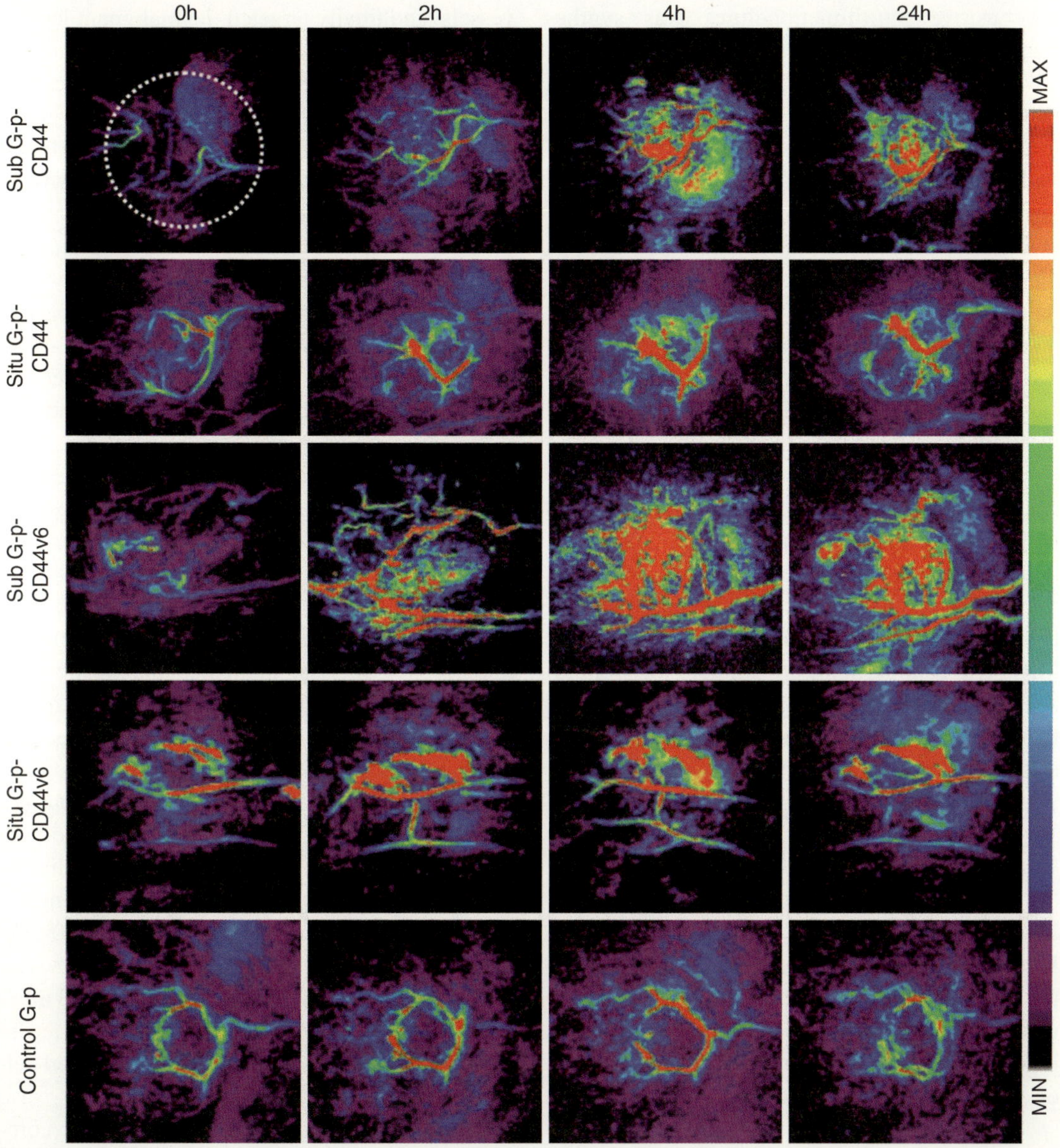

Fig. 16.3 Representative photoacoustic imaging before (0 h) and after injection (2, 4, and 24 h) of the GNS-PEG-CD44 (*first row* subtumor, *second row* orthotopic tumor), GNS-PEG-CD44v6 (*third row* subtumor, *fourth row* orthotopic tumor), and GNS-PEG (*fifth row* control) Reproduced with permission from Ref. [52]

down the migrating and invasive abilities of SGC-7901 cells. Furthermore, PEG-g-PEI-SPION itself was a highly efficient MRI contrast agent in vivo [54].

Sun et al. used magnetic nanoparticles to deliver microRNA-16 (miRNA-16), with the purpose of reversing drug resistance to chemotherapy in a mouse model of gastric cancer. The magnetic nanoparticles used in this study were PEG-coated Fe_3O_4 nanoparticles. Apart from in vivo imaging, the nanoparticles significantly suppressed SGC7901 (adriamycin-resistant) tumor growth, probably through increasing SGC7901/ADR cells' sensitivity to adriamycin [55]. In the studies of Ma et al., magnetic-polymer nanoparticles with folate receptor-targeting and pH-sensitive multifunctionalities was synthesized for DOX delivery in the treatment of advanced gastric cancer. The better efficacy of nanoparticles than free DOX was confirmed by in vitro and in vivo studies. Moreover, the accumulation of nanoparticles in the tumor site was detected by MRI [56].

Photosensitive nanoparticles are also used in the theranostics of gastric cancer. Huang et al. reported photosensitizer-conjugated magnetic nanoparticles applicated in gastric cancer imaging and therapy simultaneously. The nanoparticles were approximately 20 nm in diameter, and the photosensitizer chlorin e6 (Ce6) was covalently conjugated on the surface of magnetic nanoparticles. Therefore, the incorporated Ce6 molecules retained their spectroscopic and functional properties for photodynamic therapy, and the core magnetic nanoparticles offered the functions of magnetically guided drug delivery and MRI. The nanoparticles are suitable for simultaneous targeting photodynamic therapy and in vivo MRI of nude mice loaded with gastric cancer [57, 58].

16.5.2 Lymphatic Metastasis Imaging

Lymph node (LN) metastasis is an important factor for the prognosis of gastric cancer (GC) patients [47]. Due to the high risk of metastasis, a lymphadenectomy is the normal surgical course of treatment. However, a highly sensitive and specific pretreatment diagnosis of the LN metastatic status would be extremely helpful in better establishing individualized treatment strategies.

To this end, Qiao et al. developed a sensitive detection system for lymphatic metastasis [59] using core-shell structured upconversion nanoparticles consisting of NaGdF4:Yb, Er@NaGdF4 that had been coated with polyethylene glycol (PEG) and an antigastric tumor antibody MGb2. The upconversion nanoprobes emitted green and red light under 980 nm laser excitation. It is presumed that after injection, the sub-20 nm probes accumulated at the tumor interstitium via normal circulation, subsequently drained to the lymphatic vessels, and finally targeted the malignant lesions via antibody-antigen recognition. As a result, an orthotopic mouse model of human gastric cancer showed that this method allowed for in vivo, postinjection, optical detection of both primary and omental lymph node metastatic sites at 4 and 6 h, respectively. In particular, lymphatic metastases, which were smaller than 1 mm, were successfully detected with both high sensitivity and specificity. No detectable luminescence was obtained in benign lymph nodes, which is attributed to the specific binding affinity between the MGb2 antibody-modified nanoprobes and the tumor and lymphatic metastasis lesion.

In addition, Hironori Tsujimoto et al. used indocyanine green-loaded poly(sarcosine)-poly(L-lactic acid) polymeric nanoparticles (ICGm) to (1) image the metastatic LNs of gastric cancer and (2) perform photodynamic therapy [60]. ICG is a type of FDA-approved, infrared fluorescence dye used in medical diagnostic studies. It also has been used as a photosensitizer. In this particular study, 48 h after tail vein injection, metastatic popliteal lymph nodes (PLN) were clearly visualized in ICGm-treated mice, but not ICG-treated mice. This effect was evidence both in vivo and ex vivo. Meanwhile, photoirradiation was performed using an 808 nm laser system at a photon fluence rate of 500 mW/cm^2 for 1000s. On day 7, post-photodynamic therapy, the PLN volume of mice treated with ICGm was 3.1 ± 0.3 mm^3. This was significantly smaller than that seen in ICG-treated mice (6.8 ± 2.4 mm^3). Enhanced cellular apoptosis in metastatic LNs was also observed in the ICGm-treated mice when compared with those in the ICG treatment group. Collectively, an ICG-based theranostic system presents a promising approach for LN metastases in the treatment of gastric cancer.

16.6 Conclusion and Perspectives: From Bench to Bedside

Due to the dynamic nature and heterogeneous nature of cancer, a single therapeutic modality is unable to achieve a satisfactory and curative effect. Moreover, current treatment options often lead to drug resistance and continued disease progression. As such, the development of novel technology and combinational methods is critical to the future of clinical cancer therapies. Therefore, using a combination of drug delivery and other therapeutic agents and/or treatment to obtain synergistic effects is a promising approach. Employing nanotechnology in multimodality therapy provides significant advantages, including the controlled release of drug payloads, passive/active targeting accumulation, and normalized pharmacokinetics. However, despite the enhanced efficacy and reduced side effects established in preclinical research, taking combinational nanotherapeutics from bench to bedside is an extremely challenging task. There are still few clinical trials investigating the effectiveness of combination therapy involving drug delivery systems, with the exception of several combination, chemotherapeutic nanoparticles such as CPX-1 and CPX-351. The remaining key challenges in translating this drug delivery system include biocompatibility issues, targeting capacity, overcoming drug delivery barriers, and manufacturability [61, 62]. Despite these hurdles, we believe that with the advance of cancer biology, the growing knowledge and expertise of bioinformatics, increased genomic data, improvements to drug screening technologies, as well as increased understanding of our animal models can all be further exploited for the validation of new nanomedicine-based combination therapies. The combination of drug delivery systems and multidimensional therapies, such as gene therapy, radiotherapy, photothermal/photodynamic therapy, and immunotherapy, allows for synergistic effects to occur. Ultimately, this will translate into benefits for patients with cancer, leading to improvements in both their longevity and quality of life.

References

1. Xu HB, Huang F, Su R, Shen FM, Lv QZ. Capecitabine plus oxaliplatin (XELOX) compared with 5-fluorouracil/leucovorin plus oxaliplatin (FOLFOXs) in advanced gastric cancer: meta-analysis of randomized controlled trials. Eur J Clin Pharmacol. 2015;71(5):589–601.
2. Macdonald JS. Clinical overview: adjuvant therapy of gastrointestinal cancer. Cancer Chemother Pharmacol. 2004;54(Suppl 1):S4–11.
3. Quero L, Guillerm S, Hennequin C. Neoadjuvant or adjuvant therapy for gastric cancer. World J Gastrointest Oncol. 2015;7(8):102–10.
4. Luo W, Zhang H, Zhao Y, Wang L, Qi L, Ran J, et al. A retrospective study on intensity-modulated radiation therapy combined with chemotherapy after D2 radical surgery for gastric carcinoma. Mol Clin Oncol. 2016;4(5):740–8.
5. Hu Q, Sun W, Wang C, Gu Z. Recent advances of cocktail chemotherapy by combination drug delivery systems. Adv Drug Deliv Rev. 2016;98:19–34.
6. Ma L, Kohli M, Smith A. Nanoparticles for combination drug therapy. ACS Nano. 2013;7(11):9518–25.
7. Hu CM, Zhang L. Nanoparticle-based combination therapy toward overcoming drug resistance in cancer. Biochem Pharmacol. 2012;83(8):1104–11.
8. Ferreira RJ, dos Santos DJ, Ferreira MJ. P-glycoprotein and membrane roles in multidrug resistance. Future Med Chem. 2015;7(7):929–46.
9. Silva R, Vilas-Boas V, Carmo H, Dinis-Oliveira RJ, Carvalho F, de Lourdes BM, et al. Modulation of P-glycoprotein efflux pump: induction and activation as a therapeutic strategy. Pharmacol Ther. 2015;149:1–123.
10. Mignani S, Bryszewska M, Klajnert-Maculewicz B, Zablocka M, Majoral JP. Advances in combination therapies based on nanoparticles for efficacious cancer treatment: an analytical report. Biomacromolecules. 2015;16(1):1–27.
11. Nakahara C, Nakamura K, Yamanaka N, Baba E, Wada M, Matsunaga H, et al. Cyclosporin-A enhances docetaxel-induced apoptosis through inhibition of nuclear factor-kappaB activation in human gastric carcinoma cells. Clin Cancer Res. 2003;9(14):5409–16.
12. Takashima A, Boku N, Kato K, Nakamura K, Mizusawa J, Fukuda H, et al. Survival prolongation after treatment failure of first-line chemotherapy in patients with advanced gastric cancer: combined analysis of the Japan Clinical Oncology group trials JCOG9205 and JCOG9912. Gastric Cancer. 2014;17(3):522–8.
13. Ebert MP, Tanzer M, Balluff B, Burgermeister E, Kretzschmar AK, Hughes DJ, et al. TFAP2E-DKK4 and chemoresistance in colorectal cancer. N Engl J Med. 2012;366(1):44–53.
14. Abdelfatah E, Kerner Z, Nanda N, Ahuja N. Epigenetic therapy in gastrointestinal cancer: the right combination. Therap Adv Gastroenterol. 2016;9(4):560–79.
15. Karahoca M, Momparler RL. Pharmacokinetic and pharmacodynamic analysis of 5-aza-2'-deoxycytidine (decitabine) in the design of its dose-schedule for cancer therapy. Clin Epigenetics. 2013;5(1):3.
16. Wu FL, Li RT, Yang M, Yue GF, Wang HY, Liu Q, et al. Gelatinases-stimuli nanoparticles encapsulating 5-fluorouridine and 5-aza-2'-deoxycytidine enhance the sensitivity of gastric cancer cells to chemical therapeutics. Cancer Lett. 2015;363(1):7–16.

17. Ramanathan B, Jan KY, Chen CH, Hour TC, Yu HJ, Pu YS. Resistance to paclitaxel is proportional to cellular total antioxidant capacity. Cancer Res. 2005;65(18):8455–60.
18. Wan J, Liu T, Mei L, Li J, Gong K, Yu C, et al. Synergistic antitumour activity of sorafenib in combination with tetrandrine is mediated by reactive oxygen species (ROS)/Akt signaling. Br J Cancer. 2013;109(2):342–50.
19. Li X, Lu X, Xu H, Zhu Z, Yin H, Qian X, et al. Paclitaxel/tetrandrine coloaded nanoparticles effectively promote the apoptosis of gastric cancer cells based on "oxidation therapy". Mol Pharm. 2012;9(2):222–9.
20. Chou TC, Talalay P. Quantitative analysis of dose-effect relationships: the combined effects of multiple drugs or enzyme inhibitors. Adv Enzyme Regul. 1984;22:27–55.
21. Van Cutsem E, Sagaert X, Topal B, Haustermans K, Prenen H. Gastric cancer. Lancet. 2016;388(10060): 2654–64.
22. Liu Y, Li K, Liu B, Feng SS. A strategy for precision engineering of nanoparticles of biodegradable copolymers for quantitative control of targeted drug delivery. Biomaterials. 2010;31(35):9145–55.
23. Li W, Zhao H, Qian W, Li H, Zhang L, Ye Z, et al. Chemotherapy for gastric cancer by finely tailoring anti-Her2 anchored dual targeting immunomicelles. Biomaterials. 2012;33(21):5349–62.
24. Koizumi F, Kanzawa F, Ueda Y, Koh Y, Tsukiyama S, Taguchi F, et al. Synergistic interaction between the EGFR tyrosine kinase inhibitor gefitinib ("Iressa") and the DNA topoisomerase I inhibitor CPT-11 (irinotecan) in human colorectal cancer cells. Int J Cancer. 2004;108(3):464–72.
25. Sarkar S, Mazumdar A, Dash R, Sarkar D, Fisher PB, Mandal M. ZD6474 enhances paclitaxel antiproliferative and apoptotic effects in breast carcinoma cells. J Cell Physiol. 2011;226(2):375–84.
26. Bian X, Wu P, Sha H, Qian H, Wang Q, Cheng L, et al. Anti-EGFR-iRGD recombinant protein conjugated silk fibroin nanoparticles for enhanced tumor targeting and antitumor efficiency. Onco Targets Ther. 2016;9:3153–62.
27. Carthew RW, Sontheimer EJ. Origins and mechanisms of miRNAs and siRNAs. Cell. 2009;136(4): 642–55.
28. Dai X, Tan C. Combination of microRNA therapeutics with small-molecule anticancer drugs: mechanism of action and co-delivery nanocarriers. Adv Drug Deliv Rev. 2015;81:184–97.
29. Liu Q, Li RT, Qian HQ, Wei J, Xie L, Shen J, et al. Targeted delivery of miR-200c/DOC to inhibit cancer stem cells and cancer cells by the gelatinases-stimuli nanoparticles. Biomaterials. 2013;34(29):7191–203.
30. Mir R, Pradhan SJ, Galande S. Chromatin organizer SATB1 as a novel molecular target for cancer therapy. Curr Drug Targets. 2012;13(13):1603–15.
31. Huang B, Zhou H, Wang X, Liu Z. Silencing SATB1 with siRNA inhibits the proliferation and invasion of small cell lung cancer cells. Cancer Cell Int. 2013;13(1):8.
32. Peng Z, Wang C, Fang E, Lu X, Wang G, Tong Q. Co-delivery of doxorubicin and SATB1 shRNA by thermosensitive magnetic cationic liposomes for gastric cancer therapy. PLoS One. 2014;9(3):e92924.
33. Zhang XD, Wu D, Shen X, Chen J, Sun YM, Liu PX, et al. Size-dependent radiosensitization of PEG-coated gold nanoparticles for cancer radiation therapy. Biomaterials. 2012;33(27):6408–19.
34. Petrache Voicu SN, Dinu D, Sima C, Hermenean A, Ardelean A, Codrici E, et al. Silica nanoparticles induce oxidative stress and autophagy but not apoptosis in the MRC-5 cell line. Int J Mol Sci. 2015;16(12):29398–416.
35. Bamias A, Karina M, Papakostas P, Kostopoulos I, Bobos M, Vourli G, et al. A randomized phase III study of adjuvant platinum/docetaxel chemotherapy with or without radiation therapy in patients with gastric cancer. Cancer Chemother Pharmacol. 2010;65(6):1009–21.
36. Karasawa K, Matsumoto F, Ito S, Oba S, Furuya T, Hirowatari H, et al. Hyperfractionated radiotherapy with concurrent docetaxel for advanced head and neck cancer: a phase II study. Anticancer Res. 2012;32(9):4013–8.
37. Poudenx M, Bondiau PY, Chamorey E, Venissac N, Otto J, Pourel N, et al. Cisplatin-docetaxel induction plus concurrent 3-D conformal radiotherapy and weekly chemotherapy for locally advanced non-small cell lung cancer patients: a phase II trial. Oncology. 2012;83(6):321–8.
38. Xu WH, Han M, Dong Q, Fu ZX, Diao YY, Liu H, et al. Doxorubicin-mediated radiosensitivity in multicellular spheroids from a lung cancer cell line is enhanced by composite micelle encapsulation. Int J Nanomedicine. 2012;7:2661–71.
39. Jin C, Bai L, Wu H, Tian F, Guo G. Radiosensitization of paclitaxel, etanidazole and paclitaxel+etanidazole nanoparticles on hypoxic human tumor cells in vitro. Biomaterials. 2007;28(25):3724–30.
40. Cui FB, Li RT, Liu Q, Wu PY, Hu WJ, Yue GF, et al. Enhancement of radiotherapy efficacy by docetaxel-loaded gelatinase-stimuli PEG-Pep-PCL nanoparticles in gastric cancer. Cancer Lett. 2014;346(1):53–62.
41. Issels RD. Hyperthermia adds to chemotherapy. Eur J Cancer. 2008;44(17):2546–54.
42. Hong C, Kang J, Kim H, Lee C. Photothermal properties of inorganic nanomaterials as therapeutic agents for cancer thermotherapy. J Nanosci Nanotechnol. 2012;12(5):4352–5.
43. Chen Z, Ma L, Liu Y, Chen C. Applications of functionalized fullerenes in tumor theranostics. Theranostics. 2012;2(3):238–50.
44. Huang P, Bao L, Zhang C, Lin J, Luo T, Yang D, et al. Folic acid-conjugated silica-modified gold nanorods for X-ray/CT imaging-guided dual-mode radiation

and photo-thermal therapy. Biomaterials. 2011;32(36):9796–809.
45. Muthu MS, Leong DT, Mei L, Feng SS. Nanotheranostics—application and further development of nanomedicine strategies for advanced theranostics. Theranostics. 2014;4(6):660–77.
46. Chen F, Ehlerding EB, Cai W. Theranostic nanoparticles. J Nucl Med. 2014;55(12):1919–22.
47. Shida A, Mitsumori N, Nimura H, Takano Y, Iwasaki T, Fujisaki M, et al. Prediction of lymph node metastasis and sentinel node navigation surgery for patients with early-stage gastric cancer. World J Gastroenterol. 2016;22(33):7431–9.
48. Gobbo OL, Sjaastad K, Radomski MW, Volkov Y, Prina-Mello A. Magnetic Nanoparticles in Cancer Theranostics. Theranostics. 2015;5(11):1249–63.
49. Ruan J, Song H, Qian Q, Li C, Wang K, Bao C, et al. HER2 monoclonal antibody conjugated RNase-A-associated CdTe quantum dots for targeted imaging and therapy of gastric cancer. Biomaterials. 2012;33(29):7093–102.
50. Vinogradov S, Wei X. Cancer stem cells and drug resistance: the potential of nanomedicine. Nanomedicine (Lond). 2012;7(4):597–615.
51. Stojnev S, Krstic M, Ristic-Petrovic A, Stefanovic V, Hattori T. Gastric cancer stem cells: therapeutic targets. Gastric Cancer. 2014;17(1):13–25.
52. Liang S, Li C, Zhang C, Chen Y, Xu L, Bao C, et al. CD44v6 monoclonal antibody-conjugated gold nanostars for targeted photoacoustic imaging and plasmonic photothermal therapy of gastric cancer stem-like cells. Theranostics. 2015;5(9):970–84.
53. Chen Y, Wang W, Lian G, Qian C, Wang L, Zeng L, et al. Development of an MRI-visible nonviral vector for siRNA delivery targeting gastric cancer. Int J Nanomedicine. 2012;7:359–68.
54. Chen Y, Lian G, Liao C, Wang W, Zeng L, Qian C, et al. Characterization of polyethylene glycol-grafted polyethylenimine and superparamagnetic iron oxide nanoparticles (PEG-g-PEI-SPION) as an MRI-visible vector for siRNA delivery in gastric cancer in vitro and in vivo. J Gastroenterol. 2013;48(7):809–21.
55. Sun Z, Song X, Li X, Su T, Qi S, Qiao R, et al. In vivo multimodality imaging of miRNA-16 iron nanoparticle reversing drug resistance to chemotherapy in a mouse gastric cancer model. Nanoscale. 2014;6(23):14343–53.
56. Ma H, Liu Y, Shi M, Shao X, Zhong W, Liao W, et al. Theranostic, pH-responsive, doxorubicin-loaded nanoparticles inducing active targeting and apoptosis for advanced gastric cancer. Biomacromolecules. 2015;16(12):4022–31.
57. Huang P, Li Z, Lin J, Yang D, Gao G, Xu C, et al. Photosensitizer-conjugated magnetic nanoparticles for in vivo simultaneous magnetofluorescent imaging and targeting therapy. Biomaterials. 2011;32(13):3447–58.
58. Huang P, Lin J, Wang X, Wang Z, Zhang C, He M, et al. Light-triggered theranostics based on photosensitizer-conjugated carbon dots for simultaneous enhanced-fluorescence imaging and photodynamic therapy. Adv Mater. 2012;24(37):5104–10.
59. Qiao R, Liu C, Liu M, Hu H, Liu C, Hou Y, et al. Ultrasensitive in vivo detection of primary gastric tumor and lymphatic metastasis using upconversion nanoparticles. ACS Nano. 2015;9(2):2120–9.
60. Tsujimoto H, Morimoto Y, Takahata R, Nomura S, Yoshida K, Hiraki S, et al. Theranostic photosensitive nanoparticles for lymph node metastasis of gastric cancer. Ann Surg Oncol. 2015;22(Suppl 3):S923–8.
61. Kemp JA, Shim MS, Heo CY, Kwon YJ. "Combo" nanomedicine: co-delivery of multi-modal therapeutics for efficient, targeted, and safe cancer therapy. Adv Drug Deliv Rev. 2016;98:3–18.
62. Greco F, Vicent MJ. Combination therapy: opportunities and challenges for polymer-drug conjugates as anticancer nanomedicines. Adv Drug Deliv Rev. 2009;61(13):1203–13.

Printed by Printforce, the Netherlands